DATE DUE

JE 10 02			
FE 13 03			
AP 21 03			
NO 1 09			

RETURN TO COMMUNITY

RETURN TO COMMUNITY

Building Support Systems
for People with Psychiatric Disabilities

PAUL J. CARLING

The Center for Community Change
through Housing and Support
Trinity College of Vermont

Foreword by
JACQUELINE PARRISH

THE GUILFORD PRESS
New York   London

To Daniel Berrigan, S.J.,
who has done more than any other mentor
to help shape my views on human dignity, oppression,
and the importance of an enduring spirituality.

©1995 The Guilford Press
A Division of Guilford Publications, Inc.
72 Spring Street, New York, NY 10012

Printed in the United States of America

This book is printed on acid-free paper.

Last digit is print number: 9   8   7   6   5   4   3   2   1

Library of Congress Cataloging-in-Publication Data

Carling, Paul J.
    Return to community: building support systems for
people with psychiatric disabilities / Paul J. Carling.
       p.   cm.
    Includes bibliographical references and index.
    ISBN 0-89862-299-9. — ISBN 0-89862-323-5 (pbk.)
    1. Mentally ill—Deinstitutionalization.   2. Community
mental health services.   I. Title.
    RC439.5.C37   1995
    362.2'2—dc20   94-29724
                                                           CIP

Many people have been invaluable teachers and supporters on the path I have traveled. My mother, through both wonderful and very difficult times, has been a source of great love and of personal integrity. And the process of writing this book has, in a series of "small miracles," brought me closer to each of my brothers as well: Robert, Richard, Frank, and Jimmy.

Geri Botwinick and Tom Blatner have taught me a great deal about mental health systems and about change. In the academic world, Bill Anthony and his seminal work on rehabilitation have had a profound effect on my views. Steve Taylor's work, along with that of Mary Ann Test, Sue Estroff, Charlie Rapp, and Judith Cook, has had a strong influence. Steve Sharfstein and Judy Turner at the National Institute of Mental Health have supported my work and contributed significantly to the development of my ideas. And I must particularly thank Jacqueline Parrish, who heads the U.S. federal Community Support Program—a small but incredibly helpful and influential initiative.

At the National Institute on Disability and Rehabilitation Research, Naomi Karp and Karen Faison, tireless advocates for community integration, have both supported my work and contributed significantly to my thinking. The leaders of the Vermont Department of Mental Health have been delightful long-time coworkers in the process of change; I particularly acknowledge Rod Copeland, John Pierce, Paul Blake, and Charlie Biss.

Many professional colleagues throughout North America have contributed to my learning. Pioneering professionals like Len Stein, Ron Diamond, Elaine Stancliff, Mary Alice Brown, Tom Witheridge, Tom Fox, David Goodrich, Bev Gutray, Pam Hyde, Marti Knisley, Paul Myer, Bonnie Pape, Melodie Peet, Estelle Richman, Chris Stephens, Roger Strauss, and many others have shown that policy leadership, treatment, and empowerment can be combined into a rich recipe for reform. With regard to the specific content of this book, I should thank Marty Cohen and Leo Molinaro of the Robert Wood Johnson Foundation Program on Chronic Mental Illness; Bob Laux of Creative Management Associates in Portsmouth, New Hampshire; Susan Hasazi at the University of Vermont; and Deborah Reidy.

In this business of community integration, however, I have learned the most from consumers/ex-patients and their families. In the family movement, Agnes Hatfield, Jim and Carole Howe, Harriet Lefley, Marv Higgins, Joyce Berland, and Candy Neary have been particularly helpful in my learning. Tom Posey, an ex-patient and past president of the National Alliance for the Mentally Ill, has had the courage to bridge those worlds for me and for many others.

In the consumer/ex-patient movement, Howie the Harp, Paul (Dorfner) Engels, Dayna Caron, Judi Chamberlin, Rae Unzicker, Garrett Smith, David Gettys, Sally Zinman, Gilberto Romero, Bill Butler, Jay Mahler, Lori Shepherd, Marcia Lovejoy, Joel Slack, Marge Berthold, Susan Hardie, and many others are wonderful advocates and friends. Their movement ultimately holds the only real promise for fundamental change in our society for people with psychiatric disabilities. Pat Deegan has been an especially powerful friend, colleague, and teacher and has taught me a great deal about consumer organizing and recovery.

I am especially appreciative of the staff members, both past and present, at the Center for Community Change through Housing and Support. They have given me the time and space to write this book during periods when they would rather have had me much more readily available, and have never complained. Special thanks are due to Susan Wilson Besio, the associate director; Sinikka McCabe, formerly the director of technical assistance; and Cheryl Duncan. In addition, I thank Beth Tanzman, Jay Yoe, Annamarie Cioffari, Carole Smith, Susan Biss, Bill Montague, Jeani Beard, and Joy Livingston. Laurie Curtis deserves special attention: her valuable ideas can be felt throughout this book. I am proud of all of them, and in awe of their talents and energies.

I am grateful to Janice Ryan, O.S.M., and to Elizabeth Candon, O.S.M.—president and vice president, respectively, of Trinity College of Vermont—for their leadership in creating a new home for the Center for Community Change at Trinity. Trinity is a community of shared values that develops assertive, empowered students; that strives to include people who have been traditionally excluded from higher education; and that demonstrates its commitment to social change and social justice in a plethora of ways. Donna Dalton, my department chair, is also a partner with me in the early development of what we hope will soon be a graduate program focused on community integration throughout North America.

Several colleagues were very influential in the development of my ideas about integration and systems change: Andrea Blanch has a tireless sense of what is possible; she developed many of the ideas about choice reflected in these pages, and critiqued the first draft of this book. Priscilla Ridgway has been a major conceptualist and change agent in the emerging supported housing paradigm in mental health; many of her ideas are reflected in those sections of the book. Finally, Deborah Reidy has been a mentor in my thinking about social integration.

The assistance and encouragement of the members of my men's support group—Bill, Andy, Scudder, Harry, Howdy, and Stan—has been invaluable, as we struggle together to promote the liberation of all men. And my growing connections with people who organize support groups for people with disfiguring facial conditions hold the promise of fundamental challenge and growth. If I had not come to acknowledge my own "differentness" and the profound stigma I experienced as a child, this book, and in fact my entire career, would simply never have happened.

The staff of The Guilford Press has been magnificent throughout. Seymour Weingarten, editor in chief, saw the promise of this book years ago, and guided it through a stormy birth. Suzanne Little then helped it evolve from a massive manuscript to the final text. Through her excellent instincts, her keen sense of when to be firm and when to be soft, and her own passion for the subject, she has proven to be everything a fine editor should be. In the final stages, my son Oliver Carling proved to be an exceptional research assistant, correcting references, making many helpful suggestions about content, and critically editing the entire text.

Finally, I want to thank several of those closest to me, whose support gave me the emotional strength to put words to paper: Andy Simon and John Beattie; my sons, Nathaniel and Oliver, who remind me every day of the potential for a better world; my former wife, Anne, who supported my career in mental health in myriad ways; Cherise Rowan, my soul mate, who has been a faithful and inspired partner throughout my emergence as an adult; and Sam Dietzel, without whose advice to "just do it" this book would certainly never have been written.

People who have, or have had, a mental disorder are human beings. Beginning with this concept—an idea that is at once obvious and yet surprisingly controversial—Paul Carling, one of the leading thinkers in the mental health arena, has forged a new vision of human relations in dealing with people who have been diagnosed as "mentally ill."

I met Paul 15 years ago when we were both employed at the National Institute of Mental Health. Working with Paul was a turning point in my career as a mental health professional. He prompted me to examine my assumptions about traditional mental health services and the people they purport to serve. He enlightened me on the fundamental importance of values and the power of having a vision to guide planning. He added the word "choice" to my mental health vocabulary. Finally, he challenged me to look inward—to understand at a visceral as well as an intellectual level the importance of "home" for all people. This powerful realization is what propelled my strong commitment to developing *housing,* as opposed to mental health residential facilities, for people with psychiatric disorders.

In this book, which I view as a crowning achievement in a remarkable career, Paul Carling discloses the unhealthy aspects of current approaches to providing mental health services, including "forced help"—approaches that rob people of their dignity, self-determination, and hope for recovery and a future. He challenges many professionals' beliefs about the abilities and rights of people to make decisions that affect their lives, and about the goals of formal mental health services. He points out that participation in mental health treatment and in the formal service system too often becomes the dominant set of activities in the lives of many people with psychiatric disabilities. This is often not only unnecessary but counterproductive, if the goal is to help such people achieve full community participation and become productive members of society. From this viewpoint, the present paradigm for serving people with psychiatric disabilities is seen as perpetuating, if not actively promoting, continued dependency and separation from the rest of society.

Compounding the dependency-producing aspects of the current

mental health system are the dehumanizing effects of elements of the system. Rather than using person-preserving, person-affirming responses to help people reclaim their "selves," there is a tendency to overmedicate clients, to ignore their expressed concerns and views, and to trivialize their experiences. As a result, many people live painfully isolated lives, afraid to speak of their experiences for fear of being dealt with as *more* crazy.

I applaud Paul's vision of a time when formal services and treatment will be holistic and will be peripheral aspects rather than dominant themes of people's lives. This is not to say that formal services will not always be there when needed, but that they will be there to support the informal, natural supports in a person's life, rather than the other way around. In order to address the failings of the current system, Paul proposes a whole new way of viewing people with psychiatric disabilities and offering them services and supports—a new paradigm based on the fundamental needs and rights of all people. Paul then goes further, much further than other mental health theorists. He provides a comprehensive, detailed set of planning guidelines and practical strategies for change agents that can be used in today's (and tomorrow's) fiscal and political environments to make his vision a reality.

The need for fundamental changes to the current system and paradigm is substantiated by the growing number of people with mental disorders who are homeless or incarcerated in jails, the continuing challenges to family members, who remain the primary caregivers, and the lack of success of the current system in helping individuals achieve more independent, satisfying lives. If we consider these as the "products" of the billions of dollars being spent by our current service systems, we must conclude that our systems are doing something wrong. Our old methods, and the belief systems on which they are based, are not working.

Paul's prescription for change requires decision makers (i.e., those who control mental health service resources) to fundamentally alter their views of people with psychiatric disabilities and their approaches to offering these individuals services. They must recognize that they, their clients, the natural community supports, and the peer support groups formed by these individuals are each essential components of a system sharing a common goal of full community acceptance and participation for people with mental disorders. They must further recognize and employ the distinct but complementary roles of subjective values and objective empirical findings in bringing about needed changes.

Paul's plea for society is for community acceptance, a "willingness to embrace those with differences." I believe that this is the major challenge facing the mental health field and the consumer/ex-patient advocacy movement today. Because they sometimes look different (as a result of the unfortunate side effects of medication), relate differently, and behave differently, people with psychiatric disabilities are easy victims of stigma and discrimination. Because most are forced to live in abject poverty and have suffered multiple abuses during their lifetimes, many lack the self-worth and resources to fight back. On the positive side, these experiences have also left many with a deep sense of compassion and tolerance for others, so that, ironically, I see among people with psychiatric disabilities the strongest sense of acceptance of others with differences. I have attended their national conferences, meetings, and social gatherings, and have never witnessed greater caring for, reaching out to, and acceptance of a wider variety of people. I believe that society and the larger community could learn much about the real meaning of "community" from people with psychiatric disabilities.

In all, this book comprises a unique combination of values-based philosophy, research-based theoretical constructs, and detailed, experience-based strategies for change. It is a wonderful book that says many important things grounded in vast experience, common sense, and humanity, and shows how to apply these to every aspect of mental health, from direct services to national system change efforts. It is very simply written but contains a wealth of detail, so that it will be useful for all those who want to make a difference in the lives of people with psychiatric disabilities and those around them. Quite simply, it is the guidebook for which many in the mental health field have long been waiting.

JACQUELINE PARRISH
Director, Community Support Program
Center for Mental Health Services
Rockville, Maryland

When Paul asked me to write the preface for this book, I asked myself, "Why me?" And then I asked myself, "What's a preface?" I looked up the word "preface" and found "foreword" and "introduction." OK, so I'm introducing this book, giving it a foreword. But wait! I looked at Paul's outline and discovered that someone else is writing the foreword, and he's written the introduction! So what am I writing? The preface. So what's a preface? Who's on first?

And then it dawned on me: Paul is a professional, and I'm an ex-mental patient. What he is doing is similar to what professionals have done to me all my life—put me in a strange, confusing situation, usually one of their own creation, and expect me to fit in and adjust to it. When they finally let me out of this preface, I hope I can find a nice affordable book to live in, along with all kinds of other books in a huge library. I know that if lots of people read *this* book, then my goal can be reached.

But enough about the harsh realities of a healthy fantasy. Or is it the harsh fantasies of a healthy reality? Speaking of fantasies, I once had one: that I was one of millions of mental health clients who all lived in the communities of our choice, in our own places, with our own kitchens, our own furniture, our own bathrooms, our own food and clothing, and so forth. Of course, some of us chose to live with housemates who were friends or lovers (or both). We shared our communities with all kinds of people, of all races, religions, nationalities, ages, backgrounds, and abilities. And we did things together, helped each other, and laughed and cried with each other. When one of us had a rough time, others would respond with care and support. We all had decently paying, fulfilling jobs, doing what we did best. We had schools so that we could always learn more. And when am I going to stop prattling on about utopia? Never.

Dr. Martin Luther King had this kind of dream, and people said he was crazy too. But they were wrong. I mention Dr. King because he, more than any other person, represents the civil rights movement. For twenty years I have been active in what has been called the "mental patients' liberation movement," the "mental health consumer movement," or the "psychiatric survivors' movement." We, too, are essentially a civil rights movement. We are concerned about our rights and liberties as well as our needs—for housing, income, jobs, happiness, and well-being. Like everyone else, we want and need freedom and a good quality of life. We really want to live basically like everyone else.

After I lost my freedom for three years inside psychiatric institutions, I found that to me, freedom was the most important thing in the world. I became homeless to escape a system that again threatened to take away my freedom. I valued freedom even more than physical comfort, more than my health. This is true of most homeless people. We will not accept—and may remain homeless to avoid—any living situation, any residential facility that restricts our freedom, equality, and independence.

When we talk about independent living, we're *not* talking about leaving people alone to suffer with no help. We're talking about having freedom to make choices; to choose whom and what to be interdependent with; to choose when we need help, how it is to be provided, and by whom . . . in short, we're talking about empowerment. We're talking about independent living, with supports and services that enable us crazy folks to make a success of independent living.

The concept of "independent living" was first developed by disability rights organizations. People with physical, developmental, and other disabilities frequently face being warehoused in institutions; they are too often treated as if they are incompetent, and incapable of surviving outside of those facilities. Some of these people created independent living centers offering a comprehensive range of supportive services to enable the disabled to live on their own. The success of these centers has been proven and recognized throughout the world.

The mental health system has been slowly changing. It wasn't too long ago that the system was one of total control (and many would correctly say that it still is). It was/is too easy to force people into hospitals, and then to forcibly treat, shock, medicate, restrain, seclude, and even beat them. Physical and chemical restraints were/are the main "treatments" inside large, oppressive institutions. The system believed that this was good for us. Through the struggles of former inmates, their families, and other advocates, this began to change. The concept of the "least restrictive alternative" gained acceptance. Thus, the system was beginning to accept tentatively what consumers have always known: Freedom is good for us; restrictions are not good for us. Mental health professionals with vision began to listen to clients. The public and those they elected began to see that large institutions were bad; thus came deinstitutionalization. Although many people left those institutions, funds and resources did not. At that time, though, would it have made much difference? Were the alternatives offered at that time all that much better?

Since the 1960s, the main alternatives to large state/provincial hospitals have been smaller community-based residential facilities, including locked facilities, nursing homes, board-and-care homes, and domiciliary facilities. According to professionals, the most "progressive" of these seems to be halfway houses, which also spawned quarterway houses, three-quarterway houses, and other transitional living programs—therapeutic communities. However, many of us in the movement, and in fact most former mental patients, did not see these as progressive. I remember people referring to them as "mini-institutions," "candy-coated hospitals," and "living room jails." These were terms used by psychiatric survivors living in single-room occupancy (SRO) hotels and on the streets. True, the smaller facilities weren't as bad as state hospitals, and many people did and still do benefit from them. But most who lived in these facilities did so because the alternatives were unacceptable—the streets, SRO hotels, board-and-care homes. If they were offered a decent, affordable apartment, most would grab it. Soon, as the independent living concept seeped into the collective mind of the mental health system, we saw programs with names such as "supported independent living" or "assisted independent living." I always wondered why they didn't put the words "independent living" first. I found out when I saw how they were run—independence was not the top priority.

We could move from the state or provincial hospital ward to a quarterway facility, to a halfway house, to a three-quarterway house, to an assisted or supported independent living house, and finally (let me catch my breath) to independent living (if we could make it that far). The path along the way was fraught with difficulties, and at any time we might be sent back to the hospital. Well, hundreds of thousands of former psychiatric inmates, like myself, would not accept this. We filled up SRO hotels, emergency shelters, and the streets.

So we've gone from total control, to the least restrictive alternative, to halfway independence, to assisted independence. Now, with this book (you wondered when I would get to this), we can take that one, final, fantastic step to *independence!*

The progressive collective minds of our mental health system have slowly, by degrees, crept toward the realization that what is good for everyone—what people around the world have fought and died for, what civil rights movements have struggled for—is also good for mental health consumers. I remember a sign at one of our rallies: "Freedom Is the Best Therapy." Freedom of choice, independence, self-determination, and empowerment are what are best for us. Sure, we need supports, and not everyone can achieve the same level of independence. But we should each achieve the level and type of independence that *we* choose, using the suppports that *we* choose. And it works! People respond well to this. When people are treated like sick, dependent children, they tend to respond in a similar manner. When people are treated like capable, responsible adults, they also respond in a similar manner.

The fact is, the vast majority of former mental patients want to live independently. Ask those in the institutions, in residential facilities, in SRO hotels, in emergency shelters, and on the streets what their housing goal is, and practically all will give you the same answer: to get their own or a shared place to live. In fact, probably millions of psychiatric survivors live in their own homes, quietly and successfully. But you'll never hear about them; most will never reveal their psychiatric pasts, for fear of stigma and discrimination. So, if the majority of those who are not currently living independently want to do so, and many more are doing so, isn't it logical for most of our resources to go into those systems that help people live independently? Yes, but unfortunately most of our resources are still going into state institutions; what little is left over goes mostly into residential facilities and clinical programs. That's why deinstitutionalization has failed. It is no coincidence that the latest rankings of U.S. state mental health systems declared the one state system that is closest to having no state hospital—Vermont's—the best in the United States.

The community support model is beginning to be accepted by many mental health systems as the wave of the future. Now we hear the terms "client-centered" and "client-driven." Now we hear that client representation and empowerment are important; that people need to live in the community, integrated with everyone else; that basic human needs must be met; that the medical model is not the only way to help the "mentally ill"; that people must be able to make choices; and that housing should maximize both independence *and* interdependence. We also hear that support services should exist that are not necessarily connected to housing, but are *available, accommodating, accessible,* and *attractive* (I call this the "four-A principle"). The supports should be available to housing tenants, accommodating to each individual's needs, accessible so that clients can easily use them, and attractive so that clients *want* to use them.

How these concepts translate into housing, employment, socializing, and services is what this book is about. Paul is one of those rare visionary professionals who does something very simple: He listens to us. He cares about what we think; he knows that we *do* know what's best for ourselves. He has combined this knowledge with the technical know-how to document and research it. The results have proven that the ethics and principles our movement has stood for are not only correct, but really work! He proves this to his fellow professionals in such a way that they will listen and (I hope) learn.

Within the pages of this book are a declaration of independence and a blueprint for the future. Paul has succeeded in describing a new system for helping people. He begins with the words of former patients, which is most appropriate. He reports the need for suppportive housing, describes how to meet the need, and tells how to develop and operate supportive housing. But wait! There's more! He goes on to deal with employment and education of consumers, client and family involvement, self-help, organizing, and national trends.

If the mental health system wants to help people rather than control them—if that system truly exists for its clients rather than for itself and its own self-perpetuation—then I challenge the system to read this book, take it seriously, and follow its directions. I appeal to mental health professionals: Read this book, listen to your clients, and work with them as empowered, equal partners to plan the future mental health system. Make it a system that truly helps, not the existing one that hinders. Make it a system that reflects what is best in our society, rather than controlling and hiding away what society most fears.

This book doesn't give all the answers; no book can. There is much, much more we need to learn and develop. This book has built on other writings that have come before it; here, for the first time, are all the ingredients, the "state-of-the-art" knowledge, the practical "nuts and bolts" of implementation, put together with the needs and desires of those it will benefit. This book is part of the beginning of a new age in mental health, new concepts of helping people, and a new direction in human services. Really, it's a good book!

So, when am I gonna get out of this preface anyway???

HOWIE THE HARP
Oakland Independence Support Center
Oakland, California

CONTENTS

SECTION IV. EMPOWERING CONSUMERS
AND THEIR FAMILIES

SECTION V. CONCLUSION

Introduction:
Mental Health
and the Coming
of the 21st Century

I am a person, an individual, a human being. I happen to have
schizophrenia. For over twenty years I have lived with and in spite of it,
struggling to come to terms with my illness without giving in to it.
Although I have fought a daily battle, it is only now that I have some
sense of confidence that I will survive my ordeal.
　　　　　　　　　　　　　　　　—Esso Leete (1988, p. 67)

The problem that we're facing is that, similar to the physically disabled
and the developmentally disabled, the mental health system, and a large
part of the general public, believe that we are not capable of living independently, and believe that we must live in situations that give us care
and treatment for the rest of our lives. That's the myth we have to
debunk.
　　　　　　　　—Howie the Harp (quoted in Ridgway, 1988a, p. 24)

This book is being written in the middle of the last decade of the 20th
century. Within the lives of people who carry a label of "mental illness" or "psychiatric disability," and within mental health systems,
the past 15 years or so have been a time of profound change. In thinking about change, it is critical that we be aware of the monumental
problems we face, but also that we recognize the enormous degree of
positive change the mental health field has gone through during this
period. Although we must still confront a significant number of

1

challenges, we should also be proud of a significant number of achievements.[1]

This introduction describes the perspective I bring to this book, provides a brief synopsis of the current state of the mental health field, and summarizes the content and purposes of the book.

MY PERSPECTIVE IN WRITING THIS BOOK

This book is a product of the growing disability and civil rights movement among people with a label of "mental illness." As such, it may seem curious that the book is written by a professional, albeit one who identifies himself principally as an advocate. This is one of the many paradoxes of the current shifting sands on which we find ourselves: We are all having to redefine our roles, almost continually, as the advocacy movements of ex-patients and of their families express their voices with increasing power and effect.

Who we are, and what we choose to do with our lives, are of course profoundly shaped by our own experiences. My own path to a lifelong commitment to work related to psychiatric disabilities seems to have evolved from several profound early experiences. The first of these was growing up in poverty in New York City, and being forced to live in entire communities of people who, by virtue of their economic condition, were deemed to deserve to live only on the margins of society. As a child, I lived on the Upper West Side of Manhattan, where our block was exclusively "poor white," while the entire block across the street housed Puerto Ricans, and the next block had entirely African Americans. I then spent my adolescence and early adulthood living in one of America's great social experiments: a 1700-unit high-rise development constructed for low-income housing—one of the "projects," as we called them. My early experience in these settings with crime, with economic and racial segregation, and with the profound internalization of a sense of differentness and unworthiness that such experiences create all fueled my ambitions to rise out of poverty. However, it also left me with the struggle, on a long-term basis, to feel in any way equal to others I saw as more privileged.

I also grew up with the experience of differentness based on phys-

---

1. One indication of the pervasive change in our field is that the terms used to describe people with severe and persistent mental illnesses are themselves changing. This controversy is described in Chapter Three. My own experience, reflected in the language of this book, is that most people I meet prefer the terms "consumer/ex-patient," "consumer/survivor," or "person with a psychiatric disability."

ical characteristics. In a society that holds strong and narrow stereotypes about what constitutes beauty, the fact that I was born with a prominent facial birthmark had a profound effect on my personal and social adjustment. Living in a family whose members never talked about this, I developed the sense of "invisibility," of not mattering, and of powerlessness that many people with disabilities report. Subject to the taunts of other children, I was left with a deep sense of being not only different but inferior. Thus, in every social encounter as an adult, my first thought was characteristically to wonder what the other person thought about my birthmark, and whether he or she was uncomfortable. For someone who meets literally thousands of people a year while speaking throughout the world, this has sometimes been an excruciating impairment. It was only in my early 40s that I began to let go of that anxiety, that sense of inferiority and unworthiness, and to discover my own sense of power in social relationships—in short, to experience the business of empowerment. In the process, I began building connections with other people with disfiguring facial conditions. This prospect was initially terrifying. In talking about this with an ex-patient friend, I was struck by the similarity of our experience: the desire to dissociate ourselves from people who have had the same experience, as a way of not accepting who we are and what our communities are. At the same time, I began to understand the power of being open about my experience.

When I finally did start talking with my brothers, my sons, my friends, and my colleagues about my experience of growing up with a prominent birthmark, it became clear what a great tool this was to help others open up—to talk about their experiences of me and of themselves. So what I had always seen as a mark of shame, when held in isolation, instead became a way of joining with others. This is the same experience that mental health consumers/ex-patients report in self-help groups.

Growing up with these experiences also left me with a sense of outrage at how people who are perceived as different and/or inferior are treated in society. I can't remember a time when I was not an advocate for change, whether that was as a carpenter and general contractor working in low-income neighborhoods in Philadelphia, or as a draft counselor, civil rights worker, and peace advocate with the American Friends Service Committee during the Vietnam War. And, as a result of my upbringing, I can't remember a time when I wasn't conscious of the ways in which our society is segregated.

It was during the Vietnam War era that I first had an intense experience of community. As a high school graduate, I entered a Jesuit seminary in search of a community of shared values. Instead, I found profound disagreement about such questions as whether war and killing were moral in certain circumstances, and about whether Catholics could justify a position of conscientious objection to war. I left the seminary shortly thereafter, finding myself literally walking away from college because of my growing conviction that to be true to my values, I had to devote myself full-time to the movement to end the war. Almost by chance, I began gathering regularly with a small group of Catholics who held similar views, and who wished to integrate their moral values and day-to-day actions. We soon found a number of spiritual leaders, including Dorothy Day at the *Catholic Worker* and Daniel Berrigan. It was only through the support of that community that I was able to emerge as the first Roman Catholic in the nation to apply for—and, after an extended struggle, to be acknowledged as—a conscientious objector. As the war neared an end, I married, had children, and returned to college. It was quite a long time before I experienced that sense of community again, in becoming part of a support group of men trying to find new ways to live in a society that defines both men's and women's roles in rigid, narrow, and oppressive ways.

Like many of my contemporaries, after the Vietnam War I moved into professional training—in my case, as a psychologist. My studies and research focused on the emerging consciousness about sex roles and stereotypes in U.S. society, and on strategies for building a sense of cooperation and common ground among groups from different races, economic backgrounds, or genders. During the last semester of my doctoral program, struggling with new fatherhood and with academic and administrative duties, I delayed arranging the final internship that I would need to graduate until it was almost too late. By the time I approached my advisor, he was distressed and somewhat embarrassed, for it seemed that the only internship left was one that this distinguished graduate program had been unable to fill previously. It was a position working in a "psychosocial rehabilitation program" with ex-mental patients. At the time such programs were rare, and the dominant view in professional training programs—still very much alive today—was that such clients were simply not worth working with.

I took the internship at Horizon House in Philadelphia, one of the first psychiatric rehabilitation programs in the United States, simply because I needed it to graduate. By a stroke of luck, I thereby began what has been an extraordinary professional adventure, and one that I have never regretted. My first assignment was to work with a group of clients who had "failed in every other group in the program." Why the staff thought that a psychologist in training would have any idea how to help these individuals is still beyond me. Perhaps it mirrors the unquestioned status most of us once assigned to physicians as the holders of truth and cure, until we came to realize that many of them also had no idea what to do about many problems.

In any case, because I didn't know what to do, this became for me a profound experience of self-help, with people holding one another accountable for each other's behavior. Self-help was not an entirely new experience for me. In fact, I had held a previous internship in a rehabilitation center working with people who had undergone amputations. In that case, immediately sensing my own lack of understanding of that experience, I had invited an individual who had successfully returned to the community after such an operation to colead a recovery group with me.

After several months at Horizon House, I found myself spending more and more time with ex-patients, trying to learn what having a psychiatric disability was about from their perspective. Almost immediately, I began hearing about civil rights and involuntary treatment; the learned helplessness that so many services seemed to induce; the violations of personal dignity and choice; and the profound pessimism about ever being accepted as an equal. These issues were very different from typical professional concerns, and in fact there was surprisingly little discussion of them within professional circles. Thus, at an early stage of my career, it became completely obvious that I had to learn about two worlds: the professional world and the client world. These worlds seemed to overlap only rarely, since the power differences between those who inhabited them were so great. In fact, what I seemed to be seeing was a pervasive charade in which clients often framed their responses to professionals—and even their own internal experiences—in the professionals' terms, in order to retain access to the resources that the professionals controlled. This is certainly not a new phenomenon for those who have studied the work of Paolo Freire (1970) on the psychology of oppression, or that of Sue Estroff (1981), who has written eloquently about this process among people with a label of "mental illness." Nonetheless, it was an extremely disquieting realization for a young professional committed to helping. As such, it established within me a lifelong dissonance about the limitations of professional helping and about the capacity of systems to reform themselves.

It seems to me that throughout the time I have worked in this field, I have been aware of the need for major social change, as well as the need for profound personal change among all of us if we are to achieve true integration. It is only in the past several years, however, that such a consciousness has begun to take hold outside the ex-patient community, where the need for profound change has been obvious for at least a decade and a half.

After about 5 years, I left Horizon House. I was asked to assist in developing housing and support systems throughout the New Jersey state mental health system, learning in the process from an extremely talented pair of advocates then directing that system, Geri Botwinick and Tom Blatner. My work there was interrupted prematurely by an invitation to come to the National Institute of Mental Health (NIMH) to work with Judy Turner, Bill TenHoor, and Steve Sharfstein, who were organizing the Community Support Program, a federal program intended to stimulate the development of better community services for people with psychiatric disabilities. My job was to try to get other federal agencies to assist with the housing needs of ex-patients. In working with this program, I became aware of the growing ex-patient and family advocacy movements, and was privileged to begin traveling throughout the country, seeing many of the early attempts to support people with significant psychiatric disabilities in communities.

My specific responsibilities, however, proved far more difficult and elusive than I ever could have imagined. The intense focus in Washington on personal political advantage, the preoccupation of people in power with the opportunity of the moment (especially "photo opportunities"), and the general disregard for pursuing substantive changes in systems or in people's lives all made me realize how naive I was. Because it was clearly *right* that people should have decent housing and jobs, that the bulk of our resources in mental health should be directed to community supports rather than to state mental hospitals, and that people with psychiatric disabilities and their families should have a significant say in the systems that served them, I expected that these would be goals easily agreed upon and directly pursued by advocates and policy makers. One reality I faced, however, was that few people in Washington thought in terms of real human problems, especially if these were not amenable to a "quick fix." Another was that virtually everybody I met, even those committed to mental health reform, held deeply pessimistic views about the potential of the people who were then referred to as "*the* chronically mentally ill." This realization affected my future work in a profound way. For it was here I came to realize that the largest single barrier to change in the lives of people with psychiatric disabilities was not the lack of funding or services, but the fundamental assumptions that most citizens (including political leaders) hold, and the judgments that arise directly from those outdated assumptions.

In spite of these frustrations, I worked hard at NIMH with a very dedicated group of colleagues on the National Plan for the Chronically Mentally Ill, on a Report to Congress on Housing Needs of people with mental illness, and on a national demonstration program that linked the U.S. Department of Housing and Urban Development's

(HUD's) funding with Medicaid to provide housing and supports (albeit segregated housing).

When President Reagan was elected in a landslide and the optimism within the mental health field during the Carter years was swept away, I was invited to serve as deputy commissioner of the state mental health system in Vermont, and have made my home here since. I was fortunate to work for Richard Surles, then mental health commissioner in Vermont, during a period of profound change in the system that ultimately positioned Vermont as potentially the first state mental health system without a state mental hospital. In large part because of Richard's formative work, Vermont was recently designated by the Health Policy Research Group and the National Alliance for the Mentally Ill as the best state mental health system in the United States. It was in this context that I gained significant experience in systems change and management. The work at the state level was exciting and unbelievably challenging.

At a personal level, my most painful assignment was to be the final decision maker as to whether patients at the state hospital should be involuntarily medicated. We had all sorts of standards and procedures, but the simple and terrible "Hobson's choice" often came down to this: If individuals weren't drugged against their will, they would probably not leave the hospital for a very long time; if they were medicated, they might well experience a profound sense of violation, of anger at the system, or of helplessness to control the events around them, but at least they would get out of the hospital. In spite of the positive assistance with symptoms that medications brought to many patients, my experience was that virtually all of the patients who came before me had good reasons to refuse medications, based on their past experiences. And, too often, the system had little to offer them as an alternative. I was thus experiencing the basic dilemma of mental health systems: the perhaps irreconcilable mandates to help, but to help against a person's will; and to promote empowerment for the person, while exercising social control so as to protect society.

After several years, with a change of administration in state government, I moved on to the University of Vermont to begin developing a national program of research and technical assistance focused on the community integration of people with psychiatric disabilities. For 3 years, I was privileged to work closely with and learn a great deal from Bill Anthony, director of the Center for Psychiatric Rehabilitation at Boston University, while developing a national research and technical assistance project on housing and supports. This effort, in which Priscilla Ridgway also played a key role, drew on the experience of many forward-thinking professionals, policy makers, family members, and (most centrally) people with psychiatric disabilities; it resulted in the articulation of the "supported housing" approach, which emphasizes normal housing, consumer choice and control, and flexible supports including self-help. Following that collaboration, I organized the Center for Community Change through Housing and Support at the University of Vermont. Designated by NIMH as the national technical assistance center on housing and community support, the center developed a program of research on where and how people with psychiatric disabilities want to live, and what services and supports they and their families find helpful. The center has been privileged to provide technical assistance in nearly every U.S. state and many Canadian provinces, and as far away as Australia; it works closely with mental health systems and with ex-patient and family organizations to effect change. In 1992, the center moved to a wonderful new community at Trinity College of Vermont.

During the time that I was busy pursuing my professional career, another influence began to take shape, which has proven perhaps to be the most profound of all. My mother—a vibrant woman who worked as an executive secretary and raised five boys; who is also a talented pianist, performing as a volunteer in nursing homes and senior centers throughout New York City; and whom I always looked on as a rock of stability—began experiencing significant difficulties following the death of my father. She would become very depressed and would go to bed for weeks at a time. Then she would have periods of intense activity, in which she would not sleep at all. During these times, she would begin taking strangers into her house (some of whom were quite dangerous) and giving away her very limited income; next, just as quickly, she would demand to be rescued from the results of all of this activity. After several cycles of this, she was finally diagnosed with manic depression.

What followed that diagnosis was a series of experiences characterized by hope, despair, frustration, celebration of recovery, and despair again, not unlike those reported by many other family members of those with psychiatric disabilities. Throughout it all, my mother continued to deny that there was a problem. After repeated urging, she began to take medication, but would consistently stop doing so as soon as a particular crisis had subsided. She was assigned over the course of a decade to perhaps 10 different doctors, most of whom came to like her a great deal—a few were willing to call her on evenings and weekends and whenever she missed an appointment, and were able to make some real progress. In the end, though, the outcome always seemed the same: She would stop taking her medication, and the cycles would start again. Miraculously, she was hospitalized only rarely, perhaps because the New York City mental health system was too busy focusing on people who were in even more dire straits, and certainly because there was a family to provide intense support. It has not been uncommon, however, for one or more family members simply to give up from time to time, particularly in the face of the hopelessness generated by her denial of any real problem, and her unwillingness either to take medication or to accept responsibility for her own behavior.

There have been no easy answers in this experience, which continues as I write this book. Respecting my mother's right to make choices about her body, working to keep her out of institutions, working to get her to accept responsibility for her behavior, and continuing to work with and support my brothers in this process have not been easy tasks, but the effort has served to keep me grounded daily in the dilemmas we face in mental health systems. I continue to appreciate and celebrate the times when my mother is well and when we can share a family experience, and I miss her deeply when we cannot. I am thankful that as this book is being written, she is living with a wonderful group of elderly neighbors and is being supported by caring peers and staff members at New York's Fountain House, the oldest psychosocial rehabilitation "clubhouse" in the country. She volunteers as a pianist in local nursing homes, and is fully involved in her local community. She is looking better than she has in years—a tribute to her own persistence in recovery, and to the vital efforts of enlightened professionals and caring peers.

So, in looking over the strands of my childhood experiences; of being a family member of a person with a psychiatric disability; and of a career as a social activist in the peace and civil rights movements, a general contractor and housing developer, a service provider in a psychosocial rehabilitation program, a mental health policy maker and system manager, a researcher, and the director of a national research and technical assistance center that helps systems and communities pursue change, I am aware that the process has been above all one of a growing consciousness about the nature of oppression and the nature of change. It has been a process through which I have felt a growing personal mission to assert the right of each and every citizen, regardless of label or lifestyle, to a full and valued life in each of our communities.

Given these experiences, it seems to me to make perfect sense to try to begin this book with a spirit of openness, both to let readers know the experience base from which my views have emerged, and to encourage the same posture among all those involved in the lives of people with psychiatric disabilities. I am convinced that each of us, whether we have discovered it or not, has a mission in life—a singular contribution we can make to lift, even in small ways, the oppression of ourselves and others on this planet. It has been a singular delight to have found mine. So, having described how I came to this field and how I came to write this book, I now describe where I believe the field stands today in relation to the critical issues of community support and community integration.

THE CURRENT STATE
OF THE MENTAL HEALTH FIELD

We tend to forget that it has only been about a decade and a half since mental health professionals began entertaining the notion of a community support system for people with psychiatric disabilities. The first reference in the literature appeared in 1979 (Turner & TenHoor, 1979). This is an astonishingly short period of time for the whole field to be turned upside down in terms of mental health professionals' beliefs about people and what they need.

It wasn't that professionals did not know that a lot of things were wrong; the numbers of people in state or provincial hospitals, and where people were living in the community, indicated this. It was an outrageous situation. A major part of the problem was that no one had a way of conceptualizing or describing what needed to happen and how things needed to be different. The only things most professionals really thought about were hospitalizing people and giving them medications. It's important to understand that this is not necessarily ancient history. Some professionals and most members of the general public still think about things this way. Nonetheless, we should never underestimate the power of a simple idea to change current thinking.

The simple ideas behind a "community support system" were that people with psychiatric disabilities didn't need to languish for the rest of their lives in hospitals; that with skilled and hopeful community supports, these people could actually have lives; and that in fact some people, through self-help and other resources, could even manage to leave the mental health system. The idea of a community support system, or of a caring community, because of its sheer simplicity, has transformed the thinking and policies of mental health systems throughout North America, Europe and elsewhere in the world. That doesn't mean that people's lives in the community have necessarily gotten better. It does mean that at the policy level, in terms of where systems now say they are going, virtually every North American state or provincial mental health system has adopted a community support orientation

(National Association of State Mental Health Program Directors [NASMHPD], 1987, Pape, 1990). The issue we professionals are now struggling with is this: How do we get beyond the policy and the service system rhetoric, and really start to achieve more positive outcomes in people's lives?

In addition to policy changes, there have been enormous changes in the kinds of clinical and support services being developed in North America (Carling, 1992). The notion of a rehabilitation approach (Anthony, 1982) has been widely accepted. In this approach, services are based on what people want; service providers expect that people can actually learn and relearn skills, that appropriate supports can be developed, and that people can actually do a lot better than they have been doing. Rehabilitation is a notion that was not talked about much in the mental health field until the 1980s. Since then, it has had a profound impact on the thinking and behavior of many professionals, and on outcomes for many consumers.

We have seen day treatment programs expanding dramatically over the last decade and a half, and now we are seeing the next wave in some communities: Day treatment programs are being closed in favor of psychosocial "clubhouses," more intensive community support approaches, supported employment, and a dazzling variety of services and programs operated by consumers themselves—drop-in centers, crisis services, case management options, housing programs, and others (Carling, Wilson, McCabe, & Curtis, 1990). Residential programs, in the same way, are experimenting with "decongregation" (Nagy & Gates, 1992). So even within just this period, we are actually seeing the rise and fall of certain program models.

Historically, at a systems level, mental health organizational structures, policies, and funding priorities all appear to have been arranged on the basis of traditional notions of consumer incompetence, the primacy of professional judgment, and the central importance of institutional rather than community supports. Typically, the results of this have been that most of the money in systems has continued to support large institutions and facility-based programs, and that states or provinces rather than local governments have been seen as "responsible" for people with psychiatric disabilities. This pattern of organizing systems in a highly centralized fashion to support more restrictive settings is also giving way to a whole range of experiments with decentralization, as well as to reconceptualizations of who is responsible for services and how services should be paid for. Such experiments include "capitation funding" models, in which local communities receive a certain amount of funding based on the number of persons in need and then are accorded great flexibility in deciding how to spend that money, as long as costly institutional services are mini-mized. Other options—still rare but highly suggestive of the wave of the future—include voucher systems and even credit card systems, through which consumers can actually "purchase" the services they want. Attempts to restructure mental health systems in innovative ways began in Wisconsin in the 1970s (Knoedler, Carpenter, McCabe, Rut-kowski, & Allness, 1992), through legislation to shift the locus of re-sponsibility for hospital and community programs from a state to a local level, and to require comprehensive local community support services. As local communities discovered that costly hospitalizations could be avoided—and better quality of life promoted—through high-quality community services, they began to allocate the lion's share of mental health dollars to community programs. This Wisconsin experi-ment was widely replicated elsewhere. And in cases where this has been done well, it has been found that only the smallest proportion of a system's resources need to go to hospitalization, and that the out-comes for consumers are far more positive (Anthony & Blanch, 1989).

Because of changes in programs, organization of services, and even basic values, we are at a time in the mental health field of being able to put aside many of the obsolete assumptions we have held, based on almost no information at all. One of these assumptions was that by the late 1970s, deinstitutionalization had proceeded so rapidly that the people who were left in institutions really could not be served in our communities. But when we look at communities that have excel-lent community support services, it turns out that such an assumption is false. According to our best information, we cannot predict what the lower limit of "necessary hospital capacity" is (i.e., the minimum number of hospital beds we may need in the future).

We are on a course in Vermont, for example, of phasing down and closing our only state hospital in favor of a completely community-based service system (Carling, Miller, Daniels, & Randolph, 1987; Wil-son, 1988). It is simply not clear at this point how far the state hospi-tal census will decline. It is at a level of about 60 now for a population of about 560,000, and the census is projected to be at 30 beds shortly. There is currently no other involuntary treatment in the rest of the state outside of the state hospital. It may, in fact, be wise to take the position that no one can know exactly how much hospitalization *any* system will require in the future, because an excellent system should need very little—certainly much less than is currently used. Moreover, many of the state hospital beds we now have in Vermont can be replaced by using nonhospital alternatives and by using the services of other hospitals closer to home (Tanzman, Wilson, King, & Voss, 1990).

We have seen a real explosion of services, and service models themselves have changed enormously. The term "supported employment" has only been used in the literature since 1985 (Anthony & Blanch, 1987); "supported housing" has only been used since 1988 (Blanch, Carling, & Ridgway, 1988). Nationally, we are even engaged in a fundamental rethinking of *how* we should organize community supports.

The other dramatic change is that the whole political picture of mental health is very different today than it was even in the late 1980s. This is principally because of the growth of the family movement and the consumer/ex-patient movement (Hatfield, 1988; Leete, 1988). The existence of these two movements has fundamentally changed the nature of how we work and will work in mental health. They are becoming so powerful on a national basis that there is only one direction in which they can go: Their numbers will increase. As professionals, we have a very important set of roles to play in supporting these advocacy movements—not only by contributing time and resources and acting in collaboration with ex-patients and their families, but more fundamentally in rethinking how we behave, what we do and do not participate in, and how we can use our resources and expertise to promote the empowerment of consumers and their families. Some professionals, for example, use people with psychiatric disabilities and family members as consultants in their work. Others simply refuse to attend planning, program development, or evaluation meetings in which individuals and their families are not well represented.

At a policy level, it appears that what we are moving toward is "consumer-driven systems" (NASMHPD, 1989). We want to incorporate this as a value in our programs and systems, but the reality is that very few of us know how to put such a value systematically into practice. So we need to begin by learning together. Although I hope that the ideas in this book will be helpful, the best way to learn is by discovering a new knowledge base in partnership with people with disabilities and their families. To be sure, there will be conflict in the process, but no real change ever occurs without some conflict.

Rethinking Our Direction

So where are we now, as members of the mental health field and of society at large? We are in the midst of a fundamental rethinking of some of the most basic beliefs that have guided our behavior at both the professional and the societal levels for generations. Many people in the community support movement have come to the realization that a lot of what we have learned over the last decade and a half may not be as relevant as we thought for the future. Much of what we need to know for the next several years we simply don't know yet (Carling, 1990a). This may be the case because, in spite of all of the changes described above, far too few people with a label of "psychiatric disability" are as successful as they could be: In most U.S. communities, we still see 10–15% employment rates. And most of these people live in inadequate housing and abject poverty (Carling, 1990a).

For example, I have a friend who lives in an apartment in Burlington and receives support from outreach workers at the local mental health center. She was hospitalized as a young girl for a very long time, but is now living in the community, although she continues to have frequent crises. One day she explained to me that the reason she was so often near a crisis point was that she worried about money nearly all the time. When I asked her why, she replied: "I worry because I know that if my rent goes up only $10 a month, I will be homeless." How many of us can imagine the daily toll that living this way takes on the human spirit?

Very few people with psychiatric disabilities have decent, stable housing, or relationships with people who are not connected in some way with the mental health system. And many of them continue to cycle through a series of involuntary hospitalizations, and/or to live isolated lives at the margins of our communities. For some, their only community is the streets. Where these people are "served," it is typically in segregated facilities; their social networks are limited to other people with the same label, and to people who are paid to have relationships with them. The evidence is all around us, as we see the *New York Times* (1990) begin to refer to New York City as the "New Calcutta." And although public mental health policy increasingly emphasizes community supports and consumer and family empowerment, the majority of U.S. public funds—about 65% (NASMHPD, 1988)—are still allocated to serve small numbers of people in state institutions.

Simply put, integration has not yet really happened. Very few communities in North America are places where people with psychiatric disabilities are actually supported as regular community members—where people with and without a label of "mental illness" work side by side, live next door to one another, and enjoy friendships with one another. Most readers who look across the local communities in their area will find this to be true, in spite of the great investment in mental health services.

We do have some evidence (Hatfield, 1988) that at any given time, only a small percentage of people with psychiatric disabilities participate in *any* formal mental health program. Among those who do, many drop out after their initial experience with services. This presents us with an urgent responsibility to begin to better understand how these people are coping outside of mental health systems, and to understand why so many of them appear to find mental health services unattractive or less than helpful. One thing is clear: To survive within the kinds of deprivation described above requires a level of personal resources and resilience that should serve as an indication of the strength and potential of people with psychiatric disabilities.

Much of what we know about integration is actually little more than a series of educated guesses, since at a national level there is almost no support for research on integration. Our field does not even have basic information on where and how people with psychiatric disabilities live, work, learn, and socialize; we certainly do not have the information we need about where they *want* to live and learn and work, and on what they want in their lives (Wilson, 1992). Until we gather that information, we are not going to have much of an empirical basis with which to move forward. Although research is critically important, it's also necessary to recognize that many questions do not require empirical answers. All people have a *right* to work, to decent housing, to integration, and to respect. Those are not things we need to study.

Community Integration: Key Principles and Practical Challenges

It is clear from any discussion of community integration that we have developed an excellent conceptual framework for pursuing new approaches, but that to make these approaches a reality implies a major restructuring of the way in which both mental health systems and communities behave. Taylor, Racino, Knoll, and Lutfiyya (1987), in a seminal work on community integration (albeit one that is primarily focused on individuals with developmental disabilities) have articulated a set of basic principles, as well as the practical challenges to integration that we are now just beginning to face within mental health. The principles they describe are as follows:

- All people, regardless of any differences, belong in a community.
- People with differences can be integrated into typical neighborhoods, work situations, and community social situations.
- Support is necessary for all people and their families; this support should be offered in regular places in the community, not in specialized settings designed for people who are "different."

- The development of relationships between people with and without labels is crucial.
- People with and without labels have much to learn from one another.
- Service users and their families should be involved in the design, operation, and monitoring of all services, and should have the power to hold services accountable.

In the same way, Taylor et al. (1987) remind us that we face a series of practical challenges, not the least of which is the assertion of many professionals and policy makers that full integration of people with severe disabilities is "simply not practical." As we consider the knowledge base we will need to respond to this assertion, we may well find that the most useful knowledge will be found in the field, in communities, and in people's lives, as contrasted with traditional research approaches such as controlled studies. Reviewing successful integration attempts to date, for example, Taylor et al. conclude that preparatory programs are not effective; instead, people need to learn in community settings—in homes and jobs. Furthermore, they conclude that community acceptance of people with differences *follows* community integration; it is not a prerequisite. Taylor and colleagues find that the most effective way to meet the most complicated needs is through a highly individual approach, which includes attention to home, job, and friends; they further conclude that the major goal we should be pursuing is that of establishing long-term caring connections between people.

On the basis of this review of successful integration efforts, Taylor et al. (1987) warn that service systems appear, in fact, to have been following the most *impractical* approaches: waiting until communities are "ready" before allowing people to live there; keeping people in environments that have powerful negative effects on their functioning; trying to meet highly individual needs in programs that group large numbers of severely disabled individuals together; insisting that treatment is the primary need, and more important than a home, job, or friends; and asking people to move through multiple service environments, learning skills in each that they are then required to transfer to other settings, rather than *starting with* a home, a job, and a social network. The implications of Taylor et al.'s work for mental health systems and for the behavior of the general public are profound, since both these systems and the public seem to have assumed that the answers to people's needs lie in more and more professional services, rather than in normal community opportunities and relationships and in self-help.

A Final Word

I have a favorite *Calvin and Hobbes* cartoon (Watterson, 1988, p. 199). Calvin has said something mean to Susie and hurt her feelings. And Calvin sulks about it, as only Calvin can do. Finally, Hobbes comes up to him and says, "Maybe you should apologize to her." Calvin thinks about this for a long minute before replying, "I keep hoping there's a less obvious solution."

Like Calvin, we may well be beyond less obvious solutions. In the past, we have taken many paths in developing various societal "solutions" to the problem of mental illness. Unfortunately, the common denominator of most if not all of these paths has been a process of defining people with psychiatric disabilities principally as "mental patients," and, through the best of intentions, assuming that they have no long-term place as fully participating members of our communities. I believe that an agenda acknowledging that people are people first, and that full community integration is the only effective solution to the problem of mental illness, is the only practical course left to us as we enter the 21st century.

OVERVIEW OF THE BOOK

This book, then, is about the passing of one age and the coming of another. Its central focus is on the reality of empowerment and the opportunity for full community participation among people with a label of "mental illness." As such, it attempts to chart the directions for our collective future, as much as possible, through the words of ex-patients and family members themselves.

Section I of the book defines "community integration," and traces the history of society's and the mental health field's attempts to meet the needs of people with psychiatric disabilities, given the assumptions about these individuals that each generation has operated under. It describes the "paradigm shift" that is both challenging and energizing mental health systems, and presents an emerging model for understanding what we as professionals and advocates hope that our communities will become. Through this vision, we can begin to understand what government, the private sector, community organizations, and neighbors might do to assist in the process of integration. Finally, this section describes various definitions of "mental health consumers" and "mental illness," and discusses the burgeoning consumer self-help movement.

Section II describes the process of preparing to organize for community change, through a better understanding of the pervasive nature of stigma and how it is reflected at every level of society: among individuals, within the mental health system, and in the larger community. The section also describes the importance of people, information, and resources in the change process, with emphasis on the critical role of the change agent. Successful efforts to organize for community change are then described, along with guidelines for assembling a planning team and developing a clear mission; for gathering needed information from individuals with disabilities, their families, professionals, and other community resources; for assessing the current capacity of the community to support these individuals; for deciding which actions are most critical to pursue; for working with key constituencies; and for gathering the funding needed to accomplish community change.

Section III describes a variety of strategies for revamping existing support systems (mental health systems and higher education programs) improving access to housing, creating employment options, and promoting social integration. Section IV focuses on sharing power with people with psychiatric disabilities, as well as on working with family members as partners. A concluding chapter describes the future challenges and new directions that the mental health field faces in the 21st century.

This book is intended for all those who have begun to understand the magnitude of change that must take place in our society and in each community, if people with a label of "mental illness" are to have the option of becoming fully participating community members. Because of the broad audience for whom the book is intended, and the even broader terrain it must cover in a full discussion of integration, it can be justifiably criticized as overly ambitious. Furthermore, there are certain to be parts of the book that some readers will find too conceptual (or too practical), too professionally oriented (or too advocacy-oriented, or too family-oriented), or too heavily based on research (or not adequately supported by empirical data). It is likely that all of these criticisms and many I have not yet anticipated are legitimate, given the scope of the undertaking and the fact that integration is such a new concept in the mental health field and in our daily lives.

In response, I would simply note that it is impossible for one individual to be expert in all aspects of integration, particularly since so little real integration has actually taken place. I invite my readers, then, to see this as a series of potential ideas and strategies; to try them on for size; and most importantly, to use the ones that make sense in organizing at the local, state/provincial, or national level. In spite of its limitations, I ask readers to approach this work with the two essential tools of effective change agents: open yet critical minds, and open hearts.

REDEFINING THE NEEDS OF MENTAL HEALTH CONSUMERS

CHAPTER 1

Community Integration: The Challenge to Traditional Mental Health Services

DEFINING "COMMUNITY INTEGRATION"

As I have noted in the Introduction, the field of mental health is currently poised at a historical juncture. Its choice of direction may well determine not only whether mental health systems will be helpful or effective in the 21st century, but in fact whether these systems as we currently know them will exist at all. In fact, systems and agencies that have been professionally controlled for the last century are on a collision course with the growing consumer/ex-patient advocacy movement, which asserts quite simply that people with psychiatric disabilities are people first, with fundamental rights to control their services, their basic life choices, and their aspirations.

This movement for community integration as a *right* draws from the experience of the larger disability and civil rights movements. Because it reflects the aspirations of the "customers" of mental health systems (i.e., individuals with psychiatric disabilities and their families), it is destined to become the leading force shaping public mental health policy in the next century, just as the larger disability rights movement has become the dominant force in public disability policy. The basic belief of the community integration movement is that all people, including people with disability labels, have a right to full community participation and membership. Moreover, the movement maintains that this goal will not be achieved primarily through professional services, but rather through peer support and self-help, as well as through physical, vocational, and social integration into mainstream community activities, housing, jobs, and relationships with nondisabled peers. In short, the goal can ultimately be realized only if people with psychiatric disabilities themselves exercise full control over the services and supports they need, whether these are provided by peers or by professionals.

This movement does not assert that professional services are unimportant or unnecessary, but rather that to be effective, such services must be controlled by their users, designed specifically to achieve integration outcomes, and be organized not primarily to "fix" individuals, but instead to support those key foundations of a healthy life on which all citizens rely: a home, a job, and connections with family, friends, neighbors, and coworkers. Thus, this movement does not in any way ignore the nature or severity of an individual's disability. Rather, it approaches the person in a fundamentally new way—as an equal, and as a valued "customer" whose growing empowerment, satisfaction, and improved quality of life are the critical outcomes through which we can evaluate the success of a professional's work. And it focuses as much on eliminating societal barriers as it does on individual rehabilitation.

What then is this new concept of "community integration"? Community integration derives from various assumptions or core values about people in general, including people with labels of "differentness." Taylor et al. (1987) have articulated one set of these assumptions, which I have listed in the Introduction. To these, I would add the following:

- Success in housing, work, or social relationships is primarily a function of whether an individual has the skills and supports that are relevant to that environment or relationship.
- People's needs change over time; hence services and supports should be available at varying levels of support for as long as a person needs them, and regardless of where the person lives.
- People's relationships with service providers also change over time, so that continued access to housing, work situations, or social networks should not depend on whether or not a person is using mental health services at the time, or whether the person is "getting along" with a service provider.
- Family members of a person with a psychiatric disability require and deserve substantial support if they are to provide support to their disabled relative and meet their own needs in the process.
- Family members should not be blamed for their relative's disability, but instead should be treated with the same respect that all citizens deserve, and with the high level of involvement and support that they deserve as well.

- The legitimate target of family advocacy is for *family* needs; the fundamental power over services should rest with the individual who has the disability.

How will this vision of community integration be achieved? It will be achieved by vastly increasing the availability of stable, affordable housing that is physically integrated (i.e., not developed for any particular group, but rather for tenants both with and without disabilities). It will be achieved by creating access to employment in genuinely integrated work sites, rather than in transitional or sheltered, segregated settings. It will be achieved by arranging support through freely given, nonpaid relationships with nondisabled citizens, rather than assuming that all needs are to be met through a professional service system. It will be achieved by making services available that are both flexible and reliable, rather than forcing individuals to fit into program "slots," or even into programs at all. It will be achieved by basing all decisions about housing, work, social networks, and services on each individual's choices, goals, and needs. Finally, it will be achieved by developing and funding services operated by people with disabilities, and by transferring decision making about policies, programs, staffing, and the actual resources for services (including funding), to these people.

This view of community integration represents a fundamental shift in the way that mental health systems have "done business" over the last century or more. Therefore change will not come easily, even if it will come inevitably. Community integration stands in stark contrast to outdated views of people with psychiatric disabilities—whether held by professionals, family members, or the general public—as perennial patients, helpless and dependent, with hopeless futures. In the past, these views led us to assume that people with serious psychiatric disabilities couldn't make reasonable choices; that most of these people were too disabled to live in regular housing, work in regular jobs, study in regular academic programs, or participate in regular social relationships in the community; and that professionals had no business getting involved in housing or work, or even in the life of the community, since they were there to "fix" or "maintain" these people. In this way of thinking, individuals, rather than a complex interaction of personal and societal issues, are defined as the locus of the problem. This myth, in turn, is "validated" by the fact that "relapse" occurs periodically—a fact suggesting that these persons are perennially unstable at best, or, need continuing supervision at worst. Relapse, in fact, is a reality in living with a psychiatric disability. But it is also clearly the case that in communities in which high-quality supports are available and in which community integration is the goal, relapse is far less disruptive to housing, work, and social networks—just as we find in other long-term disabling conditions. In such cases, relapse becomes an opportunity for further recovery.

Community integration also stands in contrast to the newer assumption that people with psychiatric disabilities are essentially "service recipients" who, because of the severity of their conditions and the impossibility of recovery, are little more than commodities that justify the expenditure of large sums of public funds on supervision, a variety of facilities, and a complex industry of professional services simply to "maintain" them in the community. This assumption provides us with perhaps the most deadly of the prevailing myths about psychiatric disabilities: that recovery is impossible. This myth is held so strongly by some professionals that when they are confronted with the many ex-patients who have taken responsibility for their own healing and recovery, after years of institutionalization and homelessness, their typical response is to deny that these persons ever had serious disabilities. When confronted with that response, I am often overcome with a profound sense of both grief and anger at how difficult it must be for individuals already challenged by serious disabilities to muster up the hope to embark on the path of their own recovery, when their most trusted service providers, and in fact most of the systems that "serve" them, believe such a path to be impossible. For those who believe in community integration, it is clear that professionals who hold such beliefs have a moral responsibility *not* to work with people with psychiatric disabilities.

Finally, the community integration approach stands in starkest contrast to the traditional "medical model" ideology, which asserts that people with psychiatric disabilities are so impaired that professionals must continue to hold responsibility for controlling all key decisions that affect their lives. Challenging this myth, in effect, challenges the fundamental self-interest inherent in the status quo—whether this involves a mental health agency that owns the buildings in which a dozen "clients" live; a system of homeless shelters; a board-and-care or nursing home industry; a state hospital; certain professionals who are concerned about whether individuals with disabilities, once they control the resources for services, will continue to want their services; or some family advocates who are concerned that the growing voice of individuals with disabilities may dilute or overshadow their own growing political power in current mental health systems.

These outmoded beliefs about people with psychiatric disabilities —even though they have been overtaken by an integration approach in the case of other disability groups—will die hard in the mental health field. This will be so not only because no group with power typically

gives up that power easily, but also because so many of those currently involved (whether individuals, their families, professionals, or advocates) have come to believe these fundamental assumptions. And
yet, in spite of these formidable obstacles, it seems abundantly clear
that community integration *will* occur. In fact, it is already occurring
to an unprecedented degree. It is, in many ways, like a train that has
left the station and is hurtling down the track. The field of mental health
has three simple yet profound choices: It can get in the way, and be
run over in the process; it can step aside, and be bypassed by history;
or it can respectfully ask to be let on board, so that it can be of service
and support to those who are driving the train. Such a request holds
the promise of a very different and a much more positive future, both
for professionals and for people with disabilities.

As I write this chapter, I have just had a preview of that future.
Speaking at a conference on "consumer empowerment" in Winnipeg,
Manitoba—which was attended by mental health professionals, advocates, family members, and a relatively small number of people with
psychiatric disabilities—I had two very unusual experiences. In the first,
I was a participant in a workshop that was intended to "define the
support needs of consumers." Each person around the table, in turn,
was asked to respond to this statement: "Talk about a time in your
life when you really needed support." When all those present had
finished their stories, two thoughts struck me with great force. First,
as the stories progressed, people felt much more trusting of each other,
and expressed more and more support; second, I had *absolutely no
idea* who was an ex-mental patient and who was not. After each person spoke, the follow-up question was this: "What happened to you in
that situation?" It was then that I found out who the ex-patients were.

The second experience occurred later that day. I had just finished
giving a presentation in which I was encouraging this primarily professional audience to undertake a variety of strategies that would increase
the opportunity for consumers to take back their power. Afterward,
I found myself chatting with a man who directs a government employment and training program with a multimillion-dollar budget. We were
talking about the power of consumers speaking out about their own
needs, and he mentioned that he was going to an important government meeting the next day to present a proposal for a new program
to train ex-patients as service providers. "Why don't you have a consumer present the idea for the program?" I asked. He looked confused,
which I interpreted as resistance, so I went on to reiterate the many
reasons why this would make sense. He continued to look confused.
Finally, a light bulb seemed to go on in his eyes, and he said, laughing,
"But I *am* a consumer!"

And it occurred to me that what we are striving for in the movement for community integration is to create many such experiences: experiences in which people who are ex-mental patients and people who do not (or do not yet) have a psychiatric disability can come together and share a reality in which these differences are largely irrelevant; and experiences in which people are holding leadership positions in society, in spite of a label of "mental illness," and advocating for their own needs. This kind of successful integration is, of course, a different kind of "invisibility" than most ex-patients have experienced. Paradoxically, movement in this direction may well begin with openly acknowledging the dramatic differences in experience that people with psychiatric disabilities have had, and the value of their experience in determining mental health policies, designing and operating service programs, and training professionals.

PROBLEMS FACED BY CONSUMERS/EX-PATIENTS: BACKGROUND AND SCOPE

How Common Is Mental Illness, and How Are We Affected by It?

Serious mental illness is a major public health problem throughout the world. The federal agency responsible for U.S. mental health policy, the Center for Mental Health Services (1993), has summarized the national statistics on mental disorders as follows: More than 48 million Americans are estimated to have some mental disorder in a single year. Of these, approximately 5.5 million are disabled by severe mental illness. Estimates of the number of children with mental disorders range from 7.7 to 12.8 million, although fewer than 20% of children under age 18 with a serious emotional disturbance receive mental health services. Approximately 16.2 million Americans experience phobias; 6.4 million experience major depression; 2.9 million, obsessive compulsive disorders; 1.8 million, schizophrenia; 1.7 million, panic disorder; and 1.1 million, manic depression or bipolar disorder. At least two-thirds of nursing home residents have a diagnosis of a mental disorder, such as major depression. Up to 25% of people with AIDS will develop AIDS-related cognitive dysfunction, and two-thirds of all people with AIDS will develop neuropsychiatric problems.

The Center for Mental Health Services (1993) also notes that a majority of the 29,000 Americans who commit suicide each year are believed to have a mental illness. Suicide is the eighth leading cause of death in the United States, and the third leading cause of death among those between ages 15 and 24. Nearly one-third of those who are homeless (estimates range from 600,000 to 3 million) are believed to have a serious mental illness. More than 1 in 14 jail inmates have a mental illness. Twenty-nine percent of the nation's jails routinely hold people with mental illnesses without any criminal charges.

Moreover, according to the Center for Mental Health Services, (1993), mental illnesses have a multibillion-dollar impact on the economy each year. The total economic costs of mental illnesses amounted to $147.8 billion in 1990. More than 31% of these costs ($46.6 billion) were for anxiety disorders. Direct costs—expenditures for professional services—accounted for $67 billion, or 11.4% of all health care expenditures, in 1990. Direct treatment and support costs comprised 45.3% of the total economic costs of mental disorders. The value of reduced or lost productivity comprised another 42.7%. Paradoxically, the cost of mental health services is *not* a significant factor in rising costs of health care in the United States. Mental health, when combined with substance abuse treatment, ranks 25th in order of factors influencing the rise in U.S. health care costs (Center for Mental Health Services, 1993). Canadian research studies show that mental illness has a similarly profound impact in Canada (Pape, 1990).

The estimates above, though appearing to have a high level of precision, may mask the considerable controversy currently raging as to the numbers of people with mental illness. Until recently, for example, states and localities used widely varying estimation techniques for determining the numbers of people with mental illness within their jurisdictions. Such estimates were then used to allocate public funds for services. Advocates (e.g., M. Schneier, personal communication, September 1992) have pointed out that in some localities, these estimates were considerably lower than the national data presented above should indicate. As a result, Congress recently required the Center for Mental Health Services to develop a uniform estimation technique, and to require the use of that technique in the states as they prepare their federally mandated comprehensive mental health services plans.

Within these national estimates, researchers (e.g., U.S. Department of Health and Human Services, 1983) have estimated that among the 5.5 million individuals with significant psychiatric disabilities, roughly 25% are hospitalized or living in some other psychiatric institution, such as nursing homes, boarding homes, or group homes; 60% continue to live as adults with their families; 5% are homeless; and 10% live in their own housing. Approximately 20% of people with psychiatric disabilities consistently use professional services (Hatfield, 1988), and a roughly equal percentage are employed (Dion & Anthony, 1987).

It is important to note that these estimates differ dramatically when one compares specific states, provinces or localities. Such differences reflect diverse histories of deinstitutionalization, different availabilities of housing options, different priorities in service systems, and perhaps different attitudes among service providers (Pandiani, Edgar, & Pierce, in press).

Estimates are generally unavailable as to how many people are housed adequately, participate in educational programs, or have achieved some measure of social integration.

Problems in Housing, Employment, and Social Support

Since the late 1950s, public hospital use has been significantly reduced, and community services have been greatly expanded (Kiesler, 1982). The critical need for stable housing, employment, and social networks linked to supports, however, has only emerged in the last 15 years as a major policy dilemma (Carling & Ridgway, 1987). A majority of the 5.5 million Americans considered "long-term mentally ill" on the basis of diagnosis, disability, and duration of disorder (Center for Mental Health Services, 1993) live in inadequate housing, are unemployed, lack needed supports, or are homeless (U.S. Department of Health and Human Services, 1980, 1983). The problems are complex ones: Without active rehabilitation, many individuals lack the skills and supports needed for successful community living. In addition, the recurring nature of long-term psychiatric disabilities may result in people's losing housing and/or work as they experience repeated hospitalizations (Budson, 1981; Chatetz & Goldfinger, 1984).

However, the frequency of relapse can in fact be seriously curtailed and even prevented through a wide variety of strategies, including psychosocial services, medications, and family supports (Anthony & Blanch, 1989); high-quality case management and crisis services (Stein & Test, 1985; Fleming & York, 1989); and housing services that offer intensive supports, whether with or without medications (Mosher & Menn, 1978; P. Dupre, personal communication, August 1993). The key issue, then, is not that relapse cannot be prevented or its effects ameliorated, but that our society is failing to make the investment in known strategies for responding to and effectively reducing relapse. A second key issue involves what kinds of lives we are willing to offer people with psychiatric disabilities, apart from the intensive professional interventions that have proven effective in response to relapse. Is our goal simply to "maintain" people—to keep them out of crises and out of institutions—or to make the significant investment required for real community membership?

Housing and job discrimination based on stigma is a day-to-day reality. Landlords refuse to rent to individuals with psychiatric disabilities, and employers refuse to hire them, cutting off access to normal housing and jobs (Alisky & Iczkowski, 1990; Aviram & Segal, 1973; Segal, Baumohl, & Moyles, 1980). Moreover, many people with psychiatric disabilities live in poverty, with U.S. average reported annual 1980 incomes from $3000 to $7000, and unemployment rates as high as 85% (Dion & Anthony, 1987). Finally, people with psychiatric disabilities compete for housing and jobs with members of other low-income groups, most of whom are generally viewed as more suitable tenants or workers.

Failure to focus on people's housing and employment needs has had multiple effects. Many individuals remain in psychiatric hospitals because of the lack of housing and work (U.S. Department of Health and Human Services, 1980). Others cycle through emergency rooms and general hospitals in costly and often inappropriate stays (Chatetz & Goldfinger, 1984; Geller, 1982). Many others have been moved to "custodial" nursing and boarding homes. Most of these settings lack active rehabilitation or treatment, contribute to declines in functioning, and are often exploitative (Carling, 1981; Kohen & Paul, 1976; Segal & Aviram, 1978; U.S. Senate Special Committee on Aging, 1976). The lack of housing, work, and support options also results in substantial challenges for families (Hatfield, Fierstein, & Johnson, 1982; Wasow, 1982), who are often forced to serve as case managers, landlords, and organizers of leisure time, with little or no support or respite.

Of those with psychiatric disabilities who do find independent housing or work in the community, many live in very low-income neighborhoods where substandard housing and high crime rates are typical, or are employed in entry-level or "dead-end" jobs. "Oversaturation" of neighborhoods by people with disabilities, or unfounded fears about their dangerousness (Teplin, 1985) or about the prospect of declining property values (Dear, 1977; Sigelman, Spankel, & Lorenzen, 1979), often lead to community backlash (Coulton, Holland, & Fitch, 1984; Ridgway, 1987). Increasing numbers of people with psychiatric disabilities are homeless. Because of the decline in affordable housing, increasing unemployment, and the erosion of community services for people with psychiatric disabilities and with substance abuse problems, homelessness has become a widespread phenomenon in the United States. Estimates are that 736,000 Americans are homeless on a any given night and that 2.3 million are homeless over the course of a year. In addition, 27 million Americans are considered "shelter-poor" and at risk of homelessness (Low-Income Housing Information Service, 1988). Estimates of the proportion of homeless persons with serious mental illness range from 25% to 90% (Bassuk, 1984; Lamb, 1984; Benda & Datallo, 1988; U.S. General Accounting Office, 1988), although they have not necessarily been in mental hospitals (Baxter & Hopper, 1984). In fact, major methodological questions have been raised about estimating the size of the homeless mentally ill population (Morrison, 1989; Breakey & Fischer, 1990). Furthermore, many of these studies fail to make important distinctions regarding key subpopulations of homeless persons, such as women (Morse & Calsyn, in press; Roth, Toomey, & First, in press) and minority groups (First, Roth, & Arewa, 1988).

Although the popular press often equates homelessness with deinstitutionalization policies, there is considerable debate about the extent to which homelessness is a *consequence* of the disabling nature of mental illness coupled with mental health policies (Lamb & Lamb, 1990), or is itself a *precipitant* of psychiatric disability (Cohen & Thompson, 1992). Research studies.tend to overestimate the number of homeless people with mental illness by describing some behaviors as characteristics of mental illness rather than of homelessness itself (Koegel & Burnham, in press). Grunberg and Eagle (1990), for example, have described a process called "shelterization," which is similar to early accounts of learned helplessness in psychiatric hospitals, but which affects many homeless people and not just those with psychiatric disabilities. Shelterization is characterized by decreased interpersonal responsiveness, neglect of personal hygiene, increased passivity, and increased dependence on others.

Deinstitutionalization: A Critical Reappraisal

The United States and Canada are both in the midst of a major debate about deinstitutionalization. On the one hand, the press, researchers, and advocates debate such issues as the "failure of deinstitutionalization" and the need for "asylum" (e.g., Wasow, 1986; Zipple, Carling, & McDonald, 1988), the crisis of homelessness among people with mental disorders (Baxter & Hopper, 1984), the generally low quality of both community and hospital programs for these individuals (Torrey, Wolfe, & Flynn, 1988), and the continuing orientation of these programs toward "maintenance" rather than rehabilitation (Anthony & Blanch, 1989). Although state mental health policies stress the need for comprehensive community support systems (NASMHPD, 1986), most mental health resources are still predominantly allocated to outdated institutional programs (Carling, Randolph, Blanch, & Ridgway, 1987), and "model" community support programs appear to be relatively rare (Bachrach, 1980). We also hear of a pervasive lack of attention to mental health consumers' rights (Chamberlin, 1978; Leete, 1989). On the other hand, we also read and hear about the development of more responsive and effective community support services (Stein & Test, 1985); increased attention to consumer empowerment (Leete, 1989); more effective and respectful clinical interventions (Anthony & Blanch, 1989; Strauss, 1989); and a clearer emphasis on meeting the basic needs of people with disabilities for homes, jobs, and friends (Taylor et al., 1987; Wilson, 1992).

Considering these dramatically conflicting views, it has been suggested that the field of mental health is in the midst of a "paradigm shift" with regard to people with the most severe disabilities (Blanch, Carling, & Ridgway, 1988; Carling, 1990a; Zipple & Ridgway, 1990). We have moved from an era of institutional and facility-based thinking in which these people were seen exclusively as their illnesses (i.e., as patients), through a "transitional" period in which these individuals were seen principally in terms of their disabilities (i.e., as service recipients needing a comprehensive community support system) (Turner & TenHoor, 1979), to a world view in which these people are seen principally as citizens who happen to have disabilities, but share with all citizens the potential for, and right to, full community participation and integration (Carling, 1990a; Wilson, 1992). This conceptual shift, which has dramatic implications for how people with psychiatric disabilities are to be served, is illustrated in Figure 1.1 and discussed in more detail in Chapter Two.

PATIENT

SERVICE RECIPIENT

PERSON
(CITIZEN WITH RIGHTS)

FIGURE 1.1. Changing views of people with psychiatric disabilities.

CHANGING APPROACHES TO HOUSING, WORK, EDUCATION, AND SOCIAL SUPPORT

Housing

The Crisis in Affordable Housing

> I'm working . . . with people who are homeless, and they've been
> through the whole gamut of living in board and care homes, halfway
> houses and shelters, and everyone, without exception, says they want
> their own place or a shared place with somebody they've decided to
> share it with.
> —HOWIE THE HARP (quoted in Ridgway, 1988a, p. 26)

The housing problems faced by people with psychiatric disabilities are
compounded by dramatic changes in the current generic housing scene.
Two factors in recent years have reduced access to housing for *all* people in the United States with limited incomes: a decline in affordable
housing stock, and the rising cost of housing in relation to income.
This combination has put home ownership out of the reach of many
middle-income Americans, and decent housing out of the reach of most
of those at or below the poverty level. To make matters worse, these
trends have been accompanied by a cut of nearly 80% in federally assisted housing for low-income and special-needs groups since 1981,
and a dramatic increase in homelessness in all parts of the country
(Low-Income Housing Information Service, 1988). Kozol (1988)
describes the profound human toll these events have taken. Because
disabilities can be economically catastrophic, people with disabling
conditions are disproportionately represented in the segment of the
population that is "very poor," or well below the poverty level. A recent national study conducted by the Center for Community Change
through Housing and Support, for example, concluded that there was
not a single county in the United States in which a person with a psychiatric disability, supported by disability benefits, could afford an ef-
ficiency or a one-bedroom apartment (according to the federal standard
of "affordability"). In this study, people with psychiatric disabilities
averaged about 20% of the median incomes in their communities
(McCabe et al., 1993).

Paradoxically, because general access to affordable housing has
become in effect a national crisis, public awareness of this issue and
public support for increased federal and state spending and taxation
for this purpose are at all-time highs (National Housing Institute, 1988).
Thus, even as federal housing programs were being cut in 1988, Congress was passing sweeping new affordable housing legislation to

reverse these trends (Carling, 1990a). These developments represent an important opportunity to introduce innovative strategies for more successful community integration of mental health consumers/ex-patients through a focus on housing.

Mental Health Initiatives in Housing: Changing Models from the 1950s to the 1980s

For many decades prior to the middle of the 20th century, the dominant form of housing in North America for people with psychiatric disabilities, based on the prevailing assumptions or myths that have been described above, was the state/provincial psychiatric hospital. At midcentury, however, a variety of potent factors combined to result in large-scale releases from state institutions. These included the advent of psychotropic medications, the availability of federal funding for other institutional alternatives such as nursing homes, and the emergence of a body of case law that promoted patients' rights (Kiesler, 1982). The 1950s and 1960s abounded with rhetoric about a "community mental health" approach (Bachrach, 1980); however, I (Carling, 1978) and others have argued that deinstitutionalization to the community never really occurred. Instead, funds remained in institutions; programs needed in the community were generally not developed; and patients were "transinstitutionalized" to nursing homes, boarding homes, and foster care settings.

These outcomes make perfect sense if we understand that what fueled the deinstitutionalization movement was a variety of political, legal, and economic forces, and not a fundamentally different view of people with psychiatric disabilities. In fact, mental health legislative lobbyists continue to argue in the 1990s about how many "residential facilities" are needed, using various professional experts to support their positions. In this context, it seems clear that the mental health field will begin to shift its major focus toward integration only if the users of mental health services themselves organize to force this change. In fact, consumer and family advocacy has already begun to force a significant shift in the mental health field's view of housing and other needs in the last 15 years (as noted earlier), at least at a policy level.

Traditionally, mental health agencies have viewed housing as a social welfare problem, and have defined their roles in terms of "treatment." Public housing agencies, reflecting societal stigma, contend that mental health consumers need "specialized residential programs," and see their housing needs as a mental health responsibility (Carling & Ridgway, 1987). Thus, housing needs are often ignored: "residential services" in mental health are typically therapeutic facilities, not housing. Transitional "halfway houses" proliferated in the 1960s. In the 1970s, the concept of a "residential continuum" emerged; it included a variety of models, such as "quarterway" and "halfway" houses (Budson, 1981), "three-quarterway" houses (Campbell, 1981), "family foster care" (Carling, 1984), "crisis alternative models" (Stein & Test, 1985; Test, 1981), "Fairweather Lodges" (Fairweather, 1980), "apartment programs" (Carling, 1978; Goldmeier, Shore, & Mannino, 1977), "boarding homes" (Kohen & Paul, 1976), "nursing homes" (Carling, 1981), and "shelters for homeless persons" (Baxter & Hopper, 1984). These programs have typically been segregated, professionally staffed, and congregate in nature (Carling & Ridgway, 1987).

What do we know about these residential programs? A recent national survey of over 2500 community residential programs serving adults with psychiatric disabilities (Randolph, Sanford, Simoneau, Ridgway, & Carling, 1988) found that despite large-scale development of residential programs in the 1980s, a relatively small number of agencies were involved in providing these services in most states. In spite of the "continuum" model, few of the agencies surveyed offered more than one residential option. Fewer than a quarter of the programs were large congregate facilities, but these accounted for most of the residents in the study. The newer supervised apartment programs and supportive housing approaches, which involved standard-size housing arrangements, used larger numbers of households, each of which served a small number of people. This approach is more consistent with "normalization" principles (Taylor et al., 1987; Turner & Ten-Hoor, 1979). Intermediate care facilities, nursing homes, and shelters had few formal ties with mental health services.

Residential services, because of their cost, are generally viewed in the field as being reserved for those individuals with the most "intensive needs." In reality, however, the Randolph et al. (1988) study revealed that they typically had neither highly disabled clients nor highly professional staff. In fact, these programs were staffed primarily by paraprofessionals who had not been trained in the traditional mental health core disciplines. Follow-up services were essentially informal, suggesting that efforts to assist clients to maintain stable housing were relatively weak. Sixty thousand individuals received services from this sample of residential programs. If we extrapolate that figure to include all residential programs, it represents fewer than 5% of people in the United States with long-term psychiatric disabilities (Center for Mental Health Services, 1993). This is consistent with state estimates that between 2% and 5% of people with psychiatric disabilities are served in residential programs (Ridgway, 1986). Individuals served in these programs were primarily young adults with diagnoses of major mental disorders. Using a functional rating scale ("functional," "moderately disabled," "severely disabled," or "gravely disabled"), over one-half of the programs reported serving persons who were "moderately disabled" or "severely disabled." The remaining programs served people who were either "gravely disabled" or "functional," but surprisingly, these programs served *twice* as many persons who were "functional" as those who were "gravely disabled." This finding contradicts the popular notion that residential programs are serving only those persons with the most severe disabilities; and it raises serious concerns over whether such scarce and expensive resources should be serving so many individuals who are functioning relatively well.

Our knowledge about "what works" in residential programs is hampered by both methodological and conceptual problems. Few evaluations of community residential services have been rigorous enough for conclusions to be drawn (Braun et al., 1981; Kiesler, 1982; Test & Stein, 1978). Moreover, because the goals of community residential programs have rarely been well defined, most outcome evaluations have been conceptually flawed. The most frequently asked evaluation question has been whether or not community programs are more successful than institutional treatment in helping persons to meet basic goals of independent living. In five major reviews covering several hundred "alternatives to hospitalization," only a handful of studies met basic criteria of experimental design (Braun et al., 1981; Carpenter, 1978; Dellario & Anthony, 1981; Kiesler, 1982; Test & Stein, 1978). Taken as a whole, these studies indicated that "community-based treatment" is virtually always as effective as or more effective than "hospital-based treatment" in helping people with psychiatric disabilities to achieve employment outcomes, to gain re-entry into the community, and to reduce the use of medication and outpatient services. From these studies, we can conclude that any of a wide range of community services can assist in achieving some measure of community integration.

With regard to residential programs, Cometa, Morrison, and Ziskoven (1979) reviewed a total of 109 studies and concluded that evidence of the effectiveness of transitional halfway houses in reducing recidivism, improving economic self-sufficiency, and improving community adjustment was "highly suspect" (p. 25). Transitional residential programs may in fact be preferable to institutional care, but according to this review, they fall considerably short of helping people to achieve lasting community integration.

Several strategies for addressing the housing and support needs of homeless people with psychiatric disabilities have emerged, some

based on NIMH demonstration projects. Several studies have reported that the top priorities for most homeless persons, at least initially,
are social resources and support, rather than mental health treatment.
These studies suggest that the key interventions related to housing stability are (1) engaging an individual in a relationship focused on basic
needs, and (2) providing case management and linkages with other services (Morse & Calsyn, in press; Mulkern & Bradley, 1986; First, Rife,
& Kraus, 1990). A comprehensive outreach approach that offers health
and mental health services, and that focuses on the perspectives and
demands of clients, work options, and supported housing, has been
reported to be effective in helping most people overcome homelessness (Schutt, Goldfinger, & Penk, 1992; Culhane, 1992; Gelberg & Linn,
1988).

Goering, Durbin, Trainor, and Paduchak (1990) have summarized
essential service principles for working with people who are homeless. First, normal community living in long-term or permanent housing is the goal. Second, permanent housing with flexible supports,
rather than a residential treatment program, is the preferred model.
Third, consumer involvement in planning and governing is essential.
Fourth, a commitment to ongoing review of both the quality of housing and the adequacy of services is necessary. Despite these findings,
others continue to call for new forms of "asylum" (Drake, Wallach,
& Hoffman, 1989) or for a variety of other institutional solutions
(Belcher, 1988).

Perhaps the most intriguing findings in this area have come from
an extensive study of sheltered care environments conducted by Segal and Aviram (1978) and an analysis of the deinstitutionalization literature by Tabor (1980). Segal and Aviram's work indicated that
characteristics of the *community* were more important than characteristics of *residents* in predicting the degree to which people actually
participated in community life; specific characteristics of the facility
were the least important factor. These studies suggest that outcome
research should be reframed to include a focus on where people live
and how they spend their time, rather than focusing solely on the interventions that professionals provide.

In summary, there have been relatively few rigorous evaluations
of specific residential programs, and very few attempts to examine
professionals' success in helping people to get and keep normal housing. The lack of information on program effectiveness is a critical deficit
that can result in grossly inefficient use of resources, and, most importantly, seriously curtailed opportunities for people with psychiatric
disabilities.

Supported Housing: The Emerging Approach

One of the most important ways to find out where people want to live is
to simply ask.
                                    —Laura Van Tosh (quoted in Ridgway, 1988a, p. 26)

In recent years, as I have noted earlier in the chapter, the mental health
field has been undergoing a "paradigm shift" in its approach to housing (Zipple & Ridgway, 1990). Beginning with a series of policy statements (NIMH, 1987a; NASMHPD, 1989), U.S. national policy began
to emphasize three key emerging principles: consumer choice (Ridgway, 1988b), normal integrated housing (Hogan & Carling, 1992), and
flexible, individualized supports (Carling, 1990a). Following the development of these national policies, a large number of state and local
mental health systems began revising their goals and policies, and then
experimenting with ways to offer consumers housing and supports in
more flexible and integrated ways. Similar policy changes have occurred throughout Canada (Pape, 1990).

These policies have dramatic implications for how both housing
and services are provided and evaluated (Carling, 1990b). In the last
several years, the Center for Community Change through Housing and
Support has worked with state or provincial and local mental health
systems in 49 U.S. states, 6 Canadian provinces, and 4 Australian states
to revise their policies and funding in this new direction. The center
has also documented over 100 new local programs, some operated by
professionals and others by consumers, that conform to these new principles. Although this number represents only a very small proportion
of the total number of mental health programs nationally, supported
housing appears to represent the major future trend in the field.

Employment

The Crisis in Employment

Just as people with psychiatric disabilities are profoundly affected by
trends in affordable housing, their fortunes rise and fall as the economy experiences varying levels of unemployment. Downward shifts in
the labor market typically result in abysmally low employment levels
among people with psychiatric disabilities. Current labor market trends
include the following: There will be a dramatic decline in the need
for unskilled labor; most growth in positions will occur in small businesses, and that most new jobs will be found in the service and information sectors. Furthermore, increasing numbers of women have en-

tered the work force, in response both to the need for two incomes in two-parent households, and to the rapidly escalating numbers of single-parent households. The combined effect of these factors has been to make the total pool of jobs even smaller (Hasizi & Collins, 1988).

Within this changing labor market, many mental health agencies and vocational rehabilitation programs continue to focus on entry-level positions with no potential for substantial skills development or career advancement. For this reason, increasing numbers of consumers/ex-patients resist participation in such programs, even though they may lack the proper resources and/or skills to secure employment on their own. It is unclear to what extent the very low success rate in employment for people with psychiatric disabilities is a function of unattractive programs and lack of real job options, rather than deficits in clients (W. A. Anthony, personal communication, September 1990).

Without a significant rethinking of the field's approach, and without a significant increase in the resources allocated to strategies that produce permanent employment and progressive career options for people, it is unlikely that these success rates will change over time.

Mental Health Approaches to Meeting Employment Needs

There are a number of excellent summaries of the research on employment and psychiatric disabilities (Anthony & Blanch, 1989; NIMH, 1990). These summaries conclude that work is of profound importance from both a psychological and an economic perspective. They also indicate that although people with psychiatric disabilities represent the largest disability group served by the vocational rehabilitation system, they are the least likely to secure employment. Data on actual employment (Dion & Anthony, 1987) reveal that fewer than 25% of individuals discharged from psychiatric hospitals become employed; in the case of people with significant disabilities, that figure shrinks to about 15%.

Bond (1987) has summarized the current research on the effectiveness of mental health vocational programs. His conclusions are as follows: (1) Regardless of type, vocational programs improve paid employment rates, but not necessarily competitive employment rates; (2) sheltered settings, including hospitals, sheltered workshops, and prevocational preparation programs, are self-perpetuating and create an "institutional dependency"; (3) clients, especially those with prior work histories, benefit from rapid re-entry into community employment; (4) assessment procedures, except for situational assessments, do not predict vocational outcomes; (5) once clients terminate from a time-limited program, their progress tends to decline; (6) the length of client participation in a vocational program is correlated with client success; (7) engagement and retention of clients in vocational programs are difficult; (8) the characteristics of the provider of transitional or supported employment services are important determinants of success; and (9) clients participating in high-expectation vocational programs are at no greater risk of rehospitalization.

In a summary of the research on the predictors of vocational success among people with psychiatric disabilities, Anthony and Jansen (1984) concluded that, contrary to popular wisdom in many programs, the following factors are *not* predictive of vocational success: psychiatric symptomatology; diagnostic category; intelligence, aptitude, or personality assessments; or the ability to function in a treatment environment (e.g., a hospital or community program). Furthermore, these authors concluded that there is little or no correlation between a person's symptoms and functional skills; that the best clinical predictors of a person's ability to work are ratings done in actual work environments; that the best demographic predictor of work success is prior work history; that a significant predictor of work success is the ability to "get along" and interact socially; and that the best paper-and-pencil test predictors of future vocational performance are those that measure a person's ego strength or self-concept in the role of worker.

Just as "sheltered" approaches to housing predominated in mental health prior to the 1980s, in the vocational arena sheltered workshops and day treatment programs were seen as the major vehicles for occupying people's time. In recent years (NIMH, 1990), interest in hospital-based or even facility-based approaches has waned in favor of "real-world" approaches. Studies of sheltered workshops and of "job clubs" have not demonstrated the effectiveness of these approaches. Another approach, the Fairweather Lodge (Fairweather, 1980), involves people living and working together with minimal mental health supports in the community. A review prepared by NIMH (1990) concludes that research on this approach is "very encouraging" with regard to community employment and tenure, but that nonetheless more studies are needed. Specifically, the review asserts that research is needed into the relative effectiveness of various vocational models—particularly studies of who benefits from transitional and supported employment approaches (see below), and studies of how to effect transitions with minimal disruption and dislocation. Studies are also needed on the specific needs of women and of various racial and social class groups with regard to employment. Finally, studies are needed on the kind of employment-related services that people actually want (including services that reduce the impact of relapse on job retention), and on the specific reasonable accommodations that people with psychiatric disabilities need on the job (NIMH, 1990).

During the past decade, many rehabilitation programs have pursued a "transitional employment" approach, in which individuals work in regular industry, often with several people occupying the same position, for a limited period (generally 6 months) in order to gain work experience. This approach was pioneered by Fountain House in New York City. More recently, however, the field has begun to emphasize a "supported employment" approach. This approach differs from transitional employment in several ways. Anthony and Blanch (1989) summarize these differences as follows: Whereas the goal of transitional employment is to develop confidence and a work history, supported employment aims to produce actual goods and services and to realize the economic and psychological benefits of work; transitional employment is temporary and supported employment is permanent; transitional employment tends toward entry-level jobs with on-site support, while supported employment focuses on jobs at all levels, with variations in support both on and off site; finally, in transitional employment the employer generally knows about the disability, whereas in supported employment the employer may not know.

Supported employment was first developed for use with persons with developmental disabilities; its development was spurred by far-reaching federal special education legislation. Unlike sheltered or transitional approaches, supported employment stresses (1) a goal of freely chosen paid employment for all people with disabilities; (2) integrated work settings; and (3) ongoing support, including supervision, training, and transportation (Anthony & Blanch, 1989). Wehman and Kregel (1985) suggest that most supported employment programs should include four functions: job acquisition, job site training, ongoing monitoring, and follow-up. These functions, and strategies for developing supported employment, are described in detail in Chapter Eight of this book.

It is important to note that there have been some significant problems in adapting the supported employment approach used with people with *developmental* disabilities to the specific needs and characteristics of people with *psychiatric* disabilities. In response to these challenges, Anthony and Blanch (1989) describe several principles that, though not necessarily unique in their applicability to people with psychiatric disabilities, appear critical to these people's successful employment. These include substantial involvement of the individuals themselves in selecting the work options, based on their interests and abilities; focusing the assessment process on people's individual work goals; providing for a more lengthy pre-employment phase if needed;

assuring that there are a range of jobs with advancement potential; anticipating problems with stigma, and therefore assuring that people do not have to identify themselves as "psychiatrically disabled" in the work place if they choose not to; providing training in resume writing, interviewing, and other skill areas; planning family members' involvement with a sensitivity to the autonomy of each consumer; focusing on the application and utilization of skills, rather than only on their acquisition; and coordinating supports during nonworking hours.

Education

The Crisis in Educational Opportunities

Many people experience the onset of a psychiatric disability during their early adulthood, often before they have completed their education. It is only recently—through some of the projects throughout North America that have focused on "supported education" (Unger, Danley, Kohn, & Hutchinson, 1987),—that we have become more clearly aware of the large number of people who wish to return to school after a disability has interrupted their career planning or pursuit of a degree. Similarly, many people want further training opportunities that will prepare them for a career. Finally, people who are currently experiencing serious mental health problems in most colleges, universities, or training institutions typically have little or no access to the kinds of supports that will allow them to return quickly after a crisis, hospitalization, or other disruption. People who are able to return to school often have no access to the specific information or services they may need, such as more intensive advising, special scheduling, adjustment requirements connected with examinations, adaptations of the course registration processes or other stressors, information about the effects of medication on academic performance, and so forth. Until these needs for economic access and support are addressed, people with psychiatric disabilities are unlikely to have the same opportunities that other citizens enjoy for pursuing higher education or other training, or for enjoying the economic independence and personal satisfaction associated with careers.

Integration into Educational Settings

By contrast with their efforts in regard to housing and employment, mental health professionals have only recently begun to consider approaches that will promote career planning and re-entry into either higher education or other forms of integrated training for people with psychiatric disabilities. Innovative programs such as the one at Boston University's Center for Psychiatric Rehabilitation (Unger et al., 1987) are organized to respond to the desire of many people with disabilities to return to their interrupted college careers and/or to plan careers. This program provides the opportunity for people to participate in a career development process, including examining vocational potential, researching career alternatives, career planning, and strategic planning; it uses a self-contained classroom model. A series of observations by students in the program (Unger et al., 1987) provides an excellent description of the benefits of this approach. This program has begun to be replicated in Buffalo, New York (Buffalo State College), Toronto (George Brown College), and elsewhere.

A variety of approaches to "supported education" or "supported learning" are emerging. One is an on-site model in which students receive assistance in more integrated settings, such as Quinsigamond Community College in Worčester, Massachusetts or Mott Community College in Flint, Michigan. Other options are a "mobile supported education model," also used at Boston University's Center for Psychiatric Rehabilitation, which provides longer-term support to students participating in regular classes. Thresholds, in Chicago, is a program focused on the transition from high school to college. Finally, the state of California's community colleges, in a system-wide study, have identified major goals for increasing access to college for people with psychiatric disabilities, as well as supports focused on retention of students. Each of these innovative approaches is described in a special issue of *Community Support Network News* (1990).

Social Support

The Crisis in Social Integration

Mental health systems face the same crisis with regard to social integration. People cannot thrive or even survive in communities without a long-term network of friends and family. Furthermore, it is becoming increasingly clear that systems simply cannot afford to provide paid, long-term social relationships for consumers/ex-patients. Even if funding were available, it is doubtful they should do so, since what these people clearly need is an expanded range of freely given, voluntary relationships that are not focused on the individuals' disabilities. In the absence of real friends, many people with psychiatric disabilities experience a profound despair when they come to realize that their social networks consist entirely of people who are paid to relate to them. It is this despair, in part, that has fueled interest in the self-help and mutual support movement (P. [Dorfner] Engels, personal communication, September 1990).

Although mental health professionals have attempted to organize *programs* or *services* designed to enhance clients' social skills, in many cases they have done so in the context of refusing to develop social relationships with people with psychiatric disabilities themselves. Even today, many mental health agencies have restrictions on clients' using certain areas of the agencies, restrictions on the extent to which staff members can engage in "social activities" with clients, or even restrictions on staff members' talking with clients when they meet them on the street.

I am reminded of a recent consultation that my colleagues and I conducted in a Western state. The leadership of the mental health system, along with disability and family advocates and service providers, had gathered together for an intensive retreat designed to consider some fundamental changes in the service system, in order to increase integration outcomes and empowerment of people with disabilities. We met at a local "model program." When it came time for a break, I noticed that it took the individuals with psychiatric disabilities nearly three times as long to return to the meeting as it did anyone else. After a while, I couldn't contain my curiosity, and asked one of the disability leaders why this was the case. "Well," he said, "there are only two bathrooms in this mental health center. The one for clients is at the other end of the building."

I instantly had an image of the "colored-only" bathrooms I had seen in the South in the early 1960s. As the meeting progressed, one of the disability leaders quietly circulated a petition addressed to the executive director of the agency, who was sitting at the end of the table. We all signed it, and by the time it reached him, the policy was changed. I wondered how long it would have taken to realize the implications of "separate but equal bathrooms" if we had not scheduled a meeting there to which individuals with disabilities were invited as equals—as people, not as clients. It is hardly an authentic posture to ask the general public to embrace housing and employment integration, and to promote incorporating people with psychiatric disabilities into regular social networks, if mental health professionals are unwilling to take the lead on such behaviors in their own agencies, communities, and personal lives.

Emerging Approaches to Social Integration

Perhaps the sparsest area of mental health research related to integration is that of social networks and social integration. According to NIMH's (1990) summary of research in this area, most people discharged from hospitals spend much of their time alone; even in cases where social networks exist, they are extremely limited, often to other family members. Anthony and Blanch (1989) point out that the social networks of people diagnosed with schizophrenia tend to be smaller than average, contain fewer multiple-role relationships (e.g., people who are both coworkers and friends), and include fewer people to give support to or receive support from.

Anthony and Blanch (1989) go on to summarize a variety of approaches that the mental health field has taken to improve social networks. However, these have typically been limited to networks with others with disabilities: having people live together in residential programs, such as Fairweather Lodges; having them work and socialize together in day treatment programs; or, more recently, having them participate as members in "clubhouses." There has also been some interest in "network therapy," in which professionals attempt to augment social networks by adding members or functions, or by linking these networks to others. Self-help alternatives are increasingly seen as major components of social support; these include mutual support groups, consumer-run businesses, and drop-in centers.

Although some of the directions described above clearly have promise, it is well to remember that most of the research in this area has focused on social skills deficits, rather than on the practical impact of these deficits in actual social situations. Similarly, there has been little research on the quality or extensiveness of people's social networks, or on the strengths that people with psychiatric disabilities may bring to social relationships, such as the capacity to support others who have had similar experiences.

We know little, in fact, about the "peer culture" of ex-patients. Estroff (1981), for example, reports a rather robust social life for many young people with psychiatric disabilities, but one unknown to and often concealed from professionals. People may be reluctant to display such social skills in order to continue having access to mental health programs that, regardless of their flaws, also include the provision of concrete benefits and resources (such as housing, jobs, and entitlements). Estroff also reports significant amounts of social isolation, and concludes that loneliness may be one of the greatest barriers to community success. Clearly, much more research is needed in this area.

Aside from the need for research, it appears that mental health systems need to undergo the same kind of fundamental shift in thinking about social networks that is occurring with regard to housing, employment, and education. In this context, it is plausible to suggest that the reason professionals seem to know so little about the social networks of people with psychiatric disabilities is that their own social networks almost never overlap with those of consumers/ex-patients. If this is the case, it would be far more profitable to begin the learning process by merging those networks first.

It is also clear that consumers/ex-patients find tremendous value in peer support and in coming together as a community of people with a common experience. This experience sets them dramatically and irrevocably apart from people who have not experienced involuntary treatment, psychotropic medications, and the symptoms of severe and persistent mental illnesses (P. [Dorfner] Engels, personal communication, September 1990). Thus, peer support and a strong identification with the "mental patient community" can form a significant core of the social network of many individuals, helping to raise people's consciousness about what has happened to them. On the other hand, many individuals who are actively in the process of "recovery" may often pursue a period of work and social life outside of the peer culture and of mental health systems—perhaps in order to realize their own recovery process more fully, and to move beyond the primary cultural identity of "mental patient." After a time, some individuals may return to participation in peer support and may even take on service delivery roles, as a way of "giving back" help they have received (W. J. Montague, personal communication, September 1990). Thus, people use peer support in highly individual ways.

Those who promote social integration, then, have much to learn about balancing the changing sense of identity that characterizes the recovery process; the need and desire for peer support; the usefulness of "intentional communities"; and the need for social integration, which involves "mainstream" relationships between people with and without labels of "psychiatric disability." The key issues here, as in so many other aspects of integration, are (1) respecting the need of an oppressed group to find a collective voice and culture; and (2) respecting individuals' lifestyle differences and personal preferences, and thus promoting the availability of a variety of options for people to select from.

SHORTCOMINGS OF CURRENT MENTAL HEALTH PROGRAMS

Despite the emergence of new models and the proliferation of residential, vocational, educational, and social services, current programs do not necessarily meet the housing, work, educational, and social needs of people with psychiatric disabilities. In fact, serious questions have been raised about failing to distinguish between people's treatment needs and their needs for homes, jobs, education, and social networks. Questions are also being raised about the assumption that people need to participate in such treatment programs prior to "independent living" (Taylor et al., 1987). The growing acceptance of a rehabilitation approach (Anthony & Jansen, 1984; Blanch et al., 1988) demystifies the acquisition of stable housing, work, education, and social relationships, by defining these goals as a process of building critical skills and supports to "choose," "get," and "keep" the home, work, education, and friendships a person desires.

A range of research and training activities undertaken by the Center for Community Change through Housing and Support has revealed significant dissatisfaction among consumers, their families, and service providers with the concept of a "continuum of facilities," and with the "transitional services" model typically used to accomplish these outcomes (Carling, 1990a).

Problems with the Transitional Services Model

We (Carling & Ridgway, 1987) point out that the notion of "transitional" help through a series of time-limited stays in specialized residential or vocational settings is simplistic, and does not achieve its ostensible purpose of facilitating "independent living." Instead, it creates major difficulties for the individual, including (1) having to learn skills that are mostly relevant to group living, working, or socializing; (2) chronic dislocation through successive moves, since improvement in functioning typically requires a physical move to another setting; and (3) "discharge" or "graduation" back to the family, a boarding home, a hospital, or homelessness and unemployment, since many treatment-oriented programs do not see it as their responsibility to help people secure permanent community housing, work, education, or social relationships.

Problems with the Continuum Concept

Similarly, a "continuum" usually entails allocating resources to separate residential or vocational facilities, rather than to the services and supports that people need to function successfully in normal housing, work, and educational settings and in social networks. The "transition" and the "continuum" concepts often confuse the need for housing, work, education, and friendships with the need for specific supports; moreover, in effect, they require a person to participate in a service program in order to receive any of these benefits.

At the same time, many people are already living in community housing, are working, are in academic and other training programs, and have some social connections, but typically have little support available. Responding to the practical aspects of an individual's life, *wherever the* person is living, learning, working, or socializing, needs to become the major focus of professional concern.

Problems with Differing Perspectives between Professionals and People with Disabilities

A final area of controversy concerns the role of people with psychiatric disabilities in directly determining the need for housing, work, education, and social supports. An emerging body of research describes the preferences of people with psychiatric disabilities, and how these typically differ from the perspectives of their families and/or of professionals. In a county-wide needs assessment in Washington State, for example, we (Daniels & Carling, 1986) gathered data from both service providers and their clients about their perceptions of the need for housing and supports. Results indicated that professionals and consumers had almost diametrically opposite views about housing needs: Professionals favored transitional, highly staffed (and expensive) group residential programs for the great majority of consumers, and clients expressed preferences for normal housing with flexible supports. Most consumers preferred to live alone or with one other person, rather than in a larger group.

Recently, the first statewide study of consumers' preferences for housing and supports was undertaken in Vermont (Tanzman, Wilson, & Yoe, 1992). The study involved a random sample of individuals who were homeless, in the state hospital, or receiving community services for people with psychiatric disabilities. The results of this study have been replicated in over 50 sites in North America (Tanzman, 1993) and have direct implications for the manner in which housing and support services should be delivered. Summarizing these studies, Tanzman (1993) found that most persons would prefer to live in their own apartments or houses rather than in a facility or program run by a mental health service, in a single-room occupancy (SRO) hotel, with their families, or in a community care (boarding) home. The major barrier individuals saw to realizing their preferences was a lack of adequate income. Most respondents wanted to move in order to live in a better location, have more space in better repair, and have more freedom and autonomy. People in SRO hotels reported the least satisfaction of all respondents, including those in state hospitals and those who were homeless. The most strongly preferred characteristics of living situations were freedom and autonomy, permanence, security, and privacy.

Traditionally, mental health systems have assumed that many people with psychiatric disabilities need live-in staff members to assist them during crisis situations or to teach daily living skills. Similarly, people are often seen as needing on-the-job support from professionals. In contrast, only 10% of the respondents in the studies summarized by Tanzman (1993) reported needing live-in staff. Instead, most preferred that staff members be available by telephone, or in person if necessary, on a 24-hour basis. As contrasted with the traditional "placement" approach into congregate settings, most respondents preferred *not* to live with other mental health consumers, because they felt that it was difficult to live with other people's problems as well as their own. Instead, they wanted to live with a specific friend or romantic partner. These studies indicate that people with severe psychiatric disabilities, whether homeless, in a state hospital, or in community programs, can articulate their needs for both housing and supports, and that they generaly want the same housing as any other citizens want.

CHAPTER 2

Foundations for
a New Approach

To boldly go where everyone else has already gone.
—A popular bumper sticker in support of
the Americans with Disabilities Act

As described in Chapter One, the broader disability movement is increasingly emphasizing the importance of homes, work, education, and social integration, and is sensitizing the mental health field to the importance of separating professional support from those settings in which citizens typically meet these basic needs. Thus, it is critical that professionals avoid transforming homes, work settings, community social activities, and schools into "programs" or "service settings." Similarly, it is critical that professionals not overwhelm an individual's current or potential natural support system of friends, family members, neighbors, and coworkers in order to meet a service need, particularly in a time of crisis.

This chapter describes a community integration approach to providing services and supports, and shows how it contrasts with many service approaches in the mental health field, even the current professional model.

THE EMERGING PARADIGM SHIFT

The dramatic change in thinking that is challenging mental health systems today represents a fundamental shift in how we view people with psychiatric disabilities, what outcomes we believe are possible in their lives, and what approach to services makes the most sense in achieving those outcomes. During the 20th century, the mental health field has changed its answers to these questions in several fundamental "waves" of reform. The first half of the century could be described as the era of institutionalization—an approach that resulted in significant isolation of individuals with mental health problems from the community. These persons were cast in the role of "patients," and the predominant service approach was a traditional "medical model" one. Service characteristics included custodial care, treatment, and protection for (and perhaps from) the community. The vision of the future was one of hopelessness and lifelong dependency. From the 1950s to the present, persons with psychiatric disabilities have been viewed as "clients," or, as discussed in Chapter One, as commodities labeled "service recipients." The predominant service approach shifted during that time from the medical model to a developmental/rehabilitation model. Nevertheless, the emphasis has been on professionals' "providing services" to clients. Program characteristics have focused on the "continuum" of services, on preparing individuals for *eventual* life in the community, and on fitting individuals into program "slots." Too often, the vision of the future has been "more of the same" (i.e., long-term living in the mental health world).

By contrast, the community integration approach that is beginning to emerge in many communities in North America and elsewhere focuses on mental health consumers in the role of "citizens." It emphasizes practical supports, coping strategies, and recovery; it prioritizes networking, self-determination, and free choice. Supports that are provided are based on reciprocal, respectful relationships. The integration paradigm differs dramatically from prior service approaches in several important ways. The individual is seen as a person, rather than as a disabled client. The person's needs are defined in terms of capacities, instead of deficits. The community is viewed as a resource of possibilities, understanding, awareness, acceptance, and inclusion, rather than as an obstacle or as a source of fear, prejudice, ignorance, or rejection. In a community integration approach, power is located in the person through self-determination and through "circles of support," rather than in the hierarchical structures of service systems, in which policy makers regulate the behavior of professionals, who in turn provide services "in the best interests of" the person with a disability. The role of helpers is that of enablers and supporters, rather than that of service providers. Finally, the vision of the future is one in which every citizen pursues his or her dreams and uses his or her gifts, rather than one of continuing clienthood—a role that was in fact created directly by the service models used in the past. In an integration approach, the support role is played by a diversity of individuals, connected in freely given relationships. Even formal services are more often provided by generic community organizations and by peers.

Referring to the work of Kuhn (1970), Zipple and Ridgway (1990) present a compelling case that the integration approach represents a "paradigm shift" for the mental health field. In this shift, we can expect that national, state/provincial, and local policy changes favoring integration will be followed by an increasing intensity of change, as the old assumptions upon which traditional services have been based are seen as no longer viable, or no longer helpful in promoting the kinds of outcomes that people with psychiatric disabilities have come to value. Kuhn (1970), for example, describes the chronology of "scientific revolutions." First, "normal" science is confronted by an increasing number of anomalous observations, which lead to a crisis in the understanding of a phenomenon. "Revolutionary" science, in turn, develops competing alternative theories. The "paradigm shift" then consists of the adoption of a new theoretical framework, which is then used to resume "normal" scientific exploration. So, just as in the case of the undoing of a major scientific theory, we can expect a period of chaos until a new explanation of social reality is accepted. Thus, it is likely that the increasing conflict in the mental health field at present—conflict that primarily represents the differences in goals and power between professionals and people with disabilities—may, in fact, continue and intensify until the integration paradigm is finally broadly accepted.

In many ways, the field of mental health is in a most advantageous position to make major changes, since it has developed an excellent set of service models in recent years. To the extent that these models incorporate new assumptions about people with disabilities and transform the power relationships between professionals and individuals with disabilities, they are quite adaptable as one element (albeit not the most crucial one) in an integration approach. Thus, professional services are necessary but hardly sufficient for achieving integration. The remainder of this chapter describes the current "state-of-the-art" thinking about professional services (the "comprehensive community support systems" model), and then offers an alternative model (a "framework for support"), which views the individual within a vibrant and supportive community. The differences between these two conceptualizations are crucial: The comprehensive community support systems model is essentially a professional one, whereas the framework for support is, in essence, a self-help model. The chapter closes with a series of suggestions for incorporating mental health systems' activities into the framework for support, in a comprehensive approach to achieving community integration. Redefined processes and outcomes for research focused on psychiatric disabilities are also described.

THE CURRENT PROFESSIONAL MODEL: COMPREHENSIVE COMMUNITY SUPPORT SYSTEMS

As mental health systems began to rely less on hospitals, and began gaining valuable experience in supporting individuals with psychiatric disabilities in communities, the concept of "comprehensive community support systems" (Turner & TenHoor, 1979) emerged, primarily through the leadership of the (NIMH) Community Support Program.[1] This model, updated by NIMH as guidance for all U.S. state mental health plans (NIMH, 1987b), is described below. A word of caution is in order, however. Although the model represents the "state of the art" from a professional perspective, and it attempts to incorporate some of the new thinking about integration; the reader is advised to be sensitive to the following: a residual focus on incapacity; an emphasis on the primary need for professionally delivered services over the lifespan, rather than those offered by peers, family members and others; and assumptions about how medically oriented supports should be provided.

Client Identification and Outreach

Because many individuals are isolated or segregated, services need to locate potential clients and to offer them assistance. Outreach services, including transportation, should be offered to those who are unwilling or unable to attend formal programs or treatment centers. Outreach to shelters, soup kitchens, drop-in centers, and the streets is particularly critical for those individuals with psychiatric disabilities who are homeless.

Mental Health Treatment

Mental health treatment and clinical services include diagnostic evaluation by medical personnel; supportive counseling and psychotherapeutic treatment; medication management services; and services for those with both psychiatric and substance abuse problems.

---

1. This program is now located within the federal Center for Mental Health Services, part of the U.S. Public Health Service; it is no longer part of NIMH.

Crisis Response Services

Ongoing support and contact can prevent most crises. Because of the episodic nature of psychiatric disabilities, however, acute care and quick-response crisis stabilization services should be available to each person, to family members, and to other key members of the person's support system. These services should be available on a 24-hour basis, and should include a telephone hotline, walk-in crisis services, mobile outreach, community crisis residential options, and a small number of inpatient beds. Although there has been a virtual explosion of nonhospital crisis alternatives nationally, the continued availability of high-quality inpatient services is essential. These need to be located close to individuals' homes, and to work in close partnership with other community support services.

Health and Dental Care

Because persons with psychiatric disabilities have significantly higher rates of physical illness, they should have access to general health care and to dental services.

Housing

There should be permanent, affordable, acceptable housing available in normal community housing arrangements. Individuals should exercise choice and control over housing. Skills training, supports, and services should be available, regardless of where people live. There should also be a small number of structured supervised settings. Homeless individuals require additional living situations with varying degrees of supervision and structure.

Income Support and Entitlements

There should be assistance to help clients obtain income supports and other entitlements.

Peer Support for Clients

There should be consumer self-help groups and consumer-operated services in each locality, which are self-defined and consumer-controlled, and which supplement formal mental health services. These should include peer support groups; drop-in centers or social clubs; independent living programs that assist individuals to obtain financial benefits, housing, counseling/referral, independent living skills training, job counseling, and employment; consumer-run housing, businesses, respite care, or crisis assistance services; and community education on psychiatric disabilities and the potential of individuals with these disabilities to lead productive, satisfying lives and to contribute to the communities in which they live.

Family and Community Support

Because many persons with psychiatric disabilities reside with their families, there should be assistance to families, including education on the nature of the disabilities, consultation/supportive counseling, involvement in treatment planning, respite care, and referrals to family support and advocacy groups. Backup support should be available to landlords, employers, friends, community agencies, and others who come in frequent contact with individuals with these disabilities.

Rehabilitation Services

Social and vocational rehabilitation services are critical for most individuals living in the community.

Social Rehabilitation

In order to help each person gain or regain practical skills needed to live and socialize in the community, social rehabilitation services should include teaching clients how to cope with their disabilities; assisting them in developing social skills, interests, and leisure time activities; and teaching daily living skills.

Vocational Rehabilitation

There should be a range of vocational services and employment opportunities available to assist clients to prepare for, obtain, and maintain employment, including vocational assessment and counseling; prevocational job readiness; career development; on-the-job training; job sharing; transitional employment; supported employment; competitive employment; job development with local employers; and innovative approaches to using recovering consumers as mental health workers.

Protection and Advocacy

There should be grievance procedures and mechanisms to protect clients' rights (both within and outside of mental health and residential facilities), as well as ways to inform clients and their families of their legal rights and resources. Protection and advocacy services and the investigation of grievances against the system should be handled through various state and local agencies and voluntary organizations.

Case Management Services

There should be case management (sometimes called "community service coordination" or "resource management") services available for all clients who need these services. This involves having a single person or a team of persons responsible for maintaining a long-term supportive relationship with each client, regardless of where the client is living and the number of agencies involved. The case manager is a helper, service broker, and advocate for the client, and should function in a manner that is client-directed and client-empowering. Specific functions should include identifying clients who need and desire case management services; working with each client to develop a comprehensive service plan based on the client's needs and goals; providing information to help the client make an informed choice about opportunities and services; assisting the client, on request, to obtain needed services, supports, and entitlements; being available during and after regular working hours; and advocating at the systems level for needed systems improvements. Close contact between client and case manager during hospitalizations is essential, as are a variety of mechanisms to closely coordinate hospital and community services. For psychiatrically disabled individuals who are homeless, effective case management must be intensive and ongoing, and should take place in shelters or on the streets.

Figure 2.1, reprinted from NIMH (1987b), graphically depicts the community support systems model. Viewing this picture, one could argue that, in spite of many positive features, clients, segregated in the mental health world, are surrounded by professionals responsible for meeting their every need.

AN ALTERNATIVE TO THE PROFESSIONAL MODEL: THE FRAMEWORK FOR SUPPORT

In spite of the widespread acceptance of the community support systems perspective in the United States, Canadian mental health theorists have adopted a different and perhaps more progressive set of policies, referred to as a "framework for support" (Trainor & Church, 1984; Trainor, Pomeroy, & Pape, 1993; Pape, 1990). In this conceptualiza-

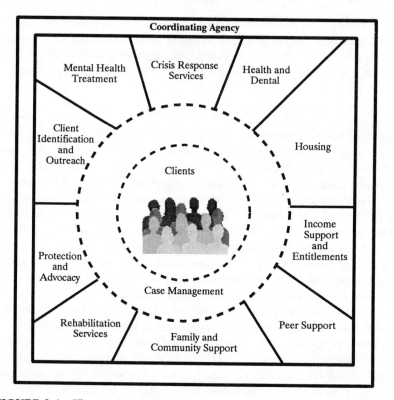

FIGURE 2.1. The community support system model. From NIMH (1987b).

tion, the core approach that is expected to lead to integration and success is not the use of professional services, but self-help. People are also expected to draw upon family, friends, and other close, freely given relationships for support. It is further assumed that people should expect support from generic community organizations and associations (e.g., churches, social clubs, and community service agencies) that are intended for all community members, not just those with special needs or labels. Lastly, people should expect services from the formal mental health service system, which is organized primarily to "support the supporters"—in other words, to bolster the efforts of self-help, natural relationships, and community resources. This conceptual approach (which is used throughout the remainder of this book) seems to be an effective way of thinking about integration, since it more closely approximates the manner in which all citizens, regardless of any special needs or circumstances, live in and expect to receive support in their communities. Within the framework for support, change will only come when powerful partnerships are developed between and among

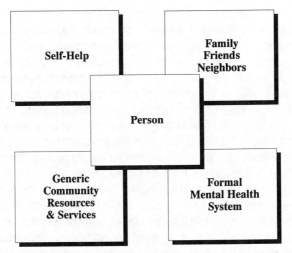

FIGURE 2.2. The framework for support. From Trainor and Church (1984). Copyright 1984 by the Canadian Mental Health Association. Reprinted by permission.

those who are involved in each part of the framework. Figure 2.2 visually depicts this model.

As suggested above, the framework for support is a model in which the major supports in a person's life come first and foremost from the person (self-help), then from friends and family (peer support and family support), then from generic community services (housing assistance, employment/training, local recreational opportunities, health care, etc.), and only then from the formal mental health system. It is within this framework that we can best examine the capacity of each of our communities to support people with psychiatric disabilities, and then to propose changes in each of these four "sectors" of support. It is important not to begin this examination from the narrow perspective of formal mental health services alone (as in the community support systems model), since the tendency in communities is always for formal services to take on the responsibilities of, or to overwhelm, the other three sectors of support. Instead of being the "backup" to those sectors, professional services then become the *only* support sector, with a person becoming increasingly isolated from natural supports. In a vicious cycle, the formal system, which is chronically underfunded, becomes too burdened to continue effective support. Thus, the person ends up isolated *and* unsupported.

The goal of the framework for support (Trainor & Church, 1984) is to ensure that people with psychiatric disabilities live rich and fulfilling lives in the community. Mental health services should be oriented toward assisting and buttressing each of the other elements of the support system in whatever ways necessary, so as to minimize the ongoing need for professional intervention. The two basic requirements for meeting this goal are (1) that individuals with mental health problems be empowered to control their own lives and to make choices about which supports to use; and (2) that the community be mobilized to use all of its capacity to welcome and support people with mental health problems. This approach has major implications for communities and for service systems, since consumer participation and empowerment are essential to successful integration. In an effective support system, all sectors are equally balanced (instead of being dominated by the formal mental health system); a legislative framework is necessary; and roles in the formal mental health system need to be redefined (Pape, 1990).

The Framework for Support Project, a pilot project incorporating the model's principles, has been tested in three communities in Canada. In a summary of the results, Pape (1990) found that achieving a balance of power is both complicated and chaotic; that consumer participation requires groundwork; that the framework cannot function without community reinvestment (i.e., shifting resources from institutional and professional services to community- and consumer-controlled services); and that there must be an articulated and explicit set of values, along with the leadership to put these values into practice. In order to understand this approach, it is necessary to describe in detail the various sectors of support in terms of their guiding principles, essential components of support, and expected outcomes.

A Focus on the Person and on Self-Help

The shift from a professional focus to one on the capacities of the person and his or her peers implies a fundamental shift in who defines the person's needs. As Judi Chamberlin has noted, "When mentally ill people are directly asked about their needs, the answers are usually no different from those of others. They want a decent place to live, a job or a productive way to spend their time, and adequate income and friends" (quoted in Ridgway, 1988a, p. 24).

Individuals with mental health problems, like everyone else, have unique strengths that can be applied to their equally unique needs. In self-help groups, these individuals use their collective strength to support one another, to reduce isolation, and to promote social change. Thus, the goal of both formal and informal support systems is to maximize the extent to which people take charge over their own lives and are able to make all substantive decisions about life goals, directions, and choices. None of us take charge of our lives without a great deal of ongoing support from others, typically from family members and friends; thus the goal is not to have a person with a psychiatric disability be "independent," but rather "interdependent," with the power to direct his or her own life. As Anthony, Cohen, and Cohen (1984) point out, sometimes an individual has to become more *dependent* on others (e.g., using a personal care attendant) in order to become more *independent* in other life areas (e.g., holding a job).

People with psychiatric disabilities move toward this degree of control over their destinies through having the support to develop clear goals, aspirations, and dreams, and through acquiring both the skills and the resources to pursue those aspirations. This focus on individual goals, skills, supports, and increased life mastery is consistent with some aspects of modern professional approaches as well, including the psychiatric rehabilitation approach (Anthony, 1979) and the comprehensive community support systems approach (Turner & TenHoor, 1979; NIMH, 1987b). Having goals, skills, and supports allows people to take personal responsibility for where they are in their lives and for where they are going. One of the pernicious aspects of "oversupporting" an individual, of course, is that all sense of personal responsibility is lost, and hence the person is consigned to the role of "terminally dependent patient." In this process, people's aspirations no longer matter. Since aspirations are irrelevant (or seemingly not achievable), they become increasingly inaccessible to the individuals, as well as to their "helpers." What follows is a claim by the "helpers" that the people are "unmotivated" or "don't know what they want"; therefore, all decisions need to be made for them. This results in a vicious, self-defeating cycle for both parties. When people try to break out of this cycle, they are often accused of being "treatment-resistant." But perhaps the real problem, as Anthony (1990a) points out, is the fact that many services are unattractive; it may be the case that "we simply haven't made people a good enough offer."

To be sure, many aspects of psychiatric disabilities themself interfere substantially with people's ability to take charge of their lives. Symptoms such as impaired concentration or judgment, difficulty in coping with feelings (including periodic despair or an intense desire to end one's life), and experiencing delusions or hallucinations are often extremely painful and pose major challenges to individuals and their families. However, to the extent that formal services and informal or natural support systems are clearly directed toward the goals of increasing individuals' control over these aspects of their disabilities, and increasing people's ability to articulate and pursue their own aspirations and self-sufficiency, the majority of individuals with serious psychiatric disabilities are able to overcome many of these challenges (Harding, Brooks, Ashikaga, Strauss, & Brier, 1987). In the process, both individuals and service providers are able to begin overcoming the negative attitudes that both groups have previously internalized about the individuals' worth and potential.

Role models are especially important in this process. Thus, contact with other consumers who have taken charge of their lives can be much more valuable than a professional's simple assertion that self-determination is possible. Individuals with psychiatric disabilities provide powerful testimony about the importance of peer modeling and mutual support:

> Mutual support acknowledges that we are all human, with strengths and weaknesses. It gives us validity as people capable of helping each other. . . . It allows us to have normal interactions in the community without someone always doing things for us, because we are perceived as too "sick" to do them for ourselves. Hence, we build self esteem and a sense of identity, dignity and inner strength. We get the good feeling of helping each other while feeling the pride of taking responsibility for ourselves as citizens of the community at large. (Zinman, Harp, & Budd, 1987, p. 48)

And Howie the Harp adds: "Who better can teach you to live independently than somebody who has learned to live independently?" (quoted in Ridgway, 1988a, p. 23).

An essential element of self-help is, of course, power. To the extent that people with disabilities have power and control in their relationships with professionals, they will better learn (or relearn) to exercise that power in ways that increase control over their lives. Thus, an important question that professionals can ask themselves after each interaction with an individual is this: "Does this person have more or less power as a result of this interaction?"

Power is also reflected in the way that a system's resources are allocated. Increasing control over those resources by people with disabilities—for instance, giving them the power to make decisions about how funds are spent, about who is hired, and so forth—provides a valuable "training ground" for increased self-sufficiency. For individuals who are living in a mental health residence or participating in a day treatment program, each of these settings represents a rich opportunity for beginning to exercise power and responsibility, thus increasing their capacity to do the same in other areas of their lives. Programs that consistently shift control of day-to-day operations, as well as long-term direction, to service users are deploying their resources most effectively for rehabilitation and integration.

Informal Caring Networks:
Friends, Families, and Neighbors

Pape (1990) reminds us that "informal caring networks of family, friends and neighbors are a major, though often unrecognized, resource. Their tangible assistance with day to day living needs, as well as the social and emotional support they often provide, may complement and often lessen the need for . . . formal services" (p. 3).

Friends and Neighbors

In the life and fabric of a community, friends are the basic support for everyone. Many people with psychiatric disabilities, for a variety of reasons, have a narrow or even nonexistent friendship network, or a network that consists almost exclusively of other mental patients (Estroff, 1981). Normal friendships, however, are developed in what McKnight (1987) calls the "associational life of a community" (p. 1)— that is, the network of voluntary activities in which community members participate simply because they enjoy them (clubs, activity groups, spending regular time at a particular night spot, etc.). Friendships are also developed through normal community participation in integrated settings, such as jobs, neighborhoods, and schools or other learning activities. Coworkers, neighbors, and fellow students become the most significant pool from which friendships develop through mutual attraction and common interests.

It makes sense, therefore, to focus the efforts of both natural supports and formal services toward maximizing the time that people with psychiatric disabilities spend in contact with a potential pool of friends. Obviously the simplest strategy is to have virtually all rehabilitation and community support efforts take place in "real" environments, such as regular work, housing, and educational settings, in ways that minimize any distinction between people with and without labels. In this respect, the best community support services are often "invisible." Services that operate in this way focus increasingly on supporting the key natural relationships in an individual's life (friends, neighbors, employer, landlord, teachers, etc.), and paying major attention to the ongoing quality and strength of an individual's natural support network. When crises occur, the focus is not only on assisting the individual but on repairing and strengthening the natural support network, so that it is increasingly able to manage and resolve future crises with a minimum of professional help.

Neighbors, in particular, can be a significant source of support for individuals with psychiatric disabilities. At times, some individuals will need help in initiating relationships with neighbors, and some support if difficulties arise in these relationships. It can be helpful for peer supporters or staff members to develop relationships with these neighbors directly, in the role of friends to the individuals with disabilities, and thus ease the transition into the new relationships. Such a strategy opens the door to providing support to both individuals and neighbors in the events that difficulties arise (such as when mental health crises disrupt their connection), as well as to celebrating these relationships as they evolve.

Families

To the extent that people are socially isolated from friends, work, housing, and normal learning opportunities, and to the extent that formal services are weak, family members tend to play the major roles of friends, landlords, and service providers. This combination of roles would overwhelm any family, and it often sets the stage for desperate and destructive situations in which institutionalization becomes the only possible "relief" for overburdened family members. The tragedy in this situation is that few families would ever seek institutionalization for individuals with psychiatric disabilities if they believed that their family member would receive adequate and reliable support in the community. Thus, a major challenge for service providers is to regain the faith of family members, many of whom have given up on the potential of service systems to adequately support people with mental health problems, and to help them achieve community integration.

Family members have specific needs for support, apart from the needs of the relative with a psychiatric disability (Hatfield, 1990). These include information about the disability; opportunities for sharing their own experiences, and for receiving support from and giving it to other families; opportunities to appreciate and cultivate the ways that an individual with a disability positively contributes to the family; assistance in helping the individual to become increasingly self-sufficient and to make the transition to his or her own home and life in the community; and support in responding to periodic crises.

Generic Community Services and Opportunities

There is a rich network of opportunities in every community through which people spend leisure time and contribute to the life of their community. Since people meet others with whom they share these opportunities on the job, in housing arrangements, and in school, the first consideration in seeing the community as a resource is the extent to which people with psychiatric disabilities have access to real jobs, integrated housing, education, and regular recreational opportunities in the community. Gaining access to such resources is a function of relationships (most jobs and homes are found through friends), as well as access to supports that are relevant to these settings.

The goal of natural support systems and of formal services should never be to create separate or parallel work, housing, educational, or recreational opportunities for people with disabilities. Rather, it should be to develop a variety of creative ways to help these individuals gain access to the richness of community life. This is done by exploring, generally through friendships, the kinds of interests individuals have in common with others in the community, and then assisting persons to build relationships with these other community members, providing friendship and support through the process. The field of developmental disabilities, which is also struggling with new approaches to social integration (see Taylor et al., 1987), is increasingly incorporating a "citizen advocacy" approach that concentrates on the development of individual friendships between people with labels and other, nonlabeled community members. This relationship provides caring companionship and, in some cases, friendly assistance. Ongoing support is provided through a committed "circle of support," consisting of friends, family members, and others. Such approaches can also be pursued by supportive professionals, as discussed below.

There are, of course, barriers to integration other than relationships, and a major one is poverty. Often people with psychiatric disabilities lack even the smallest amount of discretionary income needed to participate in a community activity, such as a recreational program or event. Helping people to increase their income and assisting them in developing money management skills can be major forms of support provided by both friends and professionals, since these resources and skills can directly enhance integration.

People often need support to build friendships with coworkers and neighbors, and then to sustain these relationships based on common interests and mutual attraction. Rather than expecting that people's social needs will be met in separate "clubhouses" where their only contact is with fellow ex-patients, professionals and others need to focus on nurturing and encouraging those long-term friendships that are part and parcel of a person's everyday life in the community.

Similarly, community members rely on regular doctors, dentists, counselors, teachers, laundries, restaurants, and so forth to get what they want and need in life. Formal mental health systems that aggressively pursue a goal of integration never develop "specialized" services that relieve community services of the responsibility for including all community members. Thus, professionals need to work more directly with those providing these community services to increase access for individuals with disabilities, rather than working only with the individuals. The strategy becomes one of supporting and changing communities themselves in order to promote inclusion of all members.

Finally, it is important to question what opportunities people with psychiatric disabilities themselves have for contributing to the community in which they live. To some extent, everyone wants to give to others and to enjoy the satisfaction of contributing. However, local fund-raising events, community volunteer activities, voting, and so forth are often not accessible to many individuals, many of whom wish to give to others and to enjoy the satisfaction of contributing. Service providers, families, and friends should be particularly sensitive to such opportunities, in that they can be tremendously healing and empowering for individuals who have come to see themselves as mere recipients of other people's kindness or even pity.

The Formal Mental Health Service System

An effective community support system is one in which professionals work with individuals (self-help) and with the natural support network (friends/neighbors, family, and generic community activities and services) to help people realize their aspirations. The components of the comprehensive community support systems model described above (NIMH, 1987b) are highly relevant, since they represent "state-of-the-art" thinking about how mental health systems can most effectively support people in the community. Unfortunately, in practice they have often been narrowly developed as only a network of formal services, instead of a network of life opportunities and of supports to the natural relationships in people's lives. In a framework for support, professional mental health services are focused on the process of self-discovery and recovery and on the outcomes of self-determination and integration, rather than only the relief of symptoms, the prevention of hospitalization, or "maintenance" in the community.

INTEGRATING PROFESSIONAL MENTAL HEALTH SYSTEMS' ACTIVITIES INTO THE FRAMEWORK FOR SUPPORT

The primary strategy for incorporating the activities of a formal mental health program or system into the larger framework for support is to systematically restructure the mission, policies, funding, operations, and evaluation of current services toward a goal of empowering individuals with psychiatric disabilities. Fortunately, there is an increasing literature on empowerment strategies in mental health to guide these efforts (Rose & Black, 1985; Zinman et al., 1987; Curtis, McCabe, Montague, Caron, & Harp, 1991). Successful strategies for redirecting mental health programs toward the empowerment perspective suggest the following systematic approach:

1. Adopt the community integration approach in all mission and policy statements, articulating values of self-determination and independent living.
2. Change the ways that professionals, agencies, and government bureaucracies relate to people with psychiatric disabilities in decisions about planning, funding, and evaluating services, and in hiring and training of staff.
3. Make the system accountable to the people it serves by asking consumers how they would like a particular service need met before starting any service or program, and by routinely evaluating all services in terms of their concrete outcomes and consumers' satisfaction.

Subsequent sections of this book describe these strategies in further detail.

CHANGING APPROACHES TO THE RESEARCH PROCESS AND TO DEFINING OUTCOMES

The approach to research and evaluation focused on psychiatric disabilities has been undergoing the same paradigm shift as the approach to services. Until recently, many researchers had low expectations for individuals with these disabilities, and thus focused on such questions as the impact of one service on the use of another (e.g., "Will the use of case management decrease hospitalization?"). In addition, traditional research has been conceptualized, conducted, and disseminated almost exclusively by professionals.

Interest in community integration, however, is spawning a new generation of research focused on (1) the lived experience of disability as the major source of the research questions to be developed; (2) full participation by people with disabilities in all aspects of research and evaluation; and (3) an emphasis on the same outcomes that are of concern to all citizens, often described as an improved "quality of life." Table 2.1 (Flanagan, 1978) summarizes the outcomes that are

TABLE 2.1. Components of Quality of Life Judged Important by Most Americans

Physical and material well-being

- *Material comforts*—things like a desirable home, good food, possessions, conveniences, an increasing income, and security for the future.
- *Health and personal safety*—to be physically fit and vigorous, to be free from anxiety and distress, and to avoid bodily harm.

Relationships with other people

- *Relationships with your parents, brothers, sisters, and other relatives*—things like communicating, visiting, understanding, doing things, and helping and being helped by them.
- *Having and raising children*—this involves being a parent and helping, teaching, and caring for your children.
- *Close relationship with a husband/wife/romantic partner.*
- *Close friends*—sharing activities, interests, and views; being accepted, visiting, giving and receiving help, love, trust, support, guidance.

Social, community, and civic activities

- *Helping and encouraging others*—this includes adults or children other than relatives or close friends. These can be your own efforts or efforts as a member of some church, club, or volunteer group.
- *Participation in activities relating to local and national government and public affairs.*

Personal development and fulfillment

- *Learning*—attending school, improving your understanding, or getting additional knowledge.
- *Understanding yourself* and knowing your assets and limitations, knowing what life is all about, and making decisions on major life activities. For some people, this includes religious or spiritual experiences. For others, it is an attitude toward life or a philosophy.
- *Work* in a job or at home that is interesting, rewarding, and worthwhile.
- *Expressing yourself* in a creative manner in music, art, writing, photography, practical activities, or leisure time activities.

Recreation

- *Socializing*—meeting other people, doing things with them, and giving or attending parties.
- *Reading, listening to music, or observing* sporting events or entertainment.
- *Participating in active recreation*—such as sports, traveling and sightseeing, playing an instrument, acting, and other such activities.

Note. From Flanagan (1978). Copyright 1978 by the American Psychological Association. Reprinted by permission.

important to most Americans; these consitute appropriate foci of integration-oriented research and evaluation.

QUESTIONS FOR THE FUTURE

Communities and service systems that are moving toward an integration approach face significant challenges. Traditional funding streams, program requirements, administrative approaches to resource allocation and management, and even staff skills are typically not oriented toward intensive support for people with psychiatric disabilities in normal housing and work settings (Carling & Wilson, 1988). Such systems, rather than developing more residential or vocational facilities, should emphasize developing better community services, using the broader community as the major resource for helping. They should focus on increasing consumers' income through employment and rent subsidies; building relationships with public and private housing agencies; and restructuring their policies, funding, and accountability mechanisms to focus on tangible outcomes. The key to the success of these strategies is a clear mission that articulates the role of consumers in this process, and specifies the types of housing, work, learning options, and services that will be made available.

Perhaps the major challenge faced by policy makers and professionals is the question of whether it is possible to construct an effective system *without* the powerful participation of consumers in all of its activities. Similarly, we need to ask how we can ensure that mental health systems will stop looking narrowly to professional solutions to the problem of integration, and instead will begin to divert major resources to services directed by consumers, to tangible resources (e.g., funding for rent, tuition), and to approaches that encourage ordinary citizens and communities to take responsibility for accomplishing the goal of integration. How can we ensure that systems will begin to base everything they do on information systematically gathered from consumers about how services should be organized and delivered, and then about consumers' satisfaction with those services? How can we ensure that systems actually use the results of this information gathering to restructure, in major ways, how business is done? How can we ensure that systems will create incentives for local programs and professionals to promote real integration outcomes? And, ultimately, how can we ensure that systems will transfer the power they hold over consumers' lives back to consumers themselves without a profound struggle? Will the political leadership in states or provinces and in communities allow this to happen? Unless consumer advocates and their allies are successful in helping policy makers and political leaders to make a fundamental shift in how they view the personhood and capacities of the people whom systems are intended to serve, this is not likely to happen easily.

CHAPTER 3

Mental Health Consumers and the Consumer Self-Help Movement

What do Abraham Lincoln, Mike Wallace, Mozart, Barbara Bush, Beethoven, Bette Midler, Rod Steiger, Leo Tolstoy, Kristy McNichol, John Keats, Tennessee Williams, Vincent Van Gogh, Isaac Newton, Ernest Hemingway, Sylvia Plath, Michelangelo, Winston Churchill, Betty Ford, Ben Franklin, Dick Cavett, Patty Duke and Charles Dickens have in common? They all had a serious mental illness.

—From a poster used in a public education campaign by the National Mental Health Association (reprinted by permission)

What do we mean when we say "people with psychiatric disabilities" or "people with long-term mental illnesses," or even "consumer/survivors"? On the surface, this appears to be a relatively simple question. In trying to answer it adequately, however, one is thrust into the heart of the general public's confusion about "mental illness," as well as a series of major controversies with which professionals, consumers, and family members are struggling in today's mental health systems. Average citizens operate under the misimpression that nearly anyone who falls into such vague categories as "homeless," "a street person," or "weird" is *de facto* someone with a mental illness; the person is then often consigned to the ranks of the serial killers or "psychos" who constitute the typical contribution of filmmakers and television broadcasters to public enlightenment on this subject.

Although it may be easy to dismiss these stereotypes as products of ignorance, it is also the case that professionals and advocates *within* mental health systems struggle mightily with such basic issues as the nature and etiology of "psychiatric disabilities," the most effective responses to the myriad conditions that are subsumed under this label, and even the numbers and locations of people who are described in this way. The resolution of these controversies is by no means an academic issue. Different assumptions about the nature of disabilities imply dramatically different approaches to treatment and support. Changing the definition of who has a psychiatric disability and who does not has a major impact on whether individuals can secure the financial benefits, services, and rights that make community membership possible. For example, when the U.S. Social Security Administration changed its criteria for psychiatric disabilities in the 1980s, hundreds of thousands of individuals lost their Supplemental Security Income (SSI) benefits until the federal courts ordered their reinstatement. Estimates of the numbers of U.S. citizens with such disabilities, in turn, drive the levels of public funding allocated to this area, the priority that these disabilities are assigned within the overall domestic agenda of government, and even the calculation of insurance benefits related to treatment services.

This chapter describes what we currently know, and what we have not yet come to agree upon, in defining who mental health consumers are and in describing the nature and etiology of their disabilities. The chapter then describes a "quiet revolution" that is taking place, even in the midst of this lack of consensus within the mental health field: a dramatic increase in the extent to which people with psychiatric disabilities are beginning to help themselves—through advocacy, offering technical assistance to one another, and developing and managing a broad range of community support services.

DEFINING "MENTAL HEALTH CONSUMERS" AND "MENTAL ILLNESS"

Chapter One has presented the latest estimates of the numbers and locations of people with psychiatric disabilities in the United States. In discussing what we mean by the term "mental health consumer," however, we need to focus first on an important topic: labels.

The Changing Nature of Labels

Label jars, not people.
—Popular disability rights slogan

Among the most striking indications of the sea change in our field are the significant conflict and confusion about what to call people who have a diagnosis of major mental illness and who have received mental health services. Terms such as "chronically mentally ill" or "the mentally ill," or even "patients," are increasingly seen as stigmatizing and connoting hopelessness. Furthermore, they reinforce the notion that the mental illness is the central feature of a person's identity. Emerging terms include "client," "consumer," and "person with a psychiatric disability." The term " person with a psychiatric disability" reflects the commonality of concerns with other disability groups; it suggests that such a person can benefit from rehabilitation and can achieve independent living. Some groups and individuals prefer the term "person with a mental illness" because it affirms their conclusion that we are essentially describing a person with a brain disease—a matter of some continuing controversy in the field. Still others prefer the term "psychiatric survivor," because it reflects either their experience in mental health systems that they view as fundamentally oppressive, and/or their "survival" of the most challenging aspects of their disabilities. Finally, a term that is gaining currency is that of "prosumer," based on Toffler's (1970) assertion that in the service sector of the global economy, producers and users of services are increasingly indistinguishable. Such a "future trend" has great appeal to those who believe that people with disabilities must operate and control their own services.

The real challenge, in my view, is to discuss common human needs first, before concentrating on special characteristics people may have. In the meanwhile, we should simply call people what they want to be called. In the short term, we can all help our language to evolve by using every opportunity to point out the damaging effects of using everyday terms that stigmatize, such as "crazy," "schizy," "paranoid," or "nuts." In the longer term, we can hope that our language will continue to evolve in the direction of greater respect and hopefulness, focusing first on people as people.

Approaches to the Explanation of "Mental Illness"

Traditional Assumptions

Historically, Western attitudes toward people with a label of "mental illness" have been almost uniformly negative. Blanch (1990) explains that the basis for these attitudes, however, has shifted dramatically over the years. And she points out that the dominant social attitudes or assumptions of a particular era have determined how people with the label are treated, as follows:

Assumption	Social response
Evil	Punish
Possessed	Exorcise
Worthless, inhuman	Abandon
Weak, vulnerable	Protect, institutionalize
Sick	Treat, medicate, hospitalize
Disturbed	Calm, pacify
Dangerous	Confine, control
Unpredictable	Supervise, watch
Incompetent	Assume responsibility

Although one may think that these negative assumptions about the nature of mental illness have long since been discarded, these beliefs are in fact prevalent today—whether in particular Hollywood films, in the teachings of a fundamentalist religious sect, or even in the popular self-help literature. As an example, Peck (1985) continues to describe people with the most serious mental illnesses as reflecting the historical essence of evil in society.

An Overview of Current Explanatory Models

Zinman et al. (1987), leaders in the mental health consumer movement, provide an overview of recent historical explanations of mental illness; they categorize these into five dominant models. First is the "medical model," which presumes a malfunction of the brain, and which is the dominant explanation of many professionals, many family advocates, and some consumers. Second is the "social/economic/political model," which assumes that people's problems are primarily attributable to the conditions in which they grew up and currently live, and which appears to be the dominant understanding of some (but certainly not all) ex-patient groups. Third is the "disability rights model," which does not necessarily presume a specific explanation for mental illness, but proposes a functional view of individuals, a rehabilitation approach to treatment with independent living as its goal, and a need for rights protection and social change. Fourth is a "nutritional/orthomolecular model," which assumes that the problems are attributable to a biological imbalance and will respond to dietary changes.

The fifth approach is, a "spiritual model," in which different states of mind are attributable to spiritual, psychic or other paranormal causes. As a final note, it is clear from the cross-cultural literature that "mental illness" has dramatically different meanings from one culture to another (Lefley, 1990a).

In point of fact, few people I have encountered in the field argue for a unitary explanation. Rather, they view mental illness as reflecting some highly individual combination of biological, social, and psychological factors, often including a heightened susceptibility to stress.

It is not surprising that there should be so many different explanations for "mental illness," since this term is used to describe a very diverse set of conditions and experiences, even by those who adhere to a view of one predominant etiology. Another confounding factor is the frequently reported lack of precision with which people are given diagnoses. Those who have been involved in the mental health field for any length of time know that it is commonplace for a person who has received services over a number of years to have also received a large number of contradictory diagnoses. Also commonplace is the tendency to see all of the individual's problems as internally based, and hence to ignore the individual's actual experience as a vital source of information about his or her current difficulties. Such a tendency leads to serious underreporting of such environmental precipitants as physical or sexual abuse, or other traumata that could lead to symptoms identical to those we currently associate with major mental illness.

Recent literature (e.g., Rose, Peabody, & Strategias, 1990) suggests widespread distortions of this type in the practice of diagnosis and assessment. A study conducted within a large New York City mental hospital, for example, found that nearly 30% of the patients admitted were misdiagnosed, partly because of language differences between staff and patients (Lipton & Simon, 1985). The results of such misdiagnoses are hardly trivial. The most common pattern reported in that study was to misdiagnose people who were experiencing major depression as having schizophrenia. These misdiagnosed patients were then treated with major tranquilizers as appropriate for schizophrenia, but since they were already struggling with a depressed mood, these drugs increased their depression and put many of them at serious risk for suicide.

The fact that people involved in developing mental health policies and programs on the one hand, and those who receive services (people with disabilities and their families) on the other, tend to hold widely differing views regarding the nature and causes of "mental illness" is no trivial issue either. Professionals, particularly those in public mental health systems, are expected by society not only to "treat" individuals with mental illness, but also to protect the public through the exercise of social control. One's understanding of the nature and course of "mental illness" has a profound effect on one's beliefs about what services should be offered; what role, if any, the person with a disability should play in the design and operation of those services; and a variety of fundamental ethical questions, including whether involuntary or forced interventions are justifiable.

Policy Perspectives in Mental Health Systems

From a U.S. federal policy perspective, NIMH (1987b) has issued an "official" definition of the "severely mentally ill adult population," which has been adopted with minor variations in virtually all state mental health systems. The NIMH definition includes individuals 18 and over, regardless of where they live (e.g., in institutions, community residences, with families, in independent apartments, in jails, or in homeless shelters); it also includes people with multiple diagnoses, such as mental illness and developmental disability, or mental illness and substance abuse. The population is defined according to three criteria: (1) diagnosis, (2) level of disability, and (3) duration of the illness.

"Diagnosis" refers to a major mental disorder included in the revised third edition of the *Diagnostic and Statistical Manual of Mental Disorders* (DSM-III-R; American Psychiatric Association, 1987). Such diagnoses include schizophrenia, major affective disorder, paranoia, organic psychosis, or other psychotic disorders, or disorders that may lead to chronic disability, such as borderline personality disorder.

"Level of disability" refers to functional limitations in at least two major life activities, on a continuing or intermittent basis. Functional limitations in major life areas include unemployment or sheltered employment; the need for financial assistance; difficulty with personal support systems; the need for help with basic living skills; and/or inappropriate social behavior of a level of seriousness that results in intervention by the mental health and/or judicial system.

Finally, "duration" refers to the extent of a person's history of receiving intensive services (e.g., crisis services, hospitalization, or extended residential services) that have disrupted the person's normal living situation.

The fact that NIMH has promulgated a "national definition," however, does not imply an absence of strong differences of opinion among U.S. national policy organizations about the nature and etiology of psychiatric disabilities. The National Alliance for the Mentally Ill, for example, takes a strong position that mental illnesses are brain diseases. The National Mental Health Consumers Association and the National Alliance of Psychiatric Survivors, two ex-patient groups, focus heavily on environmental factors and on political explanations. Most "mainstream" service provider or advocacy groups, such as the International Association for Psychosocial Rehabilitation Services, the National Community Mental HealthCare Council, and the National Mental Health Association, tend to describe the variety of needs that people with psychiatric disabilities have, without articulating a single causal explanation for such a disability.

Mental Illness as a Brain Disease

The 1990s have been dubbed by NIMH as "The Decade of the Brain" (NIMH, 1990), reflecting growing support for research into the etiology and treatment of psychiatric conditions. In fact, with advances in biochemistry, virology, genetics, and brain imaging techniques, an entirely new generation of research studies has emerged (summarized in NIMH, 1990). These studies have established, at least in preliminary findings, a broad range of links between psychiatric symptoms and such diverse aspects of human functioning as brain size and shape, endocrine and hormonal patterns, sleep patterns, neurotransmission patterns, and so forth. Although these are basic research studies and have had few clinical applications to date, the emphasis of current clinical research is on new pharmacological and perhaps genetic treatments. Many new medications are offered and gain widespread use each year. Recent examples include Prozac and Clozaril, both of which have been widely hailed as "wonder drugs." Clozaril, in early results, has been described as very effective in treating individuals with major mental illnesses who have not responded to other medications.

In recent years, the growing influence of the family movement, and the growing partnership of that movement with biologically oriented psychiatrists, have resulted in broader acceptance of mental illness as a brain disease; in turn, this has increased support for biologically oriented research. Reflecting this position, Torrey et al. (1988) conclude that "serious mental illness is composed of a series of brain diseases . . . the evidence for [which] has become overwhelming and consists of measurable differences in brain structure and function" (p. 16).

The recent resurgence of biological research has itself intensified professional debates about the exact nature of mental illness. Thus, the basic question of whether genes, viruses, other biochemical agents, or perhaps all three are implicated in schizophrenia is still very much an open one. Furthermore, this debate raises the concern that recent findings on peculiarities in brain anatomy or brain chemistry among people with schizophrenia are frequently generalized from this specific disorder to a broad variety of other "mental illnesses." In short, although research into the physical aspects of mental illness is important and useful, brain scientists are not yet in a position to definitively describe the physical characteristics of each mental illness. Hence, it is fair to conclude that such research, in its current state of evolution, does not yet support a unitary view of all "mental illness" as biological in nature.

Initially, the major support for a unitary biological view of mental illness derived from the fact that psychotropic medications did in fact reduce symptoms in a majority of cases (Anthony & Blanch, 1989). There is a growing debate, however, about the conceptual leap involved in concluding that, simply because medications affect behavior or because there are some differences between the brains of people with schizophrenia and "normal" brains, the *origin* of mental illnesses is therefore strictly biological or biochemical (Cohen, 1989; Taylor, 1989). Although there is continued debate in the field about the etiology of various psychiatric disabilities, there appears to be substantial agreement about many of the effects of mental illness. It is abundantly clear, for example, that a number of physiological and cognitive functions are dramatically affected among many individuals with psychiatric disabilities. Thus, research on the biology, biochemistry, and genetic aspects of mental illness may well lead to important findings that guide professionals, family members, and friends in designing new treatments, and in helping individuals cope with their disabilities and improve their functioning.

Practically speaking, most clinicians operate according to what is termed the "biopsychosocial approach"; that is, they assume biological, psychological, social, environmental, and historical factors are all at play in psychiatric symptomatology. Each of these factors needs to be taken into account in a highly individualized fashion with each person, along with emerging principles of empowerment, hope, and recovery. As Norman Cousins points out in *Anatomy of an Illness as Perceived by the Patient* (1979, p. 56): "Drugs are not always necessary; belief in recovery always is." The implication is that people with psychiatric disabilities need excellent medical care, provided in a holistic approach—one that begins with the needs they share with people who have not been given a label of "mental illness" or "disability."

A Disability Rights Perspective

This book takes a disability rights perspective more than any other approach since I believe that each individual is first and foremost a person, and that the equality of rights and opportunities implied in community membership is far more significant than any particular theory about the origins of a person's disability. In fact, it can be argued that historically, under the burden of various competing professional theories, individuals with psychiatric disabilities have been tyrannized more than they have been helped. Taking a disability perspective allows us to draw on the values, theory, and practice of the broader rehabilitation field, and allies mental health consumers/ex-patients with the millions of other people who carry some sort of "disability" label. This perspective also clarifies the roles of families and professionals as offering, not controlling, treatment and support. Finally, it positions people with psychiatric disabilities to take full advantage of emerging U.S. federal policy and legislation, such as the Americans with Disabilities Act of 1990 and the Federal Fair Housing Amendments of 1989, or in various federal or provincial legislation in Canada which is focused on full integration of people with disabilities.

This view, which is consistent with that of other prominent professional theorists (e.g., Anthony, 1990b), as well as consumer theorists (e.g., Deegan, 1992; Zinman et al., 1987), draws on the success of the independent living movement among people with disabilities. This movement promotes the principle that people with disabilities should be in control of the services they receive, and that such services should be operated and provided primarily by peers. Finally, this approach suggests that decisions about various supports, whether peer support, clinical services, or medications, must be made on a highly individual basis.

What Is the Experience of Mental Illness?

The lived experience of mental illness is described by individuals with psychiatric disabilities both as highly traumatic and as a source of learning and growth. Since the term "mental illness" encompasses so many diverse conditions, it is hard to generalize about characteristics and symptoms. For example, people with bipolar disorder (manic depression) generally experience wide mood swings that alternate between euphoria and significant depression. In the manic state, these people may have grandiose ideas, may exercise very poor judgment, and may experience feelings of extreme suspiciousness or paranoia. In the depressive state, the same individuals may stop eating, may retire to bed for weeks at a time, and may seriously contemplate suicide. In spite of these symptoms, however, many individuals with this condition report that they feel most "alive" during a manic phase; hence they often refuse to take medication, which levels their moods, but which they see as constraining their energy and creativity.

Individuals with schizophrenia, on the other hand, may experience powerful auditory and visual hallucinations—disturbing voices and visions commanding them to take actions that they ordinarily would not take. Many individuals experience significant confusion in sequencing and processing ideas. Often persons with schizophrenia will isolate themselves from others, feeling unable to manage the stress of maintaining interpersonal relationships.

Many individuals with serious affective disorders, such as major depression, report the incredible struggles they have with simply getting out of bed in the morning, continuing interpersonal connections, and maintaining a job or family responsibilities. Such depressions often lead to thoughts of suicide as a strategy for escaping from the pain of this condition.

Obviously, the moods, the cognitive confusion, the suspicion, and the other symptoms described above are feelings that most people without a disability label also experience, albeit with very different levels of intensity. Many people have learned to manage these feelings in a way that does not differentiate them from other community members, or they have organized supports around themselves so that if these feelings become disabling, they are hidden away within the family or in other settings. It is obvious, for example, that many great creative figures and political leaders throughout history have experienced what we now describe as "major mental illness." Many of these individuals were in situations that, in spite of the personal struggles they faced, often incorporated their differences or made allowances for them, so that they could continue to function as creators or leaders. Although these feelings and experiences appear to be far more extreme among people with psychiatric disabilities than they are among the general population, it is also becoming increasingly apparent to mental health professionals that, in some ways, the sharp distinctions we have drawn between people "with" and "without" mental illness in the past may have been somewhat arbitrary. It should also be emphasized that we need to focus on the profound diversity of "mental health consensus" in any discussion of the experience of mental illness. In fact, until recently, the literature in mental health has included very little information on the unique experiences and concerns of people of color or of women with a psychiatric disability.

Consumers and ex-patients are beginning to articulate their experiences with mental illness and with mental health treatment systems more and more clearly. All too often, they are describing this process as one of assuming the role of patients (Estroff, 1981), losing their basic rights, and ultimately developing a sense of hopelessness about the future.

Feelings of Being Invisible, Discounted

Consumers/ex-patients often report a feeling of "invisibility"; they sense that their views and desires do not matter. Esso Leete (1988) describes this well:

> I can talk but I may not be heard. I can make suggestions, but they may not be taken seriously. I can voice my thoughts but they may be seen as delusions. I can recite experiences but they may be interpreted as fantasies. To be a patient or even an ex-client is to be discounted. Your label is a reality that never leaves you; it gradually shapes an identity that is hard to shed. (p. 67)

The Struggle for Basic Rights

As we reach the end of the 20th century, individuals with psychiatric disabilities are still struggling to overcome both the societal and the internalized role of "mental patient," and to achieve the basic rights enjoyed by other citizens. Again, Esso Leete (1988) makes this point effectively:

> . . . in many places we are still fighting for basic civil rights for mental patients and an end to victimization. We are demanding such basic rights as employment (at equal pay), insurance coverage and housing. Many states still do not have laws against openly discriminating against people with mental illness, and as a group ours is possibly the most discriminated against and disenfranchised. We are therefore organizing to stop unjust and oppressive treatment, to have a voice in our own treatment, to gain mastery over our lives, and to lend much needed support to each other as we do this. (p. 66)

Status as Objects of Treatment

One reason why people with psychiatric disabilities have found it so difficult to get their basic needs met is that they have been defined, through a powerful process of societal stigma, as having fundamentally different needs from citizens without such a label. According to Wilson, Blanch, and Quinn (1987), "Individuals with the diagnosis of mental illness have been viewed as needing different things than 'more ordinary' people, and, in turn, their basic needs for respect, dignity, love, choices and environmental supports have been considered as secondary to their treatment needs" (p. 3). This reality is brought home starkly in the words of a group of ex-patients writing about self-help:

> We believe we should view our peers not as diagnostic symptoms but as people—people with real problems and with real needs—needs com-

mon to everyone. We should provide assistance and support to each other—not treatment or therapy. We believe that a person's problems are due to real causes and are not due to any fault on the part of the person. (Zinman et al., 1987, p. 5)

The Internalized Patient Role

Unfortunately, this central role as patients and treatment recipients tends to be internalized by individuals with psychiatric disabilities. Judi Chamberlin (1978), an ex-patient leader, explains:

> For too long, mental patients have been a faceless, voiceless people. We have been thought of, at worst, as subhuman monsters, or, at best, as pathetic cripples who might be able to hold down menial jobs and eke out meager existences, given constant professional support. Not only have others thought of us in this stereotyped way, we have believed it ourselves. (p. xi)

Learned Hopelessness and Helplessness

Unfortunately, internalizing the patient role can instill feelings of profound hopelessness and helplessness in these individuals—feelings that are reinforced by the catastrophic economic consequences of major mental illness, by pervasive stigma, and by the way individuals are treated within the mental health system. As Marcia Lovejoy (personal communication, August 1980) puts it, "Hopelessness is as common in mental health as salt is in the American diet." Esso Leete (1988) expands on this theme:

> In addition to psychological handicaps imposed by our illness, the mentally disabled must constantly deal with this stigma and other obstacles to empowerment and recovery erected by society. We are seen as unattractive, lazy, incompetent, unpredictable and dangerous. Although these are untrue stereotypes, admittedly we do have shortcomings. In many cases, however, our weakest attributes are those we learn in the very institutions supposedly there to help us: i.e. withdrawal, dependency, fear, irresponsibility, and lowered self-confidence, lost self-esteem and shattered personal dignity. In fact, just the label "mentally ill" is powerful enough to cause changes in our behavior and functioning. (p. 66)

This need for hope is also echoed by a prominent professional: "The central ingredient of rehabilitation is hope" (Anthony, 1979, p. 6) Another prominent researcher repeats a consumer's words: "The one thing that helped more than anything else was having just one person believe in me, believe that I could put one foot in front of the other and move forward'' (quoted by C. Harding, personal communication, April 1989).

This last quote was furnished by an author of one of the few long-term studies of the lives of people with psychiatric disabilities (Harding et al., 1987). In this study, every ''long-term'' (i.e., severely psychiatrically disabled) patient who had been discharged from the Vermont State Hospital 20 years earlier was tracked down and interviewed extensively about how his or her life had changed in the subsequent 20 years, and about what was helpful to him or her. The findings of this study were dramatic, especially to the extent that they contradicted the poor prognoses described for people with major mental illness in the psychiatric literature. In the DSM-III-R (American Psychiatric Association, 1987), for example, people with chronic schizophrenia are expected to deteriorate progressively on a downward spiraling course, and their lives are always expected to include symptoms. If such deterioration is not observed, the manual suggests that the clinician should conclude that the person has been misdiagnosed.

It now appears that much of this pessimistic prognosis is based on the experience of clinicians seeing people at their worst (i.e., during short-term acute crises). This is an especially suspect basis for predicting outcomes, since research on mental illness over the lifespan is so scant. In fact, before Harding et al.'s (1987) work, there had only been four other longitudinal studies of psychiatric disabilities—all of which, interestingly enough, had similarly positive results (Ciompi, 1980; Huber, Gross, & Schuttler, 1980; Winokur, Morrison, & Clancy, 1972; Tsuang, Woolson, & Fleming, 1979). Harding et al.'s (1987) study, in contrast to diagnostic predictions, found that fully two-thirds of those with serious and persistent mental illnesses such as schizophrenia were ''virtually indistinguishable'' from the general population after 20 years. These people were working, were living in their own housing, and had social networks comparable to those of their neighbors. Admittedly, many individuals needed intensive support, particularly within the first 5 years after leaving the mental institution. Nonetheless, this study provides strong evidence that most people with psychiatric disabilities do get much better over time.

The single most important factor in recovery, according to those Harding et al. studied (such as the individual quoted above), was ''having just one person believe in me.'' Interestingly, the findings indicated that people found pets and friends far more important than mental health professionals in their recovery (C. Harding, personal communication, April 1989).

Studies like Harding et al.'s (1987) raise major questions about the level of expectations we should hold about the potential of individuals with psychiatric disabilities for community integration. These findings counter the pervasive beliefs that many people with psychiatric disabilities are too symptomatic or too "low-functioning" to benefit from recovery and integration. To be sure, many individuals are obviously in need of intensive assistance, perhaps over an extended, or even lifelong, period, if they are to take on employment, the independent management of a household, or other comparable productive activity. But this body of research strongly suggests that, with supports that are offered within the context of choice and community participation, there is reason to hold hopeful expectations for any individual.

The Experience of Families

Lefley (1990b), Hatfield (1990), and others have described the enormous challenge that a psychiatric disability presents for others in an individual's family, particularly given the dearth of effective and reliable services, and given the larger context of "family blaming" that until recently has been so pervasive among professionals. The experience of family members, though highly individual, follows predictable patterns corresponding to the stages of acceptance of death and dying (Kübler-Ross, 1969): denial, anger, bargaining, depression, and acceptance. Family members typically experience the extreme pain involved in the loss of a "normal" relative, the loss of a set of expectations and dreams for that individual, and the painful adjustment to the reality of a very different life than they expected. Taking care of their own collective and individual needs, apart from those of the person with the disability, also presents a major challenge.

These psychological reactions are compounded by dramatic changes in family dynamics, as family members seek to continue healthy patterns with one another and to avoid focusing excessively on the individual with the disability. This is particularly challenging through repeated crises. In the all-too-frequent cases where professional services are either not available or are not "user-friendly," family members experience the isolation of coping with an unknown condition, or face being "treated" as the source of the problem. Meanwhile, they watch their relative with the disability continue to have major difficulties.

Even in service programs that are oriented toward recovery and integration, family members are often confronted with younger community support workers who assume that their desire to continue a strong connection with their relative with the disability is somehow pathological, or reflects an unwillingness of the family to "let go." In fact, deep concern about a family member, particularly one with a disability, is normal family behavior; in fact, it may be particularly adaptive in families in which a member has special needs that have only been met reliably by the family in the past.

Finally, the experience of families is often one of economic disaster: They purchase services from private hospitals and professionals, and are then shifted to the public sector when their savings or insurance runs out. As a result, many families approach community support programs already jaded by their negative experiences with professionals. Overcoming this skepticism and building trust will take time.

Families have been of great assistance to one another in providing information about psychiatric disabilities, in sharing experiences and emotional support, and in joining together to make professionals and mental health systems more accountable and responsive to their needs. It is through such activities that families can take back the power that they may have lost in their interactions with the professional world.

The Controversy over Involuntary Interventions

In North America a coherent body of law, together with powerful advocacy groups in mental health, has established a strong societal basis for providing involuntary interventions (e.g., commitment to a state/provincial hospital) when persons with psychiatric disabilities display behaviors that are "dangerous to self or others." Some states/provinces have broader standards for involuntary interventions, including "the need for care and supervision" or "personal incapacity to meet one's own needs."

Some ex-patient organizations see the state's ability to involuntarily "treat" people with psychiatric disabilities—which is based on an assumption that people lack both the competence to make their own decisions and responsibility for their own behavior—as the basis for denying these people the same civil rights that any other citizen deserve, and as a practice perpetuating the social view that people with mental illness are not responsible for their actions (Chamberlin, 1978). In this view, until such laws are changed, "mental patients" will continue to internalize the idea that they are irresponsible—a belief that is antithetical to the process of recovery, which begins with individuals' taking responsibility for their lives. These advocates therefore call for the abolition of involuntary interventions, and insist that people with psychiatric disabilities should be held to the same legal standards as any other citizen, jailed for any crimes they have committed, and offered voluntary services if their non-criminal behavior suggests that they may need help.

The polarized set of views about involuntary interventions with regard to its rationale and legitimacy, as well as its effects, is a major source of conflict among many consumers, family members, and professionals. The problem is compounded (1) by a virtual absence of basic discussion within the field as to when involuntary interventions are legitimate or helpful, and (2) by an absence of research on consumers' experience of involuntary interventions and on their long-term effects on consumers and their families (Blanch, 1993). In fact, the first national conference on involuntary interventions recently held in Houston, Texas in May 1994, began the process of building strategies among all of the key constituencies in mental health, for exploring the various perspectives of this issue, examining the effects of involuntary interventions on consumers, professionals, and family members, and developing strategies for systematically reducing and perhaps eliminating involuntary interventions in mental health systems. Leading psychiatrists (e.g., Stastny, 1994), including one who is also an ex-patient (Fisher, 1994) questioned the compatibility of "involuntary treatment" with the Hippocratic Oath. A variety of strategies to reduce involuntary interventions were summarized by Carling (1994). Such meetings hold the promise of beginning to develop very different approaches to meeting the support needs of individuals as well as the safety concerns of all community members.

Moving Forward without a Consensus

At present, the dominant view among professionals and families is that mental illness is a brain disease. It is well to recall, however, that Western society has passed through many periods of "certainty" about the origins and course of "mental illness," with such varying explanations as demonic possession, moral weakness, and so forth. Viewing the complex variety of factors that affect human behavior, many consumer advocates draw from a variety of viewpoints to develop strategies for successful community living. In the process, they adhere strongly to the principle that people with disabilities are the best judges of the particular interventions and opportunities that should be provided. At the same time, they remain intellectually open to a broad variety of possibilities for explaining and responding to these disabilities.

It is clear that there is still no complete consensus among professionals, family members, and consumers/ex-patients about the etiology of all "mental illness." All parties need to acknowledge this lack of agreement, while at the same time avoiding rigid and polarized positions. In fact, agreeing to disagree about etiology can be a major strategy for the development of a broad-based movement for community integration. This strategy can also be effective with other core issues that divide the major constituencies in mental health, such as involuntary commitment and forced medication, both of which have a profound (yet barely researched) effect on consumers and other family members. On a day-to-day basis, most professionals and advocates seem to accept the view that a complex variety of antecedents may be responsible for the difficulties an individual experiences at any given time, including the profound effects of stigma, discrimination, and social rejection. Effective clinicians remain open to new information as well. An emerging body of research (see Rose et al., 1990) suggests that a majority of people with psychiatric disabilities may have experienced some form of abuse as children. This is a critically important set of studies, since the effects of such abuse have been described as quite similar to those of schizophrenia or major affective disorders, yet the treatments of these diverse conditions are quite different.

Perhaps an analogy may be useful. For years, clinicians treated the presenting problem of depression among women primarily as an internal state, until the women's movement pointed out the clear environmental precipitants for much of this grief: abuse, powerless roles within families, systematic sexism, and patriarchal structures that denied women the opportunity for meaningful work and social roles outside the home. These realizations then changed the focus of therapy dramatically to incorporate assertiveness training and to legitimize the aspirations of women outside of their traditional roles. At the same time, therapy continues to be available to respond to depression in individuals that appears to have few, if any, environmental antecedents.

If professionals have, in effect, been misdiagnosing many individuals as schizophrenic who have actually experienced significant abuse, the focus of treatment should shift dramatically. The core principles for treatment of abuse are a recovery orientation, sharing one's experience with others who have "been there," and taking responsibility for one's situation. For women who have experienced sexual abuse, creating safe environments in which to pursue recovery and healing—environments that are often limited to other women—is critically important. Unfortunately, these program approaches are almost the opposite to those that individuals with serious mental illness are currently offered in many communities.

In the absence of consensus, then, how can we all work together? First, it is critical that we identify those issues on which all of the key constituencies do agree. As noted above, even if these are a minority of the issues, my experience is that identifying this common ground and then "agreeing to disagree" on the rest are the most powerful strategies for building coalitions for change.

Second, and perhaps more importantly, we need to begin having the perspective of consumers/ex-patients themselves form the basis of the agenda for change. In this respect, the personal stories that reflect the experience of consumers/ex-patients are the most powerful sources of knowledge about how things must change.

To be sure, the perspectives of family members are also critical. The greatest utility of family advocates—and I have learned this painfully as a family member myself—is in articulating the needs of *families,* not of consumers. Similarly, the views of professionals, and their experiences in trying to be helpful, are also critical. But these views are most helpful when they are offered through relationships that are characterized by a commitment to allowing individuals with psychiatric disabilities to make their own critical life choices. My experience, for example, is that many of the emerging ideas about consumer empowerment make the most sense to direct-service staff members, who have the most contact with consumers. These ideas, on the other hand, are often most problematic for those middle or senior managers in programs or for their counterparts in county or state mental health systems, who are most removed from their "customers," and who face the daunting task of a major restructuring of their agencies and services if truly consumer-driven systems that promote real community integration are to be achieved. Unfortunately, until recently, mental health systems have not sought or created much access to the organized perspectives of consumers/ex-patients. As this access to "consumer voice" increases, the lack of consensus in our field will take on an entirely new meaning. For as the power of people with psychiatric disabilities increases within mental health systems, it is *their* varied experiences that will increasingly form the basis for policies, programs, and funding. Similarly, it will become increasingly difficult for professionals to impose treatments or services that consumers do not want. It will also be increasingly difficult for groups representing any interests other than those of people with psychiatric disabilities to control the advocacy movement.

THE QUIET REVOLUTION: MENTAL HEALTH CONSUMERS HELPING THEMSELVES

Increasingly, mental health consumers are becoming actively involved in the mental health system by advocating for change, building coalitions, and designing and running mental health programs or self-help groups. Some have returned to school for professional training in order to better serve their communities. Others, after a period of work in the general community, have returned to the mental health field as service providers to "give something back" to other ex-patients. People with psychiatric disabilities are making contributions in significant ways at all levels of society.

Advocacy at the National, State, and Local Levels

In the United States, there is now a broad range of organizations representing mental health consumers at national, state, and local levels. At the national level, these groups include the Anxiety Disorders Association of America; the National Depressive/Manic Depressive Association; Schizophrenics Anonymous; Recovery, Inc.; and GROW, a self-help movement with over 700 chapters around the world.

National advocacy is undertaken principally by two groups: the National Mental Health Consumers Association, and the National Association of Psychiatric Survivors. The first of those groups is a network of over 500 self-help groups for ex-mental patients; it is focused on protecting people's rights, promoting consumer-run alternatives, fighting stigma and discrimination, and improving the responsiveness and accountability of mental health systems. The association's leaders testify in Congress, serve on national mental health planning bodies, bring lawsuits, and provide technical assistance to local groups. The National Association of Psychiatric Survivors is a grassroots organization that takes a strong position against involuntary interventions of any sort. It focuses primarily on supporting local membership groups, which provide a broad range of self-help and advocacy services.

The work of these national organizations has had an impact on the other national groups concerned about mental health, on funding agencies, and on policies that affect mental health systems throughout the United States. For example, these groups have been able to include a strong consumer focus within federal protection and advocacy legislation. U.S. federal and state mental health planning legislation (Comprehensive Mental Health Systems Planning Act, 1987), for example, now mandates consumer representation in all state planning, as well as the funding of consumer-operated programs. These groups have succeeded in establishing federally funded demonstration projects on self-help, as well as several national research centers with a self-help focus. They have also worked closely with the larger disability community on such key initiatives as the Federal Fair Housing Amendments of 1989 and the Americans with Disabilities Act of 1990.

Finally, these groups have been instrumental in prompting the National Association of State Mental Health Program Directors (NASMHPD, 1989) to adopt a policy supporting greatly increased consumer involvement in policy and planning activities, training, employment, and consumer-operated services within state mental health systems. As a result, many states have begun directing resources into these new activities, in some cases starting offices of consumer affairs, and in others initiating funding for consumer advocacy and service demonstration projects.

The federally funded demonstration projects that these groups have helped to bring about include such diverse services as a consumer-run model of coordinated services across an entire community (Alameda County, California); a network of consumer-operated business enterprises (Denver, Colorado); an office of consumer affairs and speaker's bureau (Indianapolis, Indiana); new administrative procedures to fund consumer services more easily (Portland, Maine); self-help-oriented case management, recreational, and information services (St. Louis, Missouri); a drop-in center, telephone support services, and assistance with the transition from hospitals (Concord, New Hampshire); a consumer-operated food bank and an outreach service for homeless people (Albany, New York); a statewide consumer network (Madison, Wisconsin); and a consumer-operated greenhouse and gardening center (Columbus, Ohio). Such projects demonstrate the effectiveness of particular service approaches, while at the same time strengthening the infrastructure of consumer organizations at state and local levels.

National Technical Assistance

A major focus of these national consumer organizations is to provide mechanisms through which local self-help groups and individual advocates can share information on successful strategies for organizing and for providing services. This is accomplished through a variety of print and electronic media. Each of these groups, for example, publishes a newsletter. Project Share in Philadelphia, through its National Mental Health Self-Help Clearinghouse, offers a wide variety of brochures that offer practical assistance to self-help groups; it also offers leadership training for these groups. The National Teleconference Project, located at Boston University's Center for Psychiatric Rehabilitation, convenes individuals and groups on a regular basis across the country in national "town meetings" to share experiences and to generate strategies for change. These teleconferences are replicated on a state-by-state basis in many areas of the country.

A pioneer in the development of such telecommunications strategies is Paul (Dorfner) Engels, president of White Light Communications, a consumer-owned and consumer-staffed national telecommunications business in Burlington, Vermont. White Light has produced a large number of videotaped interviews with key consumer leaders and professional allies across the country. These tapes are used in a variety of training and public education activities. White Light recently initiated Self-Help Live, a periodic national broadcast that links as many as 10,000 people with psychiatric disabilities at a time through a network of "downlink sites" across the country, all participating in panel discussions by consumer experts on such topics as housing, homelessness, employment, and consumer-operated services.

NIMH has recently funded a new national consumer technical assistance center, the National Empowerment Center, located in Springfield, Massachusetts. This center organizes print materials, electronic information, and conducts trainings on empowerment and recovery. The National Network for Mental Health, based in Guelph, Ontario, provides an excellent newsletter and a broad range of consumer/survivor projects, and facilitates communication among the large number of consumer/survivor groups across Canada.

Finally, an impressive number and variety of writings by consumer/ex-patients are now finding their way into the marketplace. These describe the experience of psychiatric disability; the process of recovery; strategies for coping with individual challenges; and methods of mobilizing for better services, supports, treatment, and civil rights. Deegan (1988, 1989, 1990, 1992) has been a particularly thoughtful and eloquent author on the topic of recovery.

Peers Providing Services

In addition to advocacy and technical assistance, consumers and ex-patients are increasingly demonstrating their ability to provide the full range of needed community supports to their peers (Leete, 1988; Zinman et al., 1987). Such service projects have been developed in virtually every state and province in North America.

Self-Help and Mutual Support Groups

> Everybody needs to know there is a place in society for them. That there's a place where they can belong. To be honest with you, most of us don't belong.
> —JULIE CRAFTS (quoted in Ridgway, 1988a, p. 17)

Because we humans are social animals, friendships and other close relationships are our lifeblood. Social contact is an especially urgent need for many people with psychiatric disabilities, who, as noted earlier in this book, often find themselves either completely isolated or with very restricted social networks (Estroff, 1989).

Self-help groups for people with psychiatric disabilities share a number of common characteristics, according to Zinman et al. (1987):

> . . . self-definition (define own needs); equal power of members (they are non-hierarchical in structure); respecting folks as people, not as clinical diagnoses (non-clinical, person to person); totally voluntary (non-coercive); autonomous from mental health systems and professionals; responsive to special populations (bilingual, disadvantaged, physically disabled, blacks, gays etc.). (p. 8)

These authors also address the thorny question of the role of professionals in developing self-help programs, and caution that setting up such programs within mental health systems inevitably perpetuates the power differences between staff and clients. Common pitfalls in professionally initiated self-help projects include staff members' keeping records on clients, professionals' making decisions about staff hiring, performance evaluation, and termination; and staff members' managing the budget. Self-help philosophies assume that power must rest in the hands of consumers themselves, and that support and self-advocacy go hand in hand.

Zinman et al. (1987) provide an excellent description of how self-help and mutual support efforts can provide most of the essential elements of community support, as described in Chapter Two of this book (see Figure 2.1). They can do this by offering a very strong outreach program (identification and outreach); providing experienced advice and support on "community survival" (income support and entitlement); providing crisis support, especially during times when professionals tend to be less available (crisis response services); getting together to help people to have a social life, and setting up independent living services (rehabilitation services); educating community members, and helping friends and family members to continue supporting an individual, even when the community response may be to overly control or even extrude the person (family and community support); advocating and referring people to agencies organized for the purpose of rights protection (protection and advocacy); and walking one another through the system to get what is needed (case management). The authors summarize:

> . . . mutual support acknowledges that we are all human, with strengths and weaknesses. It gives us validity as people capable of helping each other. It allows us to have normal interactions in the community without someone always doing things for us, because we are perceived as too

"sick" to do them for ourselves. Hence we build self-esteem and a sense of identity, dignity and inner strength. We get the good feeling of helping each other while feeling the pride of taking responsibility for ourselves as citizens of the community at large. (Zinman et al., 1987, p. 48)

There are now self-help organizations and activities for people with psychiatric disabilities all across North America. Examples range from a small group in Rutland, Vermont called Uptight, which meets monthly to solve problems, share concerns, and hear from consumer and professional leaders in the community, all the way to a particularly well-developed set of self-help activities offered by the Alameda County (California) Network of Mental Health Clients. Since 1984, this group has organized conferences, founded the Berkeley Drop-In Center and the Oakland Independence Support Center, created greater client representation within the county mental health system, and provided training throughout the county. Other activities of this group include Mental Health Options, which conducts peer counseling and training workshops, and the Reach Out Project, which provides information and support to patients in psychiatric hospitals. The Alameda County Network has recently created an administrative umbrella organization to share the costs of managing these diverse activities, which in turn has allowed services to be expanded in each of the individual projects.

Self-help groups, originally lacking in economic, racial, and ethnic diversity, are now proliferating among nonwhite, non-middle-class groups. The Black Mental Health Alliance in Baltimore, Maryland, for example, is creating programs to assist self-help groups to develop more culturally sensitive outreach services.

Outreach and Drop-In Centers

Two examples of an increasing number of projects focused on homelessness and psychiatric disability are Project OATS in Philadelphia, Pennsylvania, and the Ruby Rogers Drop-In Center in Cambridge, Massachusetts.

Project OATS (which stands for Outreach, Advocacy and Training Services) is a program of education and empowerment for people with mental illness who are homeless. It provides direct outreach to people on the streets; offers training in obtaining services and entitlements; and encourages the involvement of homeless people in policy development and planning in the local mental health system. The project also offers employment services and trains homeless individuals in advocacy, social service, and case management skills. Project OATS has recently initiated a housing program.

The Ruby Rogers Drop-In Center was named after the plaintiff in a famous lawsuit that established the right to refuse treatment within the Massachusetts mental health system. The center provides a range of support services, including self-help groups; basic services related to self-care; inexpensive clothing; and assistance with housing, employment, and public entitlements.

In Tennessee, an entire network of consumer-operated drop-in centers has been funded, often in conjunction with professional psychosocial rehabilitation "clubhouses" modeled after New York's Fountain House program.

Mental Health Treatment

As mental health systems begin to incorporate a higher level of "consumer voice," an interesting phenomenon has emerged: Mental health professionals who themselves have experienced psychiatric disabilities are feeling less reluctant to "come out of the closet." Moreover, they are taking advantage of their dual roles as ex-patients and as professionals to provide a different type of assistance—one based not only on treatment skills, but also on their personal experience of recovery. Such "prosumers" often have a keen awareness of the critical importance of voluntary, empowering, and respectful services.

Many organizations directed by ex-patients are moving beyond a narrow focus on self-help groups, and are beginning to provide the full range of treatment services. In a general way, this is being accomplished through an increasing emphasis in some mental health systems on hiring people with psychiatric disabilities as case managers or other service providers, working alongside other professionals who have not experienced such disabilities. In other systems, there is a focus on starting consumer-operated case management services.

One ex-patient organization that has grown into a full-service agency is Mind Empowered, Inc., in Portland, Oregon. This agency offers comprehensive case management and continuous mental health treatment to a large number of people with significant psychiatric disabilities. Interestingly enough, when the organization expanded from self-help and concrete services such as housing into the realm of treatment, the executive director, Garrett Smith (personal communication, July 1992) assumed that he would have to hire several psychiatrists and then retrain them in the consumer perspective. Instead, he found that a large number of experienced and skilled psychiatrists *who were also ex-patients* applied for these jobs, in part because they finally had the opportunity to work in a mental health agency where the experience of psychiatric disability was seen as an asset, not a source of shame to be hidden from their peers. Mind Empowered, Inc., recently embarked on a project to help a group of long-stay patients leave Damasch State Hospital and establish themselves in the community—a feat that traditional local community mental health programs had been unable to accomplish.

Consumer organizations that provide mental health treatment must eventually tackle the particularly thorny and controversial issues of medication and involuntary interventions. One source of controversy about medication lies in the very different perspectives that consumers and professionals seem to have on the subject. This difference is summarized by Deegan (1988), who points out that many professionals are primarily concerned with medication *compliance and maintenance,* since they see these as essential for continued short-term functioning. People with disabilities, on the other hand, are often primarily concerned with their own long-term recovery and with the changing role that medications play in that process over time. Therefore, they are concerned with the *responsible and informed use* of medication. On an immediate basis, consumers are also concerned about the very distressing side effects of these medications on aspects of functioning they value, such as alertness or bodily self-control.

I am reminded in this context of one of the stories that emerged from Harding and colleagues' (C. Harding, personal communication, April 1989) research, in which, as a preliminary finding, a high correlation was found between those who were doing well in the community and those who were taking medication. The young researcher, excited by this finding, mentioned it to one of her "consultants" (i.e., ex-patients). This woman, after a pause, escorted the researcher over to a dresser and opened the drawer. Inside were numerous filled but unopened prescriptions for psychotropic medications. When the researcher asked this woman (who lived in a rural area on a very low income) why she would go to the trouble and expense of showing up every month at the general store to get her prescription filled, she replied that she was convinced that if she didn't, mental health workers would put her back in the hospital. This story strikingly illustrates the lengths to which people will go to avoid the trauma of institutionalization. The story also shows how little is known about the extent to which people actually take the medications they purchase.

Although there is no question from the research literature that psychotropic medications can provide major assistance in alleviating symptoms, these chemicals are powerful, and are accompanied by many effects that consumers find distressing and negative. These effects are seen by professionals as "side effects," but by some consumers as the "main effects." They include trembling and other involuntary movements; impotence; persistently dry mouth; excessive sedation that interferes with thinking, working, and relationships; and many others. Betty Blaska (1990), an ex-patient, provides an excellent overview of many of the problems that consumers have with medications, including incorrect prescribing as a result of misdiagnosis, excessive dosages, too many drugs, downplaying side effects, ignoring the consumer's expertise, discouraging consumer education, and confining the relationship between consumer and psychiatrist to a "prescription sheet" one.

Self-help advocates and respectful professionals insist that since medication involves a very serious set of decisions for an individual, each person must be given true choice in making these decisions. If individuals want to stop taking medications, they must be given the options of reducing their use and of testing whether they can manage without any medications at all, within the context of ongoing support. It is also clear that many consumers will continue to find these medications essential in their recovery.

Crisis Response Services and Alternatives to Hospitalization

In mental health programs that are promoting consumer involvement, consumers are being hired as staff members on mental health crisis outreach teams. There are also various consumer-operated services that attempt to respond to the range of crisis needs. These include outreach crisis services, access to drop-in centers (see above), and emergency housing settings where people can go to receive support.

One example of a crisis housing alternative to hospitalization is the Center of Attention in Santa Clara County, California. This service was started by a community of ex-patients who were concerned that some members of their group had no alternative in a crisis except hospitalization. Like most self-help services, this one evolved out of the personal experience and perceived needs of the group. Group members noticed that when an individual was having a particularly hard time, he or she would ask to drop over to someone else's house. This was an unreliable system for support, however, because sometimes the person who was approached was unable or unwilling to offer help, or sometimes the crisis went on too long for the other person to cope with it. As a result, the group decided to set aside one apartment and to designate it as the "Center of Attention." Volunteers were enlisted who would agree to stay with an individual in crisis, and the list of these volunteers was posted by the phone in the apartment. A system was set up to guarantee access to the apartment. Thus, when someone had a crisis, he or she would go to the apartment and call as many of the volunteers on the list as desired; those who were available would come and spend as long as they wanted to provide support. The system worked well, and consumers reported that it resulted in a significant decrease in rehospitalization. More recently, this service has evolved into a cadre of volunteers who now go to the home of a person in crisis, so that he or she can continue functioning in as many areas as possible, while still receiving intensive support.

"Safe houses" are an attempt to provide consumers with intensive support when they cannot stay in their homes, without requiring treatment or medication. The intent is (1) to allow people to work through their psychiatric crises in a safe setting on exactly the terms they choose, thereby (2) retaining personal control of the situation and personal responsibility for their behavior. Many ex-patients see these two elements as crucial to recovery. Unfortunately, safe houses have been slow to develop in mental health systems, because of their very different approach to that used in professional services. Nonetheless, a number of such projects have been organized informally by self-help groups, and several state and provincial mental health systems plan to fund such options in the future.

Housing and Homelessness

As discussed in Chapter Two, people with psychiatric disabilities have struggled to gain access to decent integrated housing, rather than housing created specifically for mental health clients (e.g., group homes). As consumer groups organize housing services, they tend to focus on integrated settings, and on the option that most consumers seem to prefer: regular apartments in the community. In some cases, these groups are also able to arrange home ownership. Consumer-based housing efforts often start with people speaking out directly about their housing needs and preferences. Many consumer groups have become very vocal about their objections to living in group homes or other mental health facilities:

> Get twelve mental health professionals together and ask them to live in a house together, and see how well they get along. (Howie the Harp, quoted in Ridgway, 1988a, p. 7)

> I would rather be hospitalized, even with all the brutality that goes on in the hospital, than to have to exist in the demeaning condition that most group homes place their residents in. You have no rights, you have no dignity, you definitely have no privacy. (Tom Posey, quoted in Ridgway, 1988a, p. 8)

I went to this halfway house where they help people. You know how they help you? They have you sit there and do nothing all day long. They don't provide you with any case management. They didn't provide me with anyone to talk to. They didn't provide me with any structure. (Julie Crafts, quoted in Ridgway, 1988a, p. 7)

They don't want to live in a place where staff can pop in on them at any moment and say, "What are you doing, why are you doing it, and if we don't like the way you're doing it, we can kick you out!" (Judi Chamberlin, quoted in Ridgway, 1988a, p. 18)

People with psychiatric disabilities are also speaking out about their dissatisfaction with boarding homes, SRO hotels, and other environments in which they are segregated with other people with "disability" labels:

They pay . . . $300 a month to live stuck up in one raggey room. They probably make about $340 a month and they are paying . . . $300 a month for housing. (Henry Hendricks, quoted in Ridgway, 1988a, p. 10)

Some board and care houses are abusive, psychologically, verbally, physically, sexually. All of these abuses go on in board and care homes. . . . Once you're in a board and care home, you're trapped. You're financially trapped, you're economically trapped, you're socially trapped. (Howie the Harp, quoted in Ridgway, 1988a, p. 10)

I consider SRO's to be a small step above being homeless. It really isn't a decent place to live. . . . The hotels I lived in were very much vermin infested and crime infested. . . . I remember having to take a knife with me every time I went to the bathroom, just to protect myself. . . . I challenge anybody . . . to live in an SRO hotel on an SSI income and not experience paranoia, anxiety, depression, anger and all of the other symptoms of so-called mental illness. (Howie the Harp, quoted in Ridgway, 1988a, p. 12)

People are likewise speaking out about their experience of coping with homelessness and living in shelters:

I was always homeless, I was always looking for a place to stay. Ever since I was a child I was looking to get out of my mother's house. I was looking to get out of this place, get out of that place, but I always managed to find another place in society in which I stayed a little while . . . (Frances Somerville, quoted in Ridgway, 1988a, p. 14)

I had everything of mine stolen at the shelter, everything. I ended up in the Sacramento mental institute . . . and I left there with a pair of sneakers, a skirt and a shirt they gave me, a ticket to San Jose, and $1 for cigarettes. And that was all I had to my name. (Sandi DiPasquale, quoted in Ridgway, 1988a, p. 15)

I remember the first feeling I had when I moved into [my] apartment, after being homeless for quite some time, was the beauty of being able to turn on a light when you wanted to, to go to sleep when you wanted to, to watch TV when you wanted to, to eat when you want to, to go to the bathroom when you want to. Little freedoms that people normally take for granted become these tremendous, fantastic things . . . (Howie the Harp, quoted in Ridgway, 1988a, p. 16)

In response to these concerns, many self-help groups are organizing housing services, and in some cases developing housing itself. Although nearly all self-help groups, as well as many drop-in centers, focus some attention on housing, several examples of more comprehensive approaches may be useful.

First, a large number of consumer housing preference studies, whether on a statewide or a local level, have been initiated by self-help groups. Such efforts are an excellent way to focus the housing agenda—not only of the consumer movement, but often of the mental health system as well—on the options that consumers actually want. In projects of this type, consumers often design the study with the help of professional researchers; conduct interviews with other consumers in hospitals, on the streets, and in mental health programs; and formulate the findings and recommendations. Suggestions for conducting studies like this are given in Chapter Five of this book.

Second, a number of home ownership projects have been started across the country. In these projects, local consumer groups secure enough external funding to purchase property or to "buy into" a planned development. Often these projects will focus on the development of limited-equity cooperatives, in which a person with a disability is able to purchase one unit in a development, thus assuring both home ownership and physical integration in housing. An excellent example of this approach is one in which the Berkshire County Regional Housing Authority in Pittsfield, Massachusetts, arranged the development of a limited-equity cooperative. In this project, the local housing authority met with consumers to ask what type of housing they wanted. Most consumers responded that they wanted one-bedroom units that were not identifiable as "disabled" or "special-needs" housing. The housing authority then met with bankers and investors and developed a mixed-income cooperative, in which a small number of units were made available to individuals with psychiatric disabilities on SSI. Rent subsidies were used to supplement tenants' incomes as well. The majority of cooperative owners were of moderate income and had no "disability" label.

Another major housing project has been initiated by a statewide consumer organization, the Collaborative Support Programs of New Jersey. In this project, housing is developed and support services are offered through the network of self-help groups already operating in the state. The project is now in the process of developing a statewide nonprofit housing development corporation to expand housing options, all of which are designed on the basis of consumer preferences.

In Albany, New York, a group of consumers banded together to form a nonprofit housing development corporation, with the assistance of regional mental health staff. The corporation, Housing Options Made Easy, Inc., leases or purchases housing that can then be sublet or sold to consumers. Although the group does not provide mental health services, the staff of ex-patients help tenants to get the services they need, and various self-help services are offered. The emphasis is on permanent and integrated housing.

A final example of self-help housing efforts comes in the form of a recent experience I had in two different Canadian communities. I was spending a day visiting several new "clubhouse" programs, patterned after New York's Fountain House, in the Toronto area. In each of these very modern and comfortable settings, I talked with many consumers whose primary goal was to find affordable housing. The most frequent question I heard was this: "When is the staff going to get some funding for us to have the housing we need?" The staff members, who were also very concerned about housing issues, complained that government cutbacks rather than new housing were the order of the day. The situation did not seem at all hopeful.

The next day, I was attending a consumer/survivor conference in British Columbia and went to a workshop on "consumer-developed housing," presented by Unity Housing of Vancouver. The presenters described their personal experience as consumers who had very little money, but were seeking both decent housing and a sense of community. Some time ago, they decided to pool their resources and rent a small house. After sharing a very positive experience in this situation, they heard that the Canadian federal government was making some limited funding available for innovative consumer/survivor projects. They applied for a small grant and began approaching consumers they knew, asking how many would prefer to live in small communities by pooling their resources and renting houses. Within 6 months, working part-time, they were able to help 38 people find shared housing. A strong, supportive community emerged from these efforts: Tenants decided to have regular barbecues and social gatherings at the different houses, open to all of the tenants in the "program." Housemates began meeting regularly to manage the houses and to solve any problems that emerged. An expectation developed that if one individual in a household was having difficulties that required professional help, the housemates would accompany the person to the psychiatrist or other professional, and in effect would join the "treatment team" by working out a support plan. As a result, simply by acting on a desire for affordable housing and a sense of community, this group succeeded in creating a highly supportive set of social connections, organized an effective crisis response system, and even developed the self-help equivalents of such professional preoccupations as "service coordination" and "continuity of care."

As the households evolved, the tenants agreed that they wanted to increase the proportion of people without disabilities in the houses, and began to do so. In cases in which there were problems, they were dealt with by the housemates—or, in some cases, by the tenants of all of the houses. For example, one individual who happened not to be an ex-patient was living in one of the houses, and had begun to exploit and intimidate some of the other tenants. Rather than arrange a formal eviction, the tenants in the various houses agreed to have a party, at the end of which they would collectively confront the individual. They did so, and he quietly agreed to move on.

At the end of the presentation, I had a strong sense of *déjà vu* as a clubhouse member in the audience asked the first question: "That sounds great! Now how can I get the staff in our clubhouse to get a grant from the government to develop some housing for us?" The presenter responded: "Do you have a few friends who want to live together in the way we're talking about? If you do, call me tomorrow, and we'll help you find a place in about a week." He didn't say, "Sorry, we're full," or "We'll have to wait until our funding increases," or even "We'll need to assess just what housing and services would work best for you." And although this shared living option obviously might not appeal to many people, it occurred to me at that moment that a professional approach to the "problem" of finding decent housing and an effective community support system for 38 people with significant psychiatric disabilities—not to mention housing and supports that reflected their preferences—would probably take several years and 10 times as much money. Once again, I appreciated the simplicity and practicality of the self-help approach.

Employment, Training, and Rehabilitation Services

As with housing, many self-help groups and drop-in centers may focus on helping people to find and keep jobs. In this way, they are

responding to some of the primary concerns about employment, training, and rehabilitation services that consumers have articulated:

> I never really learned how to live on my own. Like what to do when
> the electricity bill is $169, and you only have $20 to pay on it? How do
> you deal with that? How do you (even) get your electricity turned on?
> How do you get your heat turned on? How do you know any of that?
> (Julie Crafts, quoted in Ridgway, 1988a, p. 23)

> I don't want you to take care of me for the rest of my life. What I want
> is for you to help me with what I don't know, so that I don't need your
> help as much anymore. . . . Don't just therapize me, give me the tools.
> (Julie Crafts, quoted in Ridgway, 1988a, p. 23)

Another concern that consumers express is having to wait for long periods of time, sometimes for years, to have opportunities for training
to pursue the work or career they really want:

> I wanted this course for a long time, for about five years. I wanted this
> course and I've been running into brick walls every time that I
> tried. . . . They said they didn't have the money to sponsor me. They said
> my name would come up but it never came up. . . . One day when I was
> at work, [they] just phoned me and told me I would start the course the
> next day. That made me really happy. (Consumer quoted in Hutchison
> et al., 1985, p. 25)

People are often asked to wait interminably just for the resources they
need to start down the path of economic self-sufficiency:

> I worked eight years as a sandblaster. There ain't anything I can't sand-
> blast. . . . I know I can get this complete sandblasting unit with . . . a com-
> pressor and two hoppers . . . all the hoses and all the nozzles and a five
> ton truck all for $5,000—the whole thing. But where could I ever come
> up with $5,000? (Consumer in Quebec, quoted in Hutchison et al., 1985,
> p. 25)

Mental health consumers are undertaking a variety of strategies
to increase employment options, including becoming involved in advisory committees for vocational rehabilitation programs, helping one
another to prepare for interviews and find jobs, and even organizing
their own businesses.

Representation on planning and advisory groups is crucial, since
until recently mental health and vocational rehabilitation systems have
focused almost exclusively on entry-level jobs now seen by many consumers as "dead-end." Participation in planning ensures that these sys-

tems will pursue the kinds of jobs and career opportunities that consumers actually want. One example of increasing "consumer voice" comes from Ohio, where the state department of mental health appointed an ex-patient, who had once been declared by professionals as incapable of ever working, to its senior management position responsible for employment services.

Drop-in centers and independent living programs operated by consumers, such as the Oakland (California) Independence Support Center, help people seek out jobs through ads and through personal networks. They also help people with self-care, inexpensive clothing, and the essential skills needed to secure work. They provide practical advice about the transition from public benefits to paid work—a transition that includes significant risk for a consumer, particularly with regard to medical benefits. They then provide peer support to help people manage the multiple demands and stresses associated with keeping jobs.

Another example of consumers addressing the need for work lies in the dozens of consumer-operated businesses that are being started across the country. Some of these include franchises, such as a Ben & Jerry's Ice Cream store in Baltimore, Maryland; and others are very successful independent businesses, often in downtown business areas, such as The Cookie Place in Providence, Rhode Island.

Finally, consumers are working to expand employment opportunities within the mental health field by writing and educating peers, professionals and employers about the kinds of reasonable accommodations that they need to succeed on the job. Howie the Harp (1991), for example, has written an especially helpful manual on this subject.

Rights Protection and Advocacy

Discrimination is a day-to-day reality for mental health consumers, both within mental health systems and in the larger community:

> I told one guy that I left my job because of mental illness, and I told him the truth. Of course, I never got hired for that job. I didn't feel like looking for a job after a while either. Yeah, really, I'm too young to retire. (Consumer quoted in Hutchison et al., 1985, p. 22)

Consumers have become very involved in the network of rights protection and advocacy groups across the United States, and in the national organizations that represent these groups: the National Association of Rights Protection and Advocacy, and the National Association of Protection and Advocacy Services. In statewide or local advocacy organizations, consumers serve as peer counselors and as monitors of services, particularly in such restrictive settings as hospitals, nursing homes, or other residential facilities. These individuals play a vital role in helping people who are institutionalized maintain connections with the outside world, giving them an avenue to express their desires and concerns about treatment, and providing them with a vehicle for pursuing grievances. In many cases, these advocates are able to identify practices in these settings that systematically compromise consumers' rights, and, through systems-level advocacy, are able to change many of these practices or to introduce further safeguards.

Case Management Services

Case management services have become accepted as among the most essential for people with psychiatric disabilities in modern mental health systems. Before I provide examples of self-help approaches to case management, a word about language is important. Many consumers find the term "case manager" itself offensive, and prefer such terms as "support worker," "resource coordinator," "individual life planner," or even "community organizer." Two consumer authors, for example, recently summarized this concern: "We're not cases and you're not managers" (Everett & Nelson, 1992, p. 49).

Consumers have become involved in the development of case management or service coordination in several ways: by being hired as adjunct staff members or aides on professional teams; by participating in academic case management training programs, and then being hired as case managers; and by organizing their own case management programs.

A number of professional case management programs across the country have begun hiring consumers to serve either as case managers or as case manager aides. One that deserves mention is the Community Support Program in Sacramento, California, which has undertaken a research demonstration project to examine the differences between professionally provided and consumer-provided case management in their agency.

Several training programs have been initiated to train consumer case managers to work in professional programs. The most famous is Denver, Colorado's Consumer Case Manager Program, started by professionals at the Psychiatric Rehabilitation Training Center, which selects, trains, and employs consumers to act as case managers for their peers across the state. Originally, this program trained consumers as case manager aides—a status to which many consumers objected. Another program that employs a more integrated learning approach is the master's program in social work at the University of Cincinnati, which trains students to become case managers. Students in this multidisciplinary program include people without a "disability" label, family members, and individuals with psychiatric disabilities. Other academic programs in New York, Maine, California, Connecticut, Massachusetts, and elsewhere are training consumers, typically in integrated classes, to provide rehabilitation, community support, or case management services.

Mind Empowered, Inc., of Portland, Oregan, has implemented a consumer-run clinical case management program, replicating Madison, Wisconsin's Program in Assertive Community Treatment model, and has been experimenting with the numerous ways in which staffing case management teams with consumers results in changes in this highly regarded professional model.

Creating Community

An early tenet of the community support systems philosophy (Turner & TenHoor, 1979) was that what people need more than anything else is a "caring community," a sense of belonging and connection to their surroundings. Increasingly, people with psychiatric disabilities are building "communities of support" themselves. In some cases, as people work to find their collective voice and to explore the many ways they can be of service to one another, these communities tend to be somewhat segregated by choice. This is not dissimilar to the collectives that emerged in the Black and Hispanic civil rights movements and in the women's movement.

An illustration from Santa Clara County, California, may be helpful. In this example, a number of consumers were assisted by several community organizers to "create" a community of interest; the consumers used their own group decision-making process to determine where they wanted to live and work, and how they would support one another. Although these organizers were "professionals," they clearly did not assume the role of helpers or treaters, but rather those of educators and community change agents. Most of the consumers chose to select housing that was very close together, while at the same time agreeing to support other group members who lived at a distance. They chose to meet frequently as a group, in order to work out how to get what they needed in the community. For the first year of their activity, the consumers' focus was relatively internal; that is, they concentrated on the group itself, and on meeting the concrete needs of group members for housing, work, and services. In its second year of activity, however, the group chose to reach out to another group located in an adjoining part of the county, and to help the new group to become organized in a similar fashion. Following this effort, several other groups representing diverse ethnic communities were given similar help. At the same time as this organizing was going on, however, people were moving into their own housing, securing work, and developing relationships with people outside of the group. Thus, although integration was not an explicit goal of the group, it evolved naturally as part of the empowerment that group members experienced through this approach. Other communities are more integrated from the beginning with people without "disability" labels. Regardless of this dimension, groups of ex-patients appear to be creating microcosms of the larger caring communities that all citizens need, and that most appear to lack. As such, this consumer movement is a powerful transformative agent that may have the potential for helping to heal our more extended communities.

Peck (1987) describes the essential characteristics of "community building" as "inclusivity," or a willingness to embrace those with differences; commitment to caring for one another; and consensus about the core values that guide action and behavior. He asserts that communities, if they are to stay intact, must be realistic, and that problem solutions developed by a community rather than by an individual are far more realistic. Similarly, community building requires a sense of contemplation or self-awareness. True communities provide a safe place for members—a place in which they can engage, in Peck's words, in "personal disarmament." Thus, true communities can fight gracefully. In such communities, according to Peck, there are no members, only leaders. Finally, he points out that true community is a spirit: the members of the group genuinely take pleasure and delight in themselves as a collective. Thus, the spirit of community, as contrasted with the competitiveness so rampant in our society, is the spirit of peace. And Peck asserts that the process of community building is one that can be organized.

> Community is integrative. It includes people of different sexes, ages, religions, cultures, viewpoints, lifestyles, and stages of development by integrating them into a whole that is greater—better—than the sum of its parts. Integration is not a melting process; it does not result in a bland average. Rather it has been compared to the creation of a salad in which the identity of the individual ingredients is preserved yet simultaneously transcended. Community does not solve the problem of pluralism by eliminating diversity. Instead it seeks out diversity, welcomes other points of view, embraces opposites, desires to see the other side of every issue. It is "holistic." It integrates us human beings into a functioning mystical body. (Peck, 1987, p. 234)

ORGANIZING FOR COMMUNITY CHANGE

CHAPTER 4

Preparing
for Organizing

STIGMA: THE CORE OBSTACLE TO CHANGE

The major challenge to integration that people with psychiatric disabilities face in most Western cultures is stigma, or social rejection. Stigma has become codified in laws, has been inadvertently used to organize helping programs, has informed social attitudes, and has promoted exclusionary and discriminatory behaviors by individuals. Because this core set of negative attitudes and beliefs has been internalized by the general public, it is a major focus of change efforts, since it serves to keep people with psychiatric disabilities in a permanently disadvantaged relationship with other citizens. The essence of stigma is the presumption of a fundamental "differentness" between people with intense, typically internal personal experiences that are not accessible to others, and other citizens who do not have these experiences—a differentness that implies inferiority.

As has been discussed in Chapter Three, traditional explanations of this differentness have ranged from characterological flaws to the presence of evil. In more recent times, individuals with a label of "mental illness" have been judged incompetent by the law and by medicine. In the larger social consciousness, people with this label are often seen today as simply not deserving the same economic benefits as other citizens—either because they are seen as not contributing to the general welfare, because they are feared, or because they are seen as incapable of benefiting from inclusion in community life. Therefore, conditions such as homelessness, life in a hospital back ward, or subsistence in a squalid boarding home are somehow tolerated by much of the general public. To many "average" citizens, these conditions are explainable wholly by the persons' "mental illness," and the only means of dealing with "mental illness" appear to be mental health treatment and/or institutionalization. In this view, the solution to homelessness becomes one of mental health professionals' providing clinical services; benevolent community groups' developing homeless shelters; and, for those who refuse either of these options, the courts' mandating involuntary treatment in institutions.

Stigma and discrimination operate at individual, community, and societal levels. It can be argued that they are perpetuated by many of the legal structures, service models, organizations, and institutions put in place by society to deal with "the problem of mental illness." Changing these beliefs and practices, and the social institutions that perpetuate them, has thus become a central goal of those working for community integration.

In order to make progress, however, change agents need to understand more about these attitudes, as well as about the process of change at the individual level, within mental health systems, and in the larger community. This chapter provides an overview of the basic building blocks for community change: understanding the effects of, and finding ways of responding to, these negative attitudes at each level of society; understanding the process of community change and the key elements in this process, especially the role of the change agent; and learning strategies for mobilizing groups to work for change.

STIGMA AT DIFFERENT LEVELS OF SOCIETY

Stigma at the Individual Level

There are three specific targets for individual change that are most relevant to community integration: "average" citizens' fear and distorted perceptions of people with a label of "mental illness"; the sense of overly developed responsibility among many professionals for the behavior of people with this label, which results in overprotectiveness and paternalism; and the internalized sense of incompetence and chronic disability among consumers/ex-patients themselves. The basic change that integration advocates are seeking is movement toward the beliefs that recovery is possible, that hope is the operative principle, and that people with psychiatric disabilities have a right to full community integration.

How then can we expect these individual negative attitudes to change? All enduring change, particularly when it is intended to improve the quality of human relationships, must be rooted in individual change. Similarly, real change, if it is to affect the actual quality of life of people with psychiatric disabilities, must occur on a person-by-person basis. Three factors related to individual change seem crucial for advocates. First, change occurs when individuals, regardless of whether they are mental health consumers, professionals, family members, or policy makers, feel a personal sense of empowerment and vision. Individuals in powerless positions must come to an awareness or consciousness of their own oppression before they can embrace change. They must understand the nature of that oppression, and then choose to assert their own power in order to resist the oppression. Therefore, change agents need to work with people to raise their consciousness and to help them reassert their sense of personal power.

Second, change occurs when individuals realize that what they are doing is not working. In science this is referred to as a "paradigm shift," during which old beliefs no longer explain current reality, and yet a new set of beliefs has not yet been formulated to replace the old ones (Kuhn, 1970). As I have noted in Chapter Two, such periods are marked by confusion, conflict, and chaos until a new view of reality is accepted. Key tools of change agents in this process are the new beliefs described above, as well as information about successful integration practices.

Change occurs when there are sufficient resources available. In the context of integration, there are two key resources: empowered people (consumers, family members, professionals, advocates) and models of behaving differently (successful integration strategies). Attitudes change as a result of behavioral changes, when people get to know one another as people in valued roles, not as stereotypes. In mental health systems, professionals, advocates, and family members can all be important allies to consumers by providing information, resources, and knowledge about mental health systems and how to influence them; by advocating for empowerment and for the services that people with psychiatric disabilities want; by accepting the personal risks involved in becoming a change agent; and by directly sharing power on a systematic, day to day basis. Change starts with individuals and then is nurtured in larger groups, as these groups develop a common vision that change is both essential and possible.

Stigma within Mental Health and Related Service Systems

Initial efforts at bringing about community integration are often focused on the practices of the mental health system, both because so many change agents work within those systems, and because the segregated patterns of settings and services within the mental health field pose a major barrier to integration. At a societal level, funding and legislation have created public mental health systems that until recently seemed to embody many negative attitudes within their programs and services. At a community level, the day-to-day practices within mental health, vocational rehabilitation, and disability benefits programs themselves have historically been structured in ways that foster segregation and dependency. By labeling all of the needs of individuals as originating with their "mental illness," and then by offering only treatment-oriented responses to such common human needs as housing, work, education, and social connections, these programs continued to reinforce the notion that their clients should be centrally defined by their impairment rather than their citizenship. Deegan (1990) describes this fundamental problem with mental health systems as a tendency to "break the human spirit" by putting staff and clients in situations where the most basic human responses are thwarted, such as a professional's or a hospital patient's inclination to reach out to another patient in pain in an isolation room. This process dehumanizes everyone involved.

Structural problems within mental health systems complicate the work of the change agent. First, there is often a lack of clarity about who is responsible for providing services to people with serious psychiatric disabilities, and fragmented authority structures and funding of programs appear to be the rule rather than the exception. Such disorganized systems of services, both among levels of government and within communities themselves, have been described for well over two decades in the mental health literature. Second, mental health services, because of the lack of an active political constituency to advocate for them, are typically underfunded. Finally, many individual programs prefer to serve people with less disabling mental health problems, or people who are more compliant with their services; such preferences exclude those individuals who are most in need, and/or those who want services on a more individualized basis.

The goal of the change agent in a mental health system is to expand the collective sense of the possible—to devise strategies for "freeing up the human spirit," so that change can be viewed as an opportunity rather than a threat. Specific strategies include creating services that are planned, operated, and evaluated by the people they serve; shifting resources to the control of service users; and focusing services on integration outcomes.

Attitudinal Barriers within Mental Health Systems

Within mental health systems, there are many myths about people with psychiatric disabilities that funtion directly to limit their life opportunities in communities. These myths are expressed in statements like the following:

> "People with mental illness need a special kind of housing."
> "They prefer to live among their own."
> "We need to 'place' people in the 'most appropriate setting' that will meet their needs over time."
> "As long as someone is 'in the community,' that's as much as we can expect."

These myths have been discussed in detail throughout Section I. Two of these myths are especially important for change agents to focus upon, since they serve as major barriers to community integration.

Myth One: People with Mental Illness Can't Make Reasonable Choices. In helping groups around North America to plan for meaningful community integration, I often hear statments such as the following. These reflect underlying assumptions either that people with mental illness can't choose where they want to live, or that, given how limited the options in the community are, their choices are a relatively unimportant consideration.

> "There's this large building that nobody wants. We could place 17 people there."
> "They're only funding transitional housing these days. Until things change, we'll just have to keep doing that."
> "If I ask my client where he wants to live, he'll probably say 'On the moon,' so I don't ask."

Many helpers and advocates within the mental health field do not believe that people with psychiatric disabilities can make meaningful decisions about where and how they should live. Although (as reviewed in Chapter Three) this myth is inconsistent with longitudinal research on mental health and rehabilitation outcomes, it continues to be part of the legacy of treatment and facility-based approaches, which assume that people primarily need protection and supervision. It is also a residue of the history of inadequate service systems in the community, in which people's failure is presumed to be confirming evidence of their incompetence—a phenomenon referred to as "blaming the victim" (Ryan, 1976).

A major effect of disregarding people's choices is the widespread pattern of "treatment resistance" reported in the literature (e.g., Bachrach, 1982). The real problem, as Estroff (1987) has suggested may actually lie in what people are offered. W. A. Anthony (personal communication, September 1990) concurs that the problem appears to be one of unappealing programs rather than of unmotivated or resistant consumers.

Myth Two: Most People with Mental Illness Are Too Disabled for Regular Housing, Work, or Social Relationships. I also frequently hear statements such as the following:

> "This is a great approach for those [few] who can live independently; it just doesn't apply to people I work with."
> "What about the client I have who has a history of self-abuse, unpredictable violence, and enjoys setting fires in his spare time? . . . So you've thought about him. So how about this other client I have who's a *real* problem?"
> "This sounds great, but not for my kid."

Section I has discussed at length the confusion that has prevailed in mental health systems between the environment in which a person resides and the supports a person receives, and describes the generally unsuccessful attempts to couple these in a single setting. When confronted with the poor outcomes among people with psychiatric disabilities who live outside of institutions, some professionals and family members may conclude: "These people are simply too ill to survive in the community." In other words, people's failures are seen as rooted in their illness, rather than in the fact that they may live almost completely unsupported lives and are often controlled by the decisions of others. As discussed in Chapter One, recent calls for reinstitutionalization and "asylum" appear to be based on that line of reasoning (Zipple et al., 1988).

Another variation of this myth is exemplified in this statement: "Most mentally ill people can't live independently." In actuality, it is probably the case that *no one* in our society can live independently. If relationships, income, a job, a home, and all of the usual supports were taken away from an individual with or without a disability, that person would be in extraordinarily difficult straits. The common thread that runs through this and similar concerns, of course, is the pervasive failure of society to help people find the places they want to be, and then to support them unremittingly once they are there.

There are also several specific challenges for change agents to face that go beyond individual attitude change: threats to the status quo, and a sense of powerlessness that seems to pervade many mental health systems.

Threats to the Status Quo

It is not uncommon, in my travels, for me to hear statements like these:

> "But I have clients who really benefitted from our group home."
> "My clients say they really like our sheltered workshop."
> "Does this mean we'll have to close all of our group homes tomorrow?"

Although it is clearly true that some individuals have found ways to use traditional programs successfully, these statements often reflect a defense of the status quo. Challenges to the status quo are rarely welcomed—not only because they assume the need for change in an accepted way of doing business, but also because they often require a "leap of faith" into new territory. Moreover, those undergoing the change rarely have all the information they need about new ways of behaving. In short, the first reaction to change is often a sense that it is harder than staying in place, and that what presently exists, though by no means perfect, may be better than some uncertain future prospect. For example, concerns expressed by program staff and managers about shifting from a facility-based approach to supporting individuals in the community often reflect the fact that service providers see themselves as caught between a known reality and an unknown future. Paradoxically, many professionals who freely acknowledge the many limitations of current approaches are at the same time strongly resistant to restructuring traditional models. A second group that frequently expresses such concerns consists of family members, who may fear that no services will be available for their relatives, particularly as parents age. Facilities such as group homes at least provide the appearance of some future support, as contrasted with a decentralized, non-facility-based community service approach.

At a more explicitly self-interested level, "industries"—such as state/provincial hospital unions, homeless shelters or transitional housing programs, organizations representing community residences, or associations of board-and-care providers—often present organized opposition to any plan to support people in regular housing, instead of in their facilities.

However professional attitudes about treatment facilities evolve, it appears inevitable that major changes are in store for facility-based programs, such as group homes or sheltered workshops. Many state/provincial and local policy makers are stressing greater accountability in these settings, and insisting that such programs either be phased out or be reserved for the most disabled individuals. Some U.S. states are refusing to fund additional facilities, and others are closing such settings (Ridgway, 1986). As one consumer leader remarked in a recent state-level meeting, "Why don't we all start by just agreeing that what we have isn't working? Then we can begin to solve the problem." (M. Finkle, personal communication, April 1990)

A Sense of Powerlessness and Hopelessness

I often hear statements that reflect a sense of hopelessness:

> "That's a great idea, but it'll never happen here: We don't have enough money; the state regulations won't let us; and besides, the local mental health center would never go for it."
> "Mental health systems are basically committed to institutions. They'll never fund the kinds of supports we're talking about here."
> "Mental health is always into fads. Today it's housing; tomorrow, who knows? I'll take the cautious approach until I see if they're really serious about this one."

A major barrier to building a vision of success for the future is the pervasive sense of failure and powerlessness in many mental health systems. These attitudes appear to be the legacy of underfunded services, ineffectively trained staffs, communities that are perceived as rejecting, and clients who are described as too disabled or unmotivated to be successful.

Such attitudes are articulated by many mental health staff members and managers. They are perpetuated by training programs that do not recognize the new focus on community integration and empowerment. Mental health professionals who graduate from these programs, for example, often lack the skills they need to help with housing needs, or to access the technical skills of those groups responsible for producing affordable housing in our communities. These attitudes also reflect the profound isolation of professionals in many programs not only from the desires of their clients, but from the rich opportunities that communities contain for housing, work, education, and social relationships. Many service providers lack knowledge of their clients' preferences, or lack connections with key community resources and/or staff members who are skilled in a community integration approach. They thus feel either skeptical or hopeless about implementing such an approach.

One of the best antidotes to such hopeless feelings is to recognize that although systems can provide powerful incentives and momentum for change, effective community integration is essentially a local community matter, and is ultimately a matter of changing individual relationships. Just as the best way for staff members to avoid "burnout" is to find an outlet for their frustration by taking an advocacy stance (Cherniss, 1980), the best antidote to this sense of powerlessness may well be for staff members to organize with a common purpose, express their frustrations with the current situation, and then move on to solutions.

The major approaches to transforming mental health systems so that they become vehicles for integration have been described in Chapter Two: adopting a community integration orientation in all policies; training staff members; sharing decision-making power with people with disabilities; and making the system accountable to the people it is intended to assist. Such changes set the stage for broader community change, since they typically provide people with disabilities with a stronger base of support, as well as a set of allies for pursuing change throughout the community.

Stigma in the Larger Community

At a community level, negative attitudes have become structured into social patterns of segregation, discrimination, and inadequate support for mental health services (particularly alternatives to institutions). Negative portrayals in the mass media reinforce these attitudes. For people with psychiatric disabilities, this results in economic marginality, segregation, repeated relapse because of the absence of supports, and living on the fringes of the mainstream culture—all of which then serve to confirm the collective negative beliefs of the public. People whose lives are disrupted by psychiatric disabilities, and who lose their homes, jobs, or status as college students, are unlikely to regain these opportunities once they are given a diagnostic label. Furthermore, since stigma is reflected in higher education training programs in the core mental health disciplines, these individuals are likely to receive treatment from professionals who are unable to see their potential for integration.

Advocates can become easily overwhelmed by opposition or bias at the community level, but change cannot be implemented in a vacuum. It is important to understand not merely how community prejudice can make people with psychiatric disabilities "outcasts," but also how these prejudices can affect the work of mental health systems, resulting in ineffective and inadequate support services. Advocates need to learn how to avoid polarized battles, and how to work collaboratively in the process of change.

Community Opposition

Stigma is a painful yet commonplace reality in the lives of people with psychiatric disabilities, often taking the form of public opposition to the inclusion of these individuals in the larger community. Concerns about stigma and "community opposition" have dominated the conversations and literature on community living for people with psychiatric disabilities for several decades. In the traditional view, advocates assume that such opposition is directly intended to exclude people with mental illnesses, and is rooted in irrational fears and hostility toward people who are "different." Thus, advocates assume that anyone who opposes a mental health facility or residential treatment program in his or her neighborhood is a "bigot" or a "redneck." Because this is a pitched battle between those with the "white hats" (advocates) and those with the "black hats" (the community), advocates often adopt strategies intended to overcome what they see as irrational and malicious resistance.

Some examples of such strategies are summarized in Ridgway (1987). One is a "low-profile" approach, in which professionals sneak facilities into communities and hope for the best, as community members come to realize what's going on after the fact. One retaliatory response of communities has been to pass legislation that requires that they be given formal notice and a role in prior approval of such facilities. A different, "high-profile" strategy used by mental health programs consists of publicly proposing the creation of a facility and then threatening to sue communities that resist. Proponents of a low-profile approach often characterize this second strategy as "organizing the opposition."

Often these strategies are defended on the basis of people's right to live in any community they choose. All citizens *do,* of course, have a right to live wherever they want to, without having to get the approval of neighbors. But even many professionals feel quite differently about having an anonymous individual move in next door than they do about having a program or facility move in next door. In fact, my experience is that most mental health professionals themselves *do not* want a group home or other treatment program sited next to their own homes. Those experienced with community zoning battles know that it is not uncommon to have local mental health professionals rise up to oppose such programs, at the same time as the local community mental health center staff members are asserting that people with psychiatric disabilities make good neighbors. In such situations, community members often complain that their rights to participate in decision making about the evolution of their neighborhood are being trampled on by professionals and/or government.

Still another strategy that advocates have used in lobbying for state-level "permissive" zoning legislation, which weakens the ability of local communities to enact zoning focused on more than two unrelated people living together, particularly those with disabilities. Finally, service systems have adopted strategies of siting facilities in marginal areas, nonresidential zones, and "transitional" neighborhoods, avoiding potential opposition by locating in communities that are too disorganized to pull together and mount such opposition. One result has been the creation of mental health and social service "ghettos" in some areas. This fuels deeply ingrained resentment among local community members against government actions that contribute to the further decline of the neighborhood; resentment against service providers, who are seen as "dumping" people with little or no support, and with no regard for the concerns of neighbors; and resentment against the consumers who live in these facilities, who, as a result, typically remain socially isolated.

So in many ways, community opposition and professional strategies for responding have represented a "lose–lose" situation for most parties involved. If advocates are truly interested in building integrated community relationships on a person-by-person basis, it hardly seems useful to start this process by engaging in direct and polarizing power struggles between the two groups of people who ultimately need to develop these positive relationships.

In order to change this somewhat discouraging scenario, however, it is important to think clearly about the different meanings of the term "community opposition." To be sure, some community opposition is rooted in irrational and oppressive beliefs about people with psychiatric disabilities. Typically, two of these beliefs are that people with psychiatric disabilities are more dangerous than other citizens, and that having a mental health residence in the neighborhood will lower property values in the area (Milstein, 1986, 1988). Research on each of these beliefs demonstrates that they have no consistent basis in fact; yet they persist, partly because of the overwhelmingly negative portrayals in the mass media of people with mental illnesses. A recent U.S. survey of public attitudes toward people with "chronic mental illness," conducted by the Daniel Yankelovich Group, found that about one-third of Americans report personal experience with mental illness or mental health professionals. Nonetheless, people still see themselves as relatively uninformed on the subject; they cite the media as their major sources of information, and believe that there is still considerable stigma. The major barrier to opportunities for people with psychiatric disabilities is seen as the "not in my back yard" (NIMBY) syndrome, in which potential neighbors resist new facilities sited near them (Yankelovich & Associates, 1990). Some ex-patient advocates refer to this as the "not on planet earth" (NOPE) syndrome (Howie the Harp, personal communication, November 1991).

Another facet of "community opposition" is the resentment of communities that have been in decline for some time, and that are just beginning to become organized, about what they see as the tendency of government to impose a whole variety of decisions on them without taking their point of view into account. Thus, government's mission of creating opportunities and empowerment for stigmatized groups often runs directly counter to the growing sense of empowerment in some local communities that are seeking to overcome social and economic marginality.

Advocates of community integration face a particularly difficult dilemma here, since they are advocates of empowering people with disabilities *through* empowerment of communities to take responsibility for all community members. It hardly seems an appropriate strategy for people with such a belief system to try to empower communities by forcing solutions from the outside, and then suing the communities when they balk. Too often, such "strategies" result in facilities that communities don't want, and that consumers themselves do not want to live in. A study by Segal and Specht (1983) describes a suit brought by residents of a shelter against the state of California because the shelter violated the state welfare code's goals of self-respect and self-reliance. Ridgway (1987), discussing this study, concludes: "It would be ironic if we were suing municipalities to establish specialized shelters and transitional group homes, and our clients were suing us for creating models that violated their rights [to stable housing]" (p. 6).

It may be helpful, in fact, to reframe the whole issue of "community opposition" as a natural and inevitable consequence of the clash between uninformed public attitudes on the one hand, and service designs that emphasize the "differentness" of people with psychiatric disabilities on the other. What's needed, then, is a "win–win" set of solutions—one that operates out of a fundamental and unwavering respect for the rights of people with labels to live, work, learn, and socialize wherever they choose to, as well as a clear recognition of the right and responsibility of communities to be fully involved in the process of meeting the housing, employment, educational, and social needs of *all* their members. A simple yet profoundly effective first step is to insist on the use of normal housing, work, and educational settings, rather than on facilities. Choosing this approach eliminates the overwhelming majority of opportunities for opposition.

Community opposition appears to have increased as homelessness and the visibility of homeless people with obvious mental health problems have proliferated, fueling fears about public safety, about people on the streets who are unserved yet obviously in need of help, and about being "hassled" in the community. The *New York Times* (1990) has described the impact on New York City by referring to the metropolis as "the new Calcutta." This perspective forms the basis for renewed calls for "asylums" (Zipple et al., 1988).

The best counter to these concerns is a strategy to increase community awareness about the true rights, needs, and potential of people with psychiatric disabilities, combined with a set of well-funded mental health services oriented to providing support to these individuals wherever they live and work, as well as a set of services to support families, police, landlords, employers, and other community members in the process. Such systems of support are described in later sections of this book.

Another essential strategy for responding to concerns about public safety is to find ways to balance the presence of a disabling condition with a clear sense of individual responsibility and consequences, rather than to excuse behavior that is legitimately objectionable to the wider community. This may involve, for example, supporting a landlord who is evicting an individual with a disability who has violated the conditions of tenancy, while at the same time working with the person to take responsibility for this behavior, and helping the person find another place to live. Although both effective mental health services and peer support can encourage the taking on of increased personal responsibility, the full implications of truly holding people responsible for their behavior are not yet clear.

Discrimination

Patterns of discrimination can of course include obvious actions, such as refusing to rent an apartment or offer a job to someone who has had a psychiatric crisis, or refusing to permit such a person to return to college. They can also include more subtle behaviors, such as discouraging membership in certain organizations or congregations, insisting that people with disabilities use certain facilities at times when professional staff members are present, or even systematically avoiding inviting coworkers with disabilities to social events after work. Changes in these patterns of discrimination are based on both formal and informal actions, including legislation that includes people with psychiatric disabilities as a "protected class," and enforcing existing federal, state/provincial and local statutes against discrimination. As word spreads among landlords and employers, behavior changes as well.

Direct action, even when no statutes seem to provide relief, can be very effective. I remember meeting a consumer advocate in New Mexico several years ago, who described a campaign her self-help group had undertaken to overturn a local public library's policy of not issuing a borrower's card to a "mental health client" unless the individual secured a second signature from a professional stating that the person was not likely to steal books. The self-help group quietly informed the librarian that ex-patients were no more likely to be negligent about their library responsibilities than any other citizens. When the librarian still refused to change the policy, the group members informed her that they planned to hold a news conference on the library steps the next morning, and to follow that with a lawsuit. That afternoon the policy was changed. Similarly, several years ago the management of Philadelphia's Public Housing Authority, concerned about the number of people with "mental health problems" in public housing projects who were apparently not receiving the services they needed, adopted a policy of not renting any more units to people with psychiatric disabilities unless professionals would guarantee services to them. A local ex-patient group organized a demonstration in which leaders chained themselves to the housing authority's office doors. The demonstration received front-page local and press coverage and made national news as well. The policy was changed.

With regard to more subtle forms of discrimination, greater visibility of people with psychiatric disabilities in public roles in the community—whether as advocates, service providers, or community leaders—tends to improve public attitudes. In the longer term, integration strategies themselves will have the most pervasive long-term ameliorative effect.

Inadequate Support Systems

The lack of adequate services in communities results from a variety of factors that go beyond mere negative attitudes. Within the larger generic network of community services and agencies outside of mental health systems, there is often an assumption that people with psychiatric disabilities should get all their needs met by specialized mental health agencies.

I remember two illustrative situations when I was managing a halfway house in Philadelphia over 20 years ago. One of the residents went down to the local grocery store to pick up some staples. While he was there, the owner called me to let me know that "one of your people is out." During that same period, there was an altercation between a rather slight staff member and a very large resident in the group home.

In spite of the efforts of other staff members to defuse the situation, the resident continued trying to assault the staff member. The police were called, since there was obvious physical danger. They were about to make an arrest for assault when the lieutenant in charge asked, "What kind of place is this anyway?" When he was told that it was a group home for people who had been in a mental hospital, he promptly instructed the other officers to leave, pointing to the resident and saying, "She's a 'mental'; we can't do anything without a court order."

Strategies for increasing the level and quality of services and supports in local communities are described in detail in Section III. To summarize, they involve systematic attempts to involve key community stakeholders—to bring them together with people with psychiatric disabilities and their advocates, in order to resolve what the larger community sees as urgent problems (homelessness and the lack of affordable housing, the level of unemployment among people with disabilities or people with low incomes, etc.). Changing the capacity of our communities to support individuals with psychiatric disabilities also requires successful strategies for changing the personal and social networks of community members.

AN INTRODUCTION TO THE PROCESS OF COMMUNITY CHANGE

At a fundamental level, communities and mental health systems begin to change when disadvantaged people become aware of their situation, organize themselves, and take collective action to demand change. Such collective action counters the twin stereotypes that people with psychiatric disabilities are incompetent, and that the role of the community is limited to providing professional mental health services for such people. Initial reactions range from denial to resentment to trying to marginalize or discount those who demand change, particularly if they do so in "inappropriate ways" (such as through expressing their anger over past treatment). However, communities that undergo sustained advocacy are often able to develop a new collective vision of supporting individuals on their own terms and in ways that promote success, both of the individuals and of the larger community. This collective vision requires leadership and organizational support for community members. It also requires resources, including a sense of hope that the goal of integration is achievable.

Put simply, communities faced with pressure to change have two options: to look to the people who are disadvantaged to define the problem and possible solutions, in which case integration will become the goal; or to look to experts or to those currently holding positions of power, in which case change efforts may well focus on the interests of the system. Lasting change in any community often involves an intense effort by citizens to tackle a problem, as well as the participation of key influential leaders or "gatekeepers." Helping to raise the consciousness of community leaders through encouraging relationships between them and people with psychiatric disabilities can be a powerful change strategy. It is, of course, also critical to know one's community—what has worked before and failed before, whose support is needed for meaningful change, and what other groups are likely to become involved in integration efforts in a positive or negative way.

Conflict is both to be expected and welcomed in the process of change; it arises simply because each person has experienced a different reality and has a different set of self-interests. The key to a positive change effort is to manage the process so that conflict does not become an excuse for personal insult, injury, or inaction, but instead is used as an opportunity to resolve important community problems. People who are temporary adversaries can still be approached with respect. Groups that attempt to avoid conflict are also avoiding the potential for change. The assumptions about change inherent in this book are that it can be a profoundly human and open-hearted process, and that we can all operate with the same integrity and decency when pursuing change on a broad scale that we expect of each other in any mutually respectful relationship.

In summary, then, social structures are changed when people gain power to direct their own lives. Sufficient numbers of individuals must be politically active to create a movement that is perceived as politically powerful. The power of the movement can be strengthened through coalitions or alliances with other groups, such as disability rights organizations, and other groups within the mental health arena that share a common agenda. Chapter Five describes specific change strategies in more detail.

THE KEY ELEMENTS IN CHANGE: PEOPLE, INFORMATION, AND RESOURCES

The Role of the Change Agent

In essence, *anyone* can choose to become a change agent—a person with a psychiatric disability who has rediscovered a sense of personal power, a family member who wants a better network of supports in the community, or a professional who has come to the conclusion that traditional approaches have outlived their usefulness. Change agents are found in self-help groups, among professionals, in family support groups, in government, and in higher education. Change agents are essentially people whose consciousness has been raised to the extent that they are no longer willing to support old "solutions." The good news is that there are large numbers of change agents emerging who are focused on community integration and self-determination for people with psychiatric disabilities. These individuals are discovering many allies among the variety of mental health constituencies. A change agent is not only a person with expanded consciousness, but also an individual with the motivation, drive, and organizational know-how to make change happen.

The Importance of Leadership

The community problems described in this book will not come as news to many North Americans, and certainly not to many mental health professionals. Why then have these problems not been addressed more successfully in more communities? The critical ingredient required to initiate any change effort—whether in changing policies and funding at a state/provincial level, in helping a local mental health program to become more directed by its clients, or attempting to include people with disabilities within a local congregation or other community group—is a single individual who is able to see that things can be different. This person is willing to take on a leadership role: to raise the issue, to mobilize support for change, and to persevere through the inevitable resistance—in other words, to make the change happen. Unfortunately, when an individual takes on leadership in this way, it often allows people who are generally unhappy about some aspect of this problem to focus their unhappiness on the leader. Assuming leadership, particularly within a culture of negative attitudes and self-interest, requires courage, intelligence, and the ability to avoid the isolation and discouragement that consistently threaten to undermine a leader's effectiveness. Strategies to organize support for leaders and leadership are described below.

Sustaining Leadership:
Developing a Personal Support System

Change agents, above all, must be persistent. The major barrier to "hanging in there" over the long haul of change is the level of discouragement that can be induced by powerful and what seems like equally persistent resistance to change. The best strategy the change agent can employ to overcome this isolation and discouragement is to organize a personal support system. Often the most critical initial question any change agent can ask, when faced with an intractable, long-standing, and seemingly overwhelming social problem, is this: "What will *my* support system be for tackling this problem and trying to make a difference over the long haul?" Identifying a few friends or a support group, and making them aware of the leadership and commitment that is being undertaken, can provide the basis for receiving support and avoiding isolation when the going gets tough.

Change as a Personal Commitment

Change agents are most helpful when they have a strong personal commitment to change, whether because they have been directly affected by how people with disabilities are treated, or because of their own experience of social marginalization, empowerment, healing, and recovery. They are most effective when their work is motivated by a strong commitment to social justice, a high level of personal integrity, and a sense of deep respect for all other people, regardless of whether they agree or not on particular issues. Change agents need to be excellent listeners. They need to be willing to embrace the major personal changes that appear to accompany involvement in this particular struggle: the willingness to become part of a community of people who have been socially marginalized, and, in the process, to experience social rejection themselves; the willingness to experience the extent to which people have been mistreated, and to witness the level of rage that such mistreatment engenders; and the willingness to practice real integration throughout their own communities and lives—in their work, their friendship networks, their churches or synagogues, their schools, and their neighborhoods.

Change Agents as the Vehicles for Community Action

In spite of the difficulties of making change, I have been consistently impressed with the fact that in communities throughout North America and elsewhere, small groups of individuals who are willing to assume leadership are solving community problems. They are creating recycling systems; bicycle paths; voter registration drives; political reform efforts; shelters for victims of domestic violence; peer counseling programs for gay, lesbian, and bisexual youths; "sweat equity" housing renovations; alternative schools; and a thousand other community improvements. As far as the needs of people with psychiatric disabilities are concerned, there is an equally impressive flowering of successful self-help and community organizing efforts. In each case, the change agents are the ones who are able to move the larger community from a sense of confusion, anger, or hopelessness about an issue toward constructive action.

Change agents committed to integration are most effective if they are already active and involved members of their local community, because they have inside knowledge of how things get done there, and because they have a network of relationships with which they can influence the process of change. Effective change agents conduct their activities in concert with other members of the local community, while working at the same time to increase the community's willingness to include *all* of its members. In this way, solutions to these problems are "homegrown," and can reflect a strong sense of ownership and pride within the community.

Key Constituencies to Consider

Change agents are only as effective as the individuals and groups they work with. Once the purpose of the group's effort is clear (see Chapter Five), it is then important to ask this question: "In order to create a more inclusive community (or a more integration-oriented mental health system or program), whose involvement, commitment, and sense of ownership are essential?"

Major changes in communities require not only planning, but also the full participation of some key "gatekeepers"—people who control access to the material resources and often the social opportunities in a community. In organizing for change, it is critical to move beyond "preaching to the choir," and to reach out to those who, though they may be inclined to work in partnership, are unfamiliar with the needs of people with psychiatric disabilities, and are currently not involved in solutions to the problem of community integration. The major strategy used to get these key people involved is to increase the contact between these individuals and people with psychiatric disabilities. This is the core of the community integration change process.

In general, there are several groups that ultimately will need to be involved regardless of the uniqueness of a particular community. These include a diverse group of consumers/ex-patients, family members, other advocates, mental health professionals, housing and employment professionals (in both the public and private sectors), key political leaders, and ordinary citizens. Of course, who becomes involved at what time depends on the particular focus of community organizing that the group settles on (see Chapter Five).

Information as Power

In addition to people, information is a critical tool for change agents. The basic information that has the most power to effect change is knowledge of what has happened to people and of how people define their own needs and desires. Chapter Five describes a number of strategies to gather information on consumer preferences; on family perspectives; on the capacity of the community to support individuals with psychiatric disabilities; and on such key issues as housing, work, education, and social networks.

Resources

Funding and other resources are also critical to any community change effort. Chapter Five describes a variety of strategies concerning resources for change efforts; these include deciding whether the group should seek funding to provide actual services (as opposed to serving principally as an advocacy organization), practicing grantsmanship, and obtaining no-cost and low-cost resources.

ORGANIZING A PLANNING GROUP

Ralph Nader was once approached by a woman in Orlando, Florida who, frustrated in her efforts to change public consciousness on the issue of nuclear power, told Nader, "I wish we could clone you." Nader's reply shows a depth of wisdom about the process of change:

> Listen, we all have to do our part. There are enough people out there, they've just got to be connected. It's all organization. My dad once told me, 'You know the difference between people who treat people unfairly and people who are victims? Organization.' It's how so few can exploit so many. (Nader, 1990, p. 42)

Thus, before decisions are made about any formal structures through which better housing, work, and social supports can be planned and developed, it is first of all critical to think about what small group of individuals will be willing to make a long-term commitment to this issue over an extended period. Who are the key individuals who seem particularly concerned about these issues, open to new ideas, and able to proceed with hope? Are these people who project positive energy and ideas, people with a sense of possibilities? Are these people with a sense of perspective, a sense of humor? Above all, are these people with a strong and unwavering respect for other people, especially for consumers/ex-patients and their families? Some of these may be friends or associates who are local consumer advocates, family members, service providers, neighbors, local business people, church members, sympathetic realtors, employers, or neighbors.

Often a group comes together around a common theme or problem it wants to address, such as the lack of housing options or employment for people with psychiatric disabilities. The process of change typically starts by convening a small group of these individuals, and asking them to make a commitment to begin working on a particular aspect of community integration. The initial purposes of the group can be (1) For individual members to help one another do what they are already doing, but more effectively and with more satisfaction; and (2) for all members to learn new information and perspectives that will allow the group to have a larger impact on the community.

Even coming together for mutual support, however, may invite resistance. Often, an initial reaction to such an invitation may be something like this: "But I already work all day in mental health [or as an advocate], and I'm nearly burned out. The last thing I want to do is to spend more of my time on this." My own experience, however, is that "burnout" more often results from a dedicated person's trying to help one individual at a time within a system or a community that does not effectively support those efforts. The most effective antidote to such burnout can be to become involved in addressing some of the root causes of those problems and frustrations. In this process, it is often possible to reframe these daily frustrations as mental health system, community, or societal problems that require different interventions than those used in supporting individuals.

Once a group is formed, members can begin simply by sharing their experiences, being careful to balance the discussion between successes and frustrations; gripe sessions, in themselves, are ultimately discouraging. It will soon become apparent that each member has a very different perspective on some of the issues the group is concerned about (e.g., on the role and value of professional vs. self-help approaches; on the extent to which consumers/ex-patients should control services and resources; on the role of families in advocacy and services; or on such thorny issues as medication and involuntary interventions. It is important to recognize from the outset that working with these differences is essential if the group is to come up with new solutions to the problem of community integration.

The task of the group throughout its work is not to come up with the "right view" on all of the issues, but to identify those perspectives with which everyone can agree, and then to "agree to disagree" on the rest. As noted in Chapter Three, this has been the most powerful strategy in communities in which consumers/ex-patients, family advocates, and professionals have been able to jointly develop and advocate for a unified agenda for change. The only way to preserve the value and usefulness of each of these different perspectives, and to keep them available as learning material for the change process, is to treat each person's views with attention and respect. However, the emphasis should be on trying to proceed as thoroughly as possible from the perspective of consumers/ex-patients themselves. The best way to accomplish this latter objective is to be sure that the group contains a majority of people with psychiatric disabilities.

CHAPTER 5

Strategies
for Change

In the nuclear age, we have changed everything about our world except the way we think about the world, and thus we drift toward unparalleled disaster.

— ALBERT EINSTEIN (quoted in Lapp, 1964, p. 16)

Once a group has been formed to work toward change, it is helpful to develop a systematic approach that will sustain the group over the extended period required to achieve broad change. This chapter describes strategies for achieving community integration that have proven successful in a number of state/provincial mental health systems and local communities. These strategies include developing a mission (i.e., a clear image of the kind of community or system the group is trying to achieve); deciding on the group's specific priorities for action by taking a hard look at the opportunities and concerns of the community; collecting information that will be helpful in achieving the group's goals; considering whom to work with and to involve; and figuring out financing.

DEVELOPING A MISSION

Why Clarifying the Group's Mission Is Important

Achieving a fully integrated community is a long-term process, perhaps even as lifelong one, with fresh challenges emerging from even the most decisive victories. Thus, there are compelling reasons to focus first of all on the larger outcomes the group is trying to achieve, and specifically on the kind of community the group is trying to promote. Over time, the specific focus of the group's work may change greatly, but what is needed throughout is an enduring vision of the kind of community the group is moving toward—a vision that embodies the group's long-term goals and the principles that will guide its work. In fact, the experience of planning experts in systems undergoing major change related to community integration (Carling & Wilson, 1988; Carling & Ridgway, 1987) indicates that the greatest stumbling blocks the mental health field faces may well be the pervasive confusion and conflict about what specific outcomes it is trying to accomplish in people's lives, what strategies are most effective in achieving these outcomes, and what values should guide the development of these strategies. Once a mental health system or organization has clarified those outcomes in the form of a mission statement, there is evidence that the expectations of consumers, families, and professionals all improve, as do the actual outcomes in the lives of consumers (Pandiani, Edgar, & Pierce, in press).

A mission statement describes a clear vision of success—an ideal community. As such, it provides a "road map" that places the group's specific projects or activities within a larger, more long-term context. Practically speaking, it is a tool through which the group can evaluate the inevitable compromises it must make within the context of movement toward this ideal community. A mission statement is also useful in that it suggests the kinds of information the group should gather, and can serve as a philosophical "guidepost" for critical decisions the group will have to make in the process of actually implementing its plans. Such a statement essentially summarizes the group's most closely held values about people with psychiatric disabilities, the life opportunities they should have and the responsibilities of the community. Therefore, it needs to be constructed with care.

The process of developing a mission statement is one of re-examining how the local community should change to become more inclusive. The statement should specify where people with psychiatric disabilities will be living, learning, working, and socializing; how they will be supported; and on what basis decisions will be made about their lives. There are several effective strategies for developing a mission statement:

- Providing the group (especially its nonconsumer members) with an opportunity to hear directly from consumers/ex-patients about their needs and desires.
- Centrally involving families.

- Expanding the group's consciousness about housing, employment and social needs through readings and films.
- Being willing to reappraise current approaches, and to acknowledge openly what is not working.
- Promoting an environment in which constructive disagreement is encouraged, and in which the group will take the necessary time for consensus building.
- Avoiding superficial agreement or technical solutions to basic needs, and focusing instead on key differences in values or expectations, which if unaddressed may re--emerge and undermine the group's efforts later.
- When the group does reach agreement on a particular value, making its specific implications clear to all participants is important so that the value can be used to guide concrete actions and decisions.

A mission statement, then, represents an ideal by which to gauge the group's actions. As such, it may reflect a variety of values, some of which will inevitably come into conflict when they are applied to real problems. For example, whereas the group may value housing that is physically integrated, a small group of ex-patients may ask for assistance in finding a house in which they can live together. In this case, the values of free choice, self-determination, community building, and peer support may outweigh the value of physical integration. A mission statement provides a context in which to discuss the particular balance that the group achieves between and among competing values in each action it takes. It is, in effect, a mechanism for keeping the group grounded in the core values on which it will base all of its future decisions.

Key Elements of a Mission Statement

It is useful for the group to include in the mission statement the outcomes it desires, as well as some guiding principles.

Desired Outcomes

- *Stable, affordable, integrated housing.* Endorsing this outcome implies that the group will need to take action to help increase consumers' income so they can have access to housing. It may also imply working with other groups to make rent subsidies routinely available. And the group will have to consider the "transitional" nature of any current mental health residential programs, and to decide whether these should be considered treatment settings or housing options. The group may need to become involved in housing development, negotiate with landlords in the local area to improve consumers' access to rental housing, combat discrimination, or become part of the larger housing advocacy network in the community.

• *Real work.* This outcome typically implies a concerted effort to work with local employers to gain access to existing job opportunities and create new ones; to assess consumers' interest in work; to adapt work environments as necessary; and to support consumers in their employment over time.

• *Educational opportunities.* This outcome implies assessing consumers' educational aspirations, and working with the various education and training organizations in the community to identify opportunities for inclusion.

• *Social networks.* This outcome anticipates full inclusion in the "affiliational" life of the community (McKnight, 1987), including the variety of community organizations and activities structured to support people on the basis of shared interests, not special needs. The entire process of planning for community integration should be a model for how communities should include people with special needs, characteristics, or labels, so that ultimately those labels become insignificant.

• *Successful coping with psychiatric disabilities, and progress in recovery.* The movement to define outcomes in terms of tangible benefits to consumers is long overdue, but should not obscure the need to include outcomes related to the psychiatric disabilities themselves and their responsiveness to treatment. Also of critical importance are outcomes such as consumers' personal satisfaction with their lives, feelings of personal power and effectiveness, the development of successful coping strategies to manage disabilities over time, and learning to take charge of the recovery process.

Guiding Principles

The group will want to articulate the principles or core values that will be used to inform its actions or projects. These might include values like the following:

• *Basing housing, work, education, social networks, and services on consumer self-determination.* This principle implies that the group must continually assess consumers' collective choices about the kinds of housing, jobs, educational options, social connections, and services that should be developed; plan for a broad range of options; and advocate for restructuring services and benefit programs so that they come under consumer control.

• *Making flexible and reliable services and supports available.*
This principle implies that natural supports, generic community services, and peer supports will be given greater emphasis in the future than in current professional programs. It also implies that professional services themselves will be restructured to conform to consumer preferences, as well as to strengthen natural support systems (such as those provided by family, friends, and coworkers). This will typically involve shifting funding and responsibility away from professionally controlled programs, and toward individualized services reflecting consumers' desires.

A Sample Mission Statement

The following mission statement, focused on housing as well as broader community integration outcomes, was developed in a 2-day intensive planning retreat for the leadership of the Virginia mental health system (state mental health and housing staff, consumers, families, and other advocates):

> All individuals, including those with mental disabilities, should live in stable, decent, affordable housing of their choice. People should choose their housing from that available to the general public throughout the community. To ensure choice, the mental health system has the responsibility to assure availability and access to existing housing, and to stimulate the preservation and development of housing. The mental health system should also assure that the necessary supports will be available to secure adequate housing, meaningful work, education, personal relationships and community participation regardless of where people choose to live. (Virginia Department of Mental Health, Mental Retardation and Substance Abuse, 1990, p. 1)

Once the group has articulated a vision of the ideal inclusive community it wants to work toward, it is ready to apply the mission to its own community, and to begin making decisions about specific desired changes.

DECIDING ON SPECIFIC PRIORITIES FOR ACTION

The group is now ready to make decisions about the particular activities it wants to take on first. Three questions can guide the group's work on this important task:

> "What changes in this community would make the most difference in the day-to-day lives of people with psychiatric disabilities?"

"Where are the opportunities for change in this community right
now—what is most ready to change?"

"What actions are we as a group most interested in and most pas-
sionate about taking?"

Examining each of these questions thoughtfully will allow the group
to formulate a set of actions in the community that will not only reflect
the group's interests, but also catalyze support for a broader culture
of inclusiveness in the community, and therefore will pave the way
for subsequent projects.

Changes That Would Make the Most Difference in the Community

The first thing to do is to examine the major barriers to integration
in the community. Typical obstacles that the group may want to consider include the lack of consumer choice and involvement; the lack
of effective services and supports; the need for redirecting and restructuring the financing of services and supports; the need to increase
consumers' income; a lack of mechanisms, relationships, and resources
for accessing preserving, and developing affordable housing; difficulties in accessing and developing jobs; barriers to educational and training opportunities; and social isolation.

It is not unusual for a group to feel overwhelmed by the enormity
of the problem of integration and empowerment, and by the multiple
challenges the group will face in pursuing these goals. What the group
will find as it moves along, however, is that many of the fundamental
barriers are attitudinal in nature. Once the group moves forward with
a project, the impact on the community will inevitably be greater than
the project itself: Any such project represents increased positive visibility for people with psychiatric disabilities, which in turn tends to
improve public attitudes. Furthermore, it is important to remember
that it is not solely the group's responsibility to overcome all of these
challenges; it is a community's responsibility. The task of the group
is simply to act as a catalyst for change, which includes making people in responsible positions aware of how the failure to address these
community problems is curtailing the life opportunities of citizens, and
assisting those responsible persons in figuring out how to "do business" differently.

After examining the specific obstacles to integration, the group
can then brainstorm practical strategies for overcoming these
challenges (e.g., "What would be in place if that barrier no longer ex-
isted?"). For example, one challenge related to the lack of consumer
income is that there is no funding to help consumers get housing while

they are on the waiting list for a rent subsidy. In that case, the desired outcome might be to develop funding to subsidize consumers' rents, and to help them with startup costs (furnishings, deposits) until they receive a federal subsidy. This money could be repaid by individuals as their circumstances permit, thus creating a "revolving loan fund."

Developing concrete, practical ideas like these helps the group to create a manageable agenda, while maintaining its focus on those actions that are most likely to lead to the greatest change. Many such practical ideas are described in Section III.

Key Community Concerns as Opportunities for Change

In any community, certain issues are "hot" or "on the front burner" as far as the public consciousness is concerned. If the community is concerned about public safety, then it may be appropriate to mount a campaign to decrease the victimization of people with psychiatric disabilities as targets of crime. If the community is concerned about the high cost of rental housing or about homelessness, it may be appropriate to develop some projects focused on affordable housing, such as a campaign for a rental subsidy program or a home ownership initiative targeted broadly to low-income individuals. If there is concern about "street people," developing outreach services may be the logical place to start. In other words, the group should identify those issues about which the community as a whole is concerned, and then take action in such a way that people with psychiatric disabilities are seen as contributing to the solutions. Throughout this process of selecting actions, of course, the group is guided by the priorities of consumers/ex-patients and their families.

Becoming involved in broader community issues often requires the group to conduct a variety of educational activities. Such educational efforts reframe the stereotypes commonly held in the larger community. These efforts, however, appear to be far more effective if they are tied to particular issues in which the general public has a strong interest. More generalized stigma reduction educational campaigns run the risk of perpetuating "we–they" thinking.

Chapter Four has reviewed a number of the critical community concerns that underlie patterns of community opposition, discrimination, and unwillingness to fund or politically support the services and benefits needed by many people with psychiatric disabilities for success in the community. Effective strategies for responding to these typical community concerns include the following: focusing on community organizing and community development; using integrated settings to meet consumers' housing, work, and support needs, and aggressively developing mental health services and other supports to promote consumers' success in these settings; promoting consumer and family "voice"; directly and forcefully countering any efforts to deny consumers their rights to integration; and promoting positive attitudes toward integration by building relationships one at a time. These strategies are now discussed.

Focusing on Community Organizing and Community Development

The group should emphasize seeing the community as part of the solution rather than as part of the problem. Typical strategies include viewing the community as a resource; seeing all people, including consumers, their families, other advocates, and service providers, as equally valuable members of the community; identifying key potential supporters of integration in the community; and involving a broad range of community members in integration projects. To the extent that change agents are sensitive to the needs and concerns of their community, and make sure that each of their actions serves to benefit the community as a whole rather than only one of its constituent groups, the larger community is likely to support these change efforts.

Using Integrated Settings to Meet Consumers' Needs and Developing Relevant Supports

Choosing relevant approaches to providing mental health services and other supports that will respond to people's needs in housing, employment, and educational settings, not only may be goals in themselves for a group; they may be the means of achieving further goals. When it becomes evident that these objectives are being fulfilled and are meeting with success, much of the community opposition to "those people" (a nameless, faceless group), to "facilities" (segregated work and housing settings), and even to "government imposing its will on us" (forcing a community to accept a large group home) can be diffused or avoided all together.

Promoting Consumer and Family "Voice"

A powerful strategy for building individual relationships between people with and without labels, and for avoiding community discussion that emphasizes the "differentness" of people with disabilities, is to promote every opportunity for consumers and their families to speak out about their experiences and needs. Change agents also know that community change often brings deep prejudices to the surface and involves significant conflict. Thus, it is important to anticipate the support needs of people who have the courage and determination to stand up and publicly identify themselves as having psychiatric disabilities, or as being family members of individuals with disabilities.

Often consumers, family members, and advocates are overwhelmed with anger and frustration at the grim reality that what should be basic human rights must be fought for on a daily basis, person by person. Such anger is a normal response to an intolerable situation; it can be a productive tool if it solidifies a commitment to change and spurs the group into action. I am reminded of a recent observation by William Sloane Coffin, nuclear freeze activist and former chaplain at Yale: "You cannot experience true compassion for those who are oppressed without experiencing, at the same time, anger at that which oppresses them" (personal communication, October 1990).

By making sure that organizing efforts and all other community change strategies are undertaken by integrated groups, change agents become a proactive force for change, rather than merely reacting to the occasional zoning hearing or other public meeting called to try to exclude people with psychiatric disabilities from a neighborhood. To be sure, advocates must organize vigorously to be well represented and effective at such meetings; however, these meetings should be the exception to advocates' work in communities, rather than their primary focus.

Directly Addressing Efforts to Deny
Consumers' Rights to Integration

Respecting the rights of communities and working as community members to create change in no way implies that advocates should be naive about the level of antagonism within most communities toward people with psychiatric disabilities. In spite of all their organizing efforts, these individuals are often forced to confront individuals (e.g., landlords, employers), or members of organized community groups who continue—out of prejudice—to deny them their right to full community participation. In such cases, advocates need to be firm in countering such actions: first through attempts to educate and persuade, then through legal action.

Tools for legal action are growing. In the United States, the Federal Fair Housing Amendments Act of 1989 prohibits discrimination against people with a label of mental illness in the sale or rental of housing. The Americans with Disabilities Act of 1990 extends such protection to employment, public facilities and services, and other aspects of community life. Excellent materials are now available that describe the specific provisions of these laws, and suggest effective strategies for countering community opposition. The Bazelon Center's Community Watch Program (2021 L Street N.W., Suite 800, Washington, DC 20036) is an excellent source of assistance in designing legal strategies to respond to community opposition. A newsletter, *Action Line,* is also available from this group.

Promoting Positive Attitudes through Relationship Building

Through building relationships one at a time between people with and without special labels, attitudes can be changed. In spite of several major public relations campaigns against stigma by such diverse organizations as the National Alliance for the Mentally Ill and the NIMH, as well as statewide antistigma efforts in New York, Ohio, Illinois, California, and elsewhere, a recently completed U.S. survey funded by the Robert Wood Johnson Foundation (Yankelovich & Associates, 1990; see Chapter Four) confirms that attitudes toward people with psychiatric disabilities are still quite negative and are based primarily on ignorance.

These findings are consistent with the literature on attitudes of people toward disabilities in general (Anthony, 1979), which suggests that improving attitudes is not a function of information alone, but rather of personal contact with individuals with labels. Contact alone is not likely to improve attitudes, however, particularly in settings where people are devalued or functioning poorly (e.g., in institutions). It is for this reason that many students who complete internships at state hospitals, as well as many staff members who work for a short time in low-quality community mental health programs, leave those experiences with poorer attitudes than those with which they began (Carling, 1990c). What is especially effective in improving attitudes is contact that occurs in normal, integrated settings, in which a person with a label is seen *as a peer in a valued role.* The best examples of such contact are those between coworkers on a job, tenants in a housing situation, members of a social or other community group, planners of community or mental health systems change, or service providers.

Thus, advocates of community change need to be vigilant in identifying opportunities for people with labels to participate in community life in ways that will promote the kinds of contact described above. Helping people to obtain the supports they need allows them to operate from a position of strength and to participate fully in these opportunities.

In the long term, building the kind of framework for support that emphasizes personal responsibility, self-help, the support of family and friends, and full participation in the community is the best strategy for overcoming community concerns. As Taylor et al. (1987) have pointed out, community acceptance is not a *prerequisite* for community integration; it is an *outcome* of successful integration.

Actions the Group Is Most Interested in Taking

Having reviewed those actions that are likely to have the most impact, and the opportunities for change in the community, the group is ready to make a decision about the specific actions or projects with which it wants to begin. It is helpful to be as specific and concrete as possible at this stage. Often, individual group members have difficulty giving up a "pet project" that the majority may feel is less of a priority. In this case, it is helpful to understand that the first set of group activities is simply a way to get started and to accomplish some small victories in what will essentially be a longer-term effort.

After deciding on a specific project, the group can identify those smaller steps that are most likely to "get the ball rolling," since change rarely occurs in large increments. To take the example of trying to establish a rent subsidy program, one initial step might be to begin exploring funding sources, such as community foundations or a local congregation. Another might be to meet with mental health and housing officials or a local legislator, in order to explore the possibility of allocating public funds for this purpose. A third step might be to begin negotiating with the local low-income housing coalition to get this initiative onto its agenda, in order to broaden the base of support for such a program. A fourth step might be to explore the feasibility of conducting a community-wide assessment of consumers' housing needs and preferences, since such an assessment will undoubtedly document the need for rental assistance.

Once the group has decided upon the specific project it wants to undertake, it is now ready to draw upon three important tools in the process of community change: gathering relevant information; deciding whom to work with and to involve; and figuring out financing.

GATHERING THE INFORMATION
NEEDED FOR CHANGE

There are many sources of information relevant to community integration. The group will obviously only be interested in those that are directly relevant to the project at hand. Since such projects can vary greatly, this section describes a variety of these information sources, as well as strategies for gathering information.

At one level, "assessing needs" can be a profoundly simple process. I remember helping Priscilla Ridgway a number of years ago with a needs assessment manual she was developing. The manual (Ridgway & Carling, 1988) was intended to provide a comprehensive approach to determining what people with psychiatric disabilities need. Priscilla found that the literature in this area was already voluminous, and she spent a great deal of time in the library as we began work on the project. After some time, she appeared in my office and announced that, having reviewed what all the experts had to say about needs, she was finished. I suggested that the next step was a detailed outline, but she pointed out that she had already captured the essence of needs assessment; in fact, she had finished the manual. Delighted, I asked to see it. She then showed me a *very* thin volume containing only three pages. The first page said simply: "Find the people." The second said: "Ask them what they need." And the third page said: "Give it to them." The actual manual we produced (Ridgway & Carling, 1988) was of course considerably longer; still, I hope it remained faithful to that gem of wisdom.

Because a group may concern itself with a broad range of issues, the following material is rather extensive and detailed. The reader, therefore, will want to select from this material only those sources and strategies that will be most helpful to the success of a particular project.

Once the group has settled on a specific project, individuals and subgroups can begin to gather necessary information. Is there information, for example, on the income levels of people with psychiatric disabilities in the local community or in the state or province? Have any prior planning efforts produced information on housing, work, education, social networks, or services and supports? What is known about the issues of homelessness and unemployment in the community, county, or state/province?

Obviously, the group will want to carefully evaluate the usefulness of existing information, particularly assessments of needs. These assessments frequently lack a clear focus on empowerment or community integration outcomes; therefore, they may well contain assumptions about what people need that are based on some of the myths described earlier in this book or they may simply be based on professionals' opinions, rather than on information gathered from people with disabilities. The group's task here is to answer these questions:

"Is this information relevant to the outcomes we are seeking?"
"How will this information be useful in helping others become

aware of the problem we're concerned about, and in enlisting their support?"

"What questions does this information raise that the group will need to answer, or even counter with information that the group gathers itself?"

Assessing Consumers' Preferences

Freud spent years agonizing over the question of what it is that women really wanted. He would have had a much easier time of it if he had simply asked them.

—BETTY FRIEDAN (1963, p. 68)

In each community change effort, participants must continually make hard decisions about resources and about the breadth of their work, particularly when the group is working on a problem of significant scope. The most valuable source of knowledge for such decisions consists of the wishes of people with psychiatric disabilities themselves. Unfortunately, little information is typically available to policy makers or funders that is based on consumers' own preferences. To frame needs in terms of what consumers want cuts short a great deal of the debate involved in trying to reconcile the perspectives of various constituencies (e.g., professionals and families). Consumer preference information also represents a very powerful political tool, since it encourages different kinds of decisions about how resources will be allocated in a system or a community (who is responsible for meeting housing, work, and support needs; what key opportunities consumers need; etc.).

As recently as 1987, there were no documented studies in the United States, published or unpublished, that systematically described where and how people with psychiatric disabilities want to live. With the development of a consumer housing and supports preference methodology (Ridgway & Carling, 1988; Tanzman et al. 1992), the number of such studies has increased dramatically; the Center for Community Change through Housing and Support has now reviewed over 60 of them. A recent manual on this approach, and a summary of these studies, have been prepared by Tanzman (1990, 1993).

Conducting a consumer preference assessment can be as easy as convening a set of focus groups, or as complicated as designing an in-depth, scientifically valid study. Space does not permit a detailed description of the variety of these approaches, but the reader will find the manual by Tanzman (1990) an excellent resource for practical ways to gather this type of information.

Depending on the particular interests of the group, consumer preference studies can be used to document many important aspects of consumers' lives, such as the following:

- Social aspirations and the extent to which consumers are socially integrated (friendship networks, family relationships, and relaionships with coworkers, neighbors, and those with whom they share an avocational interest).
- Current and preferred participation in generic community services and activities.
- Characteristics of consumers' current and preferred housing situations (cost, quality, location, with whom they live, and what they like and dislike about their housing).
- Consumers' current and preferred employment situations (including the reasons they work, career aspirations, types of jobs, location, wages, and preferences for education and training).
- Consumers' educational levels (including other types of nonacademic training they have received).
- Consumers' current and needed incomes, and use of public benefits.
- Consumers' access to, use of, and satisfaction with mental health services, as well as preferences for services in times of crisis or other needs.

The basic method for conducting a consumer preference study involves assembling a team; deciding on the purposes/use of the information, and on a dissemination strategy; conducting the assessment; summarizing the findings; and using the results.

With regard to a team, the group will want to involve local consumer groups; family groups; state/provincial or county mental health officials; local mental health professionals, and those responsible for housing, employment, and educational opportunities in the community. The team may also include key decision makers, such as legislators. The team then needs to decide on the purposes and audiences for the study, as well as on how the results will be used. They may be used in proposals for funding from state/provincial or federal mental health, housing, or rehabilitation agencies; as part of ongoing planning within local, county, or state government; and directly in advocacy efforts.

After reading over the descriptions of other such studies, and studying the manual by Tanzman (1990), the team may wish to draft an initial description of the survey project to be used in soliciting both funding and cooperation from key groups whose help will be needed.

Because there are at present no comprehensive instruments to assess preferences across *all* aspects of community integration, the team will need to spend some time formulating questions that are specifically relevant to its goals.

In actually conducting the assessment, the team will need to decide whether to focus on all people with psychiatric disabilities, or only on one subgroup (e.g., people currently living in psychiatric hospitals, people who are homeless). The team must also define the range of content (housing, work, education, social networks, and/or support systems). Finally, the team must decide on the practical details of identifying and training consumer interviewers; specifying the role of professionals and system planners in the study; developing or adapting a survey instrument; collecting the information; and analyzing the results. Although detailed strategies for each of these activities are beyond the scope of this book, some general guidance may be helpful.

It is important for consumers to serve as interviewers in preference studies, since respondents appear to be much more comfortable about providing information to someone who has "been there." Professionals, no matter how well intentioned, may have their own preconceptions about what persons with psychiatric disabilities need, or about who should control or develop the resources related to housing, work, education, social or service opportunities. Moreover, consumer interviewers often have access to other consumers that professionals do not, particularly those who are currently not involved in mental health programs. The reliability of studies using consumer interviewers is typically in the upper 90% range (Tanzman et al., 1992).

Throughout the survey process, the team will need the cooperation of a variety of people in the mental health system. Often someone at the state/provincial level who oversees the mental health management information system will be needed to generate a list of clients who currently receive services in community mental health agencies or in the state/provincial hospital. Assistance may be needed from hospital, community, and shelter staffs to secure access to those clients who are currently being served.

An excellent survey instrument has been developed (Tanzman, 1990), drawing from the earlier work of Ridgway and Carling (1988), so there is no need to "reinvent the wheel." The team may need to adapt it, since it focuses particularly on housing and support issues. Once the instrument is adapted, it should be reviewed by the consumer interviewers to assure ease of administration and clarity of language, and then it should be pilot-tested. Respondents should, of course, be paid for participating.

It is critical that a plan for analyzing the results be developed. The best way to develop such a plan is to answer these questions: "What are the three (or four or five) most important pieces of information the team wants to provide about people's lives?" "What are the three (or four or five) most important questions the team is trying to answer about where and how consumers want to live?"

In summarizing the findings, the rule is to keep things as straightforward as possible. The group can then report a simple series of findings that can be readily understood by policy makers or citizens with no background in research (e.g., a finding that "People generally prefer 'normal housing' as contrasted with group homes or SRO lodgings, regardless of whether they are homeless, in a state hospital, a group home, or living with their families"). It is usually helpful to prepare a summary of no more than two or three pages of these major findings for broad distribution. Often results are reported to the mass media; the state or county mental health, housing, and employment authorities; the legislature; and other advocacy groups. The brief summary of findings is a helpful tool for disseminating information about people's needs to those who are involved locally in housing, employment, or educational activities, or those who are interested in reorganizing local mental health services. The variety of uses for such findings is nearly endless; specific decisions about how to use it depend on local circumstances and the group's goals. The group should be aware, however, that the findings can constitute a very powerful political tool, since they often represent the *only* such comprehensive information on consumers' needs in a service system or community.

Assessing the Needs and Perspectives of Families

> For too long, families have been the major landlords, case managers and crisis workers for their mentally ill relatives. And when there's a problem, their needs for support are ignored, since professionals are too busy blaming them for creating the problem in the first place.
> —Mother of a son with a psychiatric disability in Tennessee
> (personal communication, September 1991)

Families of people with psychiatric disabilities are the second most ignored source of knowledge about the experience of such disabilities, and about what can be done both to support families and to help individuals to move on to greater self-sufficiency (Hatfield, 1988). Families should have the primary voice in determining what kinds of supports they need. In designing a strategy to gather information from families on their perspectives, the key questions become "What issues are families most concerned about?" and "What do families want?"

Various methods have been used to solicit information from consumers' families, such as mail surveys, telephone surveys, and "focus groups." A grant awarded by the MacArthur Foundation to the National Alliance for the Mentally Ill is being used to collect data from families throughout the United States on service availability and needs (Kasper, Steinwachs, & Skinner, 1992). It is useful to involve the local chapter of the Alliance for the Mentally Ill as a coordinator for the collection of this information. Overlapping strategies for collecting information may also be important, however, since some local chapters have been less than successful in involving people of color and people with low incomes. The Federation of Families for Children's Mental Health is a key group concerned about "transition issues" among adolescents and young adults with serious emotional disturbances who are "graduating" into the adult service system.

As a first step, the group needs to clarify the purpose and scope of this information-gathering effort by asking, "What is the most critical information that the group needs from families to achieve its mission—that is, to promote integration of people with psychiatric disabilities?" The group then needs to decide on a limited number of specific questions, the best approach to gathering the information, and the number of respondents who should be involved. This is primarily a question of human and fiscal resources, as well as of the level of access to the family network. Strategies can range from a large survey (e.g., all known family members in the state or province) to a series of small focus groups geographically spread out across an area.

Whether the group will use a mail survey, an individual interview approach, or a series of focus groups, it is very important to have developed and tried out a series of clear questions in advance. Several useful instruments are available for this purpose from the Center for Community Change through Housing and Support as well as extensive materials related to their use. These include Edgar (1989) and Housing Committee of the California Alliance for the Mentally Ill, Casteneda, and Sommer (1986). The group can also request the most recent set of studies of family needs, or instruments used in those studies, from the National Alliance for the Mentally Ill (2101 Wilson Boulevard, Suite 302, Arlington, VA 22201).

As is true of consumers' interviewing consumers, it is preferable to use family members to gather information from other family members. This is also an excellent way to get more family members involved in the community integration agenda. The results should be summarized by describing the family members from whom the information was collected, any relevant subgroups, and the major themes emerging from the findings.

Assessing the Community's Current Capacity to Support People with Psychiatric Disabilities

For groups that are interested in improving support for consumers through regular community relationships, as well as support from peers and from professionals, it is important to gather information about the community's capacity to provide these types of support. In order to do this, the group needs to have a clear idea about what constitutes "effective" community support for people with psychiatric disabilities. The model suggested in Chapter Two is that of a "framework for support," in which the major supports in a person's life are identified as (1) the self; (2) friends, family members, and neighbors; (3) generic community services (housing assistance, employment training, local recreational opportunities, health care, etc.); and (4) the formal mental health system. It is through a comparison with such a model that the group can best examine the capacity of its own community to support people, and can identify and call for specific changes in the professional service system that will more directly support the self-help, social networks, and generic community services that sustain people. Specific questions of interest to the group might include the following:

"In what ways do people meet one another in this community?"

"How and where do people spend their time in this community— as workers, as homeowners/tenants, at play, as learners?"

"In what areas of community life are people with psychiatric disabilities still most segregated or excluded (work options; integrated housing; coworker relationships; neighbor relationships; community service participation; use of generic service providers; recreational and avocational activities; education and training options)?"

"In what areas of community life are we seeing increasing integration, and what is fostering success in those areas?"

"Which key individuals and groups in this community, were they to become involved in the integration agenda, would make the greatest difference?"

"To what extent do current mental health services promote integration, and help people to achieve real jobs, integrated housing, and a network of social relationships?"

"Which new services are needed, and how should existing services be changed so as to support integration and empowerment?"

After the group has formulated the most critical questions it wants to answer, it is helpful to identify a list of key informants who are most likely to be able to answer each of these questions. The best informants about self-help are likely to be people with psychiatric disabilities themselves, who can share information about the barriers to articulating their goals, to getting assistance with skills training, and to getting help organizing the resources they need. This information can easily be elicited as part of a consumer preference study (see above). The best informants about social networks are also consumers themselves, although it can also be helpful to query friends, family members, neighbors, coworkers, and other community members. Members of these latter groups can be asked about the positive contributions of these relationships in their lives, and about the supports that are important to maintain them.

Various informants about generic community opportunities and services are appropriate: employers; landlords; those who provide professional services to the community (e.g., physicians); and those involved in community organizations, such as churches, synagogues, recreation centers, community clubs, and associations. Lists of such resources can be found in the "Welcome Wagon" or "Community Happenings" listings in newspapers, or in community centers.

In assessing the adequacy of professional mental health services, the essential components of community support systems (see Chapter Two, Figure 2.1) constitue a useful organizing tool. In order to document the extent to which these services are actually available in the community, and the extent to which they are oriented toward integration, the group should identify such key informants as state/provincial and county mental health officials, local mental health service providers, and especially those who are responsible for working directly with people with psychiatric disabilities. One excellent resource for assessing the professional community support system in a local area is a method devised by Ridgway and DeSisto (1987), which has been used in a number of communities across North America. The group will also want to examine the extent to which individuals with psychiatric disabilities are involved in planning and policy development within the formal system; in training events as both learners and teachers; in the provision of services as staff members of mental health agencies; and in the operation of consumer-run service alternatives.

Strategies for collecting information will vary from sitting down with individuals for informal discussions, to focus groups, to public forums and mail surveys. One resource that reviews many such practical information collection methods is the needs assessment manual described earlier (Ridgway & Carling, 1988). After gathering information, it is best to summarize the broad themes that have emerged among each separate informant group in response to each question. The group will then want to prepare a brief statement about the following: the current capacity of the community to support people with psychiatric disabilities; key barriers to integration, and emerging strategies for overcoming them; and the current state of mental health services, and how they need to be augmented and changed to promote successful community integration. This information will put the group in a powerful position to influence political leaders at various levels of government, as well as other policy makers in the community.

Housing Needs

If a group is primarily interested in housing issues, it will want to examine current information on the availability of affordable rental housing, as well as housing available for ownership by individuals with very low incomes, in order to compare the community's housing stock with the housing consumers want, and to begin to develop strategies for bridging the gap. Because of the national crisis in affordable housing, it is important, both in the collection of information and in the development of strategies, to work in close partnership with other advocates interested in affordable housing in the community. Working this way will directly increase access to needed information, and ultimately to more integrated housing for people with disabilities.

Each community generally has a municipal office responsible for housing and community development, which can be a useful source of information on that community's housing stock. Such offices often have extensive information (including census data), on the number, type, quality, and cost of current housing units, as well as vacancy rates for those units; often this information is broken down by neighborhoods. These data generally reveal a severe shortage of affordable housing. In communities that receive any funding from the U.S. Department of Housing and Urban Development (HUD), a local Comprehensive Housing Affordability Strategy Plan is required, Such a plan describes the needs of the community for affordable housing, including the needs of people with disabilities, and articulates the ways in which the community intends to meet those needs. In many of these plans, however, the needs of people with psychiatric disabilities are ignored, although homelessness has become a more prominent element.

What does the community intend to do about affordable housing? Often the plan required by government agencies will project fair-ly limited goals for housing preservation and development, since these are based in part on available federal funds, which have been reduced dramatically in recent years. Many communities have also done more extensive planning for affordable housing and have separate plans or reports that describe the problem and propose short- and long-term solutions. Many U.S. states have reports on affordable housing and homelessness that can be obtained from the state office of housing and community development, the state housing finance agency, or the state's coordinating office on homelessness.

The group will want to gather and read as much of this information as is available, and consider certain questions: "What are the opportunities in this plan for increasing access for people with psychiatric disabilities to affordable housing?" and "Would the housing described as 'affordable' in this plan be affordable to people on a limited income (i.e., SSI)?"

It is also important to gather information through the group's network of local contacts in the housing field about which organizations are most concerned about affordable housing in the community, and which would be most receptive to collaborative action. Examples might include the local public housing authority, community land trusts, neighborhood development groups, landlord associations, or certain housing developers. Gathering information from this network is primarily a matter of meeting with people to get their perspective on the affordable housing situation in the community, on what they see as opportunities to become involved, and on what they see as emerging trends.

Once the group has gathered all of the available information, it will want to compare findings about housing availability with those about consumer preferences. This will both provide an idea of the *specific* housing access and development strategies the group will want to devise, and target the individuals and groups it will work with to make that housing a reality.

The issue of income is critical here, since most "affordable housing initiatives" in the United States today, whether funded by federal, state, or local government, continue to target individuals or families who earn between 50% and 80% of the median income in a community. The problem is that people with psychiatric disabilities and others on SSI tend to earn about 20% of the U.S. median income, making this "affordable housing" too expensive for them (McCabe et al., 1993). Ideally, however, the group's contacts with the housing network should have given it some ideas about strategies for overcoming this "affordability barrier."

The group should then prepare a brief summary of its findings.

This will be very useful in communicating about the "market" it represents in discussions with those in the public and private housing sectors. It will also be very useful in applications for funding to government agencies, foundations, and others. In any case, once the information on housing has been reviewed, the group can decide on a format for presenting it, based on the actual project it is undertaking.

Employment Needs

If a group's primary focus is on work, it will naturally want to concentrate its information-gathering efforts in that area. As noted in Chapter One, people with psychiatric disabilities have among the lowest employment rates of any group in the United States, averaging between 10% and 20% (Dion & Anthony, 1987). Most local communities have municipal offices responsible for employment and training. They also often have information (which sometimes includes specific information on people with disabilities) regarding the number, type, location, and pay level of jobs in the local area for a given period of time, as well as sectors of the local economy in which the availability of jobs is likely either to increase or to decrease. State-level employment and training offices are often very useful sources of similar information, including information on training opportunities. Virtually all U.S. states have convened a governor's commission on the employment of people with disabilities, or a similar body, which may have information relevant to the group's work. Other sources of information are the state office of vocational rehabilitation and the state department of mental health.

It is important to develop a network of key community leaders—including business leaders, individual employers, and staff members of vocational rehabilitation and local employment offices, as well as of mental health agencies—to begin to understand their perspectives on the employment barriers faced by people with psychiatric disabilities. They can also identify employment opportunities in the community, can help develop ideas for strategies to increase employment, and can determine the potential for funding employment initiatives. Local mental health agencies can be helpful by hiring consumers as service providers or in administrative or support positions, and by supporting consumers once they are working.

Once the group has reviewed all of this material, it can contrast what it has found with information about consumer preferences and can summarize the employment opportunity picture in the community. Such a summary should include the kinds of jobs that consumers want, the jobs that tend to be available, where they are and how much they pay, which sectors of the employment market are increasing, which employment areas contain opportunities for career advancement, the unemployment and underemployment problems in the community, and what the community is doing to meet employment needs. The group can then begin to develop specific strategies for meeting consumers' needs for employment.

Educational Needs

As I have noted throughout Section I, psychiatric disabilities often disrupt the normal career development, educational, and training experiences of young people. Groups that are primarily interested in educational initiatives will want to focus on two aspects of this problem: the kinds of supports necessary to include people whose participation in higher education or other training settings has been disrupted; and the kinds of supports helpful for people who are currently participating in an academic or other training program, but who are at risk of having that participation interrupted or terminated because of psychiatric disabilities.

The group will want to identify the variety of educational and training organizations in the community that could provide greater access to people with psychiatric disabilities. It will also want to document the extent to which any of these organizations have been actively involved with community integration efforts, and whether they have any support services available for students with "special needs." If so, are these services relevant to the needs of people with psychiatric disabilities? In many cases, building relationships with sympathetic faculty members and administrators can be of major assistance in this effort. Some of these individuals, for example, may have family members with psychiatric disabilities, or may have had prior experience as mental health service users themselves.

Once the group has gathered the information, it will want to compile it into a profile of local educational and training opportunities, and to compare this profile with the information on consumer preferences. This will allow the group to begin developing concrete strategies for creating more educational opportunities.

Needs Related to Social Networks

Understanding the opportunities for and barriers to social integration in the community requires, first and foremost, active membership and participation in the life of the community. It also requires a clear sense of the kinds of social opportunities in which people with psychiatric disabilities are most interested. And social interests are, of course, highly individual. Groups that are primarily interested in social integration will want to focus their work on gathering information on consumer preferences (see above), and on the practical opportunities that consumers are looking for to increase their social connections in the community—whether with peers, within local community organizations, or within churches and synagogues. It is also important to understand the barriers that consumers identify to increased social connections: a lack of material resources, such as money or appropriate clothing or transportation; inexperience, shyness, or feelings of being seen as different; not having the requisite skills to participate in an activity; concerns about discrimination and social rejection; a lack of companions to accompany one to social activities; and so forth (Reidy, 1992). What specific supports do consumers feel they need in order to become more socially active? Finally, it is important to understand consumers' current social networks and how they would like to expand them.

The group then needs to investigate the extent to which community organizations, such as activity centers, adult education programs, and religious congregations, already actively include individuals with psychiatric disabilities. They also need to find out which organizations have special rules that exclude or segregate people with differences. Finally, at a more fundamental level, group members need to ask themselves the extent to which their own social networks are fully integrated.

Once the group has gathered this information, it will want to develop a brief report of its findings; these findings should be used to develop specific projects and activities, and to solicit support for the group's efforts.

DECIDING WHOM TO WORK WITH
AND TO INVOLVE

As noted in Chapter Four and throughout this chapter, there are a number of key constituencies whose involvement in change is critical. These include people with psychiatric disabilities themselves, family members, other advocates, mental health professionals, housing professionals, employment professionals, educational leaders, and community political leaders. Issues related to involving each of these constituencies are discussed below.

Consumers/Ex-Patients

If group members have done a good job of forming an initial support group so that it includes a good many people with psychiatric disabilities, it will probably already have access to other consumers/ex-patients in the community. As the group develops a clearer concept of its aims and of who needs to be involved, it will be important to think about the places where people with psychiatric disabilities live or work that might not be immediately accessible to the members of the group. For example, significant numbers of people with a history of mental health problems may live in the local homeless shelter, in boarding homes or nursing homes, in public housing, in jails or prisons, or in the public mental hospital. What is the range of consumer groups in the local area? Do these include members of a psychosocial rehabilitation clubhouse, a peer support group, or a local "liberation," "ex-inmate," or "psychiatric survivor" group? How can the group reach people who are participating in community mental health treatment programs? In the effort to involve people, the group needs to be sure to include individuals from a variety of backgrounds, including current service users; those who no longer receive services; those who have found help through nontraditional sources; those with little education and those with higher education; and those who are now successful community members.

Often groups that seek to involve consumers/ex-patients in their efforts forget about the kinds and levels of support that are necessary to get people with psychiatric disabilities involved and to keep them involved. There are two excellent manuals that will help here (Zinman et al., 1987; Rose & Black, 1985), as well as a broad variety of materials available from the Center for Community Change through Housing and Support and from Project Share in Philadelphia. Focusing on the practicalities of transportation, food, and other such details is very important. People may need to be paid if they have to miss work to attend a planning meeting. It is important to avoid tokenism (i.e., inviting just one or two people from a particular constituency), which can be threatening and isolating. Some people can be invited just to observe; with time, they will become fuller participants. Each group member who is a professional or nonconsumer advocate can routinely be asked to arrange transportation for one other member who is a consumer, thus meeting a basic logistical need and building a personal relationship at the same time.

Also, it is important to provide an orientation to anybody who is becoming involved. The language of mental health and that of planning can be completely unintelligible to the layperson, and all too often people will opt to stop coming to group meetings, rather than admit they don't know what others are talking about. My own experience is that the real problem when someone doesn't understand what is being discussed is typically not a technical one. Rather, it is that the discussion has stopped focusing on people and their needs, and has drifted into comparing theories, abstract ideas, or technical issues that may often not be terribly relevant to meeting those needs. So all group members should be encouraged to trust their feelings of boredom; these are often a sign that the group has gotten off track.

It is also important to remember that for many consumers it is a painful experience to recount their "stories," as valuable as these may be to the group. It can also become very frustrating for consumers to come together with much more privileged people to talk about solving their own problems and those of their peers, only to find at the end of the discussion that some members of the group must return to a shelter or group residence, and others go home to comfortable houses or apartments. The discouragement that all group members experience periodically is particularly difficult for consumers, given these realities. I remember Harold Mayo, an ex-patient advocate in Florida, telling me: "It feels wonderful to come and give a keynote speech at this conference, to feel all of this concern, and to meet all of these kindred spirits. But it is heartbreaking to have to return to my own world: a world of complete isolation" (personal communication, January 1990).

Having an organizing effort that is composed of a majority of consumers keeps the process grounded in consumers' experiences. Recently, I was finishing a 4-day intensive planning process focused on housing with key leaders and advocates in a Southern state. The group was tired and began getting sidetracked into a discussion of whether it should be "planning for a variety of housing options," instead of focusing on integrated housing. The former is usually a code phrase for planning to develop more group homes and other treatment settings instead of, or in addition to, normal housing. People began articulating different theories about whether patients should stay in the hospital until housing was ready for them in the community, or whether they had a right to leave, or if they had the right to refuse a group home even if it was the only option. The level of irritation in the group grew. At that moment, a young ex-patient began to cry. Everyone else stopped talking, and she said, with great effort:

> Don't make us stay there any longer than we have to. I'm crying because I was just remembering how painful it was to be a very young woman, admitted for the first time to a state hospital, and to be asked to strip

and shower with 40 other women. It was so humiliating that I wished I were dead.

The personal meaning of institutionalization for this young woman, in contrast to the hypothetical situations that others were raising, had a very sobering effect on the group. Several of the woman's friends moved in to support her, and when the discussion resumed, the question was posed to the consumers in the room: "What do you think should happen for people who are ready to leave the hospital, when there's no housing for them?" It immediately became a much more respectful and practical discussion.

Family Members

The family movement has become an increasingly powerful force in communities and mental health systems. This development is long overdue, since family members have a critically important perspective on needs. The family movement itself is changing. Initially, family advocates saw themselves as the major spokespersons for the needs of individuals with psychiatric disabilities. As the primary consumer movement itself grows more powerful, however, family members are moving to a position of speaking for *themselves* and their own needs. In some cases, they are joining with the psychiatric disability movement to promote the realizations of consumers' goals. Thus, it is critically important to understand that although the advocacy agenda of families and individuals with psychiatric disabilities may overlap at points, the needs and perspectives of the two groups are often quite distinct. As a result, many differences of perspective and opinion exist between the organized family movement and parts of the consumer/ex-patient movement.

Often family members are referred to as "secondary consumers," in that they are affected by psychiatric disabilities and by how systems do or do not respond to these disabilities much more directly than any other "constituents" involved, except, of course, for consumers/ex-patients themselves. Families have made significant progress in having professionals see that they are not to blame for the problem of psychiatric disability, and that they are important partners in the process of treatment, rehabilitation, and systems change. Recently, families have begun to develop effective partnerships with consumer/ex-patient groups. The major national family group in the United States, the National Alliance for the Mentally Ill, now has a "Client Council" that provides advice to the organization. A past president of the National Alliance, Tom Posey, is both an ex-patient and a family member.

The involvement of family members can be sought through local family groups, state chapter affiliates of the National Alliance for the Mentally Ill, and the Federation of Families for Children's Mental Health, as well as through advertising. Like consumers, families often need support in attending meetings, becoming knowledgeable about the system, learning terminology, and so forth. Many family members need assistance with transportation, and may need to be compensated when they take time off work to attend meetings. It may be best to schedule meetings during evenings or weekends to be sure that a larger group can attend.

Often family members—because of their negative experiences with the mental health or health care systems—are highly skeptical about the ability of formal and natural support systems to help people with serious disabilities to successfully integrate themselves into the community. An advocate active in Vermont's family movement describes this phenomenon:

> The problem that many family members have is one of "visioning": they've had such a bad time in systems that they simply can't imagine a world in which people are getting the kind of supports they need, even though we'd all prefer that they have these supports in the community, rather than in some institution. (C. Neary, personal communication, September 1989)

Therefore, it is critical to keep families closely involved as the group gathers information, makes decisions about what changes are needed, and builds trust among members. It is particularly valuable to visit communities in which very positive developments are occurring (e.g., where people with very serious disabilities are being routinely assisted in their own homes and jobs, rather than in quasi-institutional settings).

Other Advocates

The problems of housing, unemployment, and social isolation among people with psychiatric disabilities are fundamentally community problems, not merely problems for a service system. To the extent that these problems are seen as, or worked on as, mental health problems, change efforts may only serve to continue patterns of isolation and segregation, and may promote the continued unwillingness of community members to assume greater responsibility for inclusion. Therefore, it is critical to involve those individuals and groups who are vitally concerned about integration opportunities in the broader community, and to ensure that all approaches taken on behalf of people with psychiatric disabilities occur within the larger context of overall solutions to the community's housing, employment, and social problems. There is no more effective strategy for pursuing integration than to involve, from the beginning, those groups and coalitions that are already concerned about housing, homelessness, unemployment, and related needs in the community.

Such groups consist of low-income housing coalitions; homelessness coalitions; boards that operate neighborhood housing development corporations or land trusts, or services for people who are homeless; community action agencies and other antipoverty programs; disability rights groups; independent living centers for people with severe disabilities; and so forth. Unfortunately, such groups often share the mistaken impression of the general public that people with psychiatric disabilities need specialized kinds of housing, work, and relationships, and that only mental health professionals have the expertise to provide these. It is tremendously liberating for advocates and professionals outside the mental health field to come to the realization that they have *precisely* the skills needed to meet the needs of people with psychiatric disabilities: the skills of housing planning, financing, and development, and of job development and training. Admittedly, individuals with psychiatric disabilities typically have special needs for certain kinds of supports. From "housers" and employers, this may include financing approaches that respond to the very low incomes of many members of this group, or reasonable accommodations on the job site. Strategies for responding to these needs are described in Section III of this book.

Mental Health Professionals

In any community, there are mental health professionals strongly committed to consumers' right to, and ultimate capacity for, community integration. The group will want to involve as many mental health leaders as possible who share this view. It is best to involve people who are eager to learn more about creative and respectful ways to provide professional supports for consumers in their own work, housing, and educational settings, and who are keenly interested in stretching the boundaries of natural support systems and peer supports in ways that replace professional services with long-term caring relationships.

Often such professionals are those who are working directly with clients with significant disabilities, whether in psychosocial programs, in residential settings, in community support services, or in employment programs. In some cases, they are "alternative" practitioners in the community, who are willing to work with individuals with less professional control than is characteristic of some formal mental health services, and with a much more flexible attitude toward the use of medications. Some policy makers and system leaders fall into this category as well. Finally, some professionals have direct experience as consumers, and their perspective is especially valuable. In spite of the real contributions of these professionals, it is important to ensure that they are not elevated by members of the group to the status of "experts" with more knowledge about the "mysteries" of mental illness than nonprofessionals in the group. The reality is that even the best mental health systems have been largely unsuccessful in achieving true integration. Thus, the fact of the matter is that the group should be composed of people whose expertise and views are varied, and that no background is as valuable as the direct experience of mental health systems that consumers/ex-patients and their families possess.

Housing Professionals

In every local community, various individuals and organizations in both the public and private sectors are responsible for housing planning, financing, development, and management. Some of these networks are large, and others are quite small. They may consist of a complex array of local public housing authorities, community development offices, neighborhood development corporations, community land trusts, nonprofit housing development corporations, government lenders, local banks, developers, builders, realtors, landlords, and others. In small communities, they may consist of one local official, a few planning board members, a developer, and a few landlords. In either case their participation is essential, since they represent the basic capacity of a community to respond to the housing needs of all of its citizens. Much of this capacity can be enhanced simply by getting people to work in a focused way on a problem, and by bringing in a limited set of additional resources as encouragement and "wherewithal" to make something happen. The individuals from the housing community who become involved in a group's efforts should be those who can influence their peers, and thus pave the way for the support of the larger housing community for the group's goals.

The first step in involving these "housers" is to understand the network itself. As the group was forming, it may have invited one or more of these housing representatives to provide information on the "lay of the land." Through meeting with these individuals, the group can find out who in the community is interested in affordable housing, local housing politics, and so forth. Eventually, members may want to work with a broad range of these housing organizations; initially, however, depending on the focus of the organizing effort, the group may want the involvement of a small number of these individuals who are well respected and who seem to share the group's values.

It is important for the group not to limit itself to the public sector. Some of the most creative housing initiatives involve a mix of private and public resources. Such projects tend to get moving much faster than those that involve only public money; they often cost less to accomplish; and they involve far fewer rules, regulations, and built-in inflexibilities.

Employment Professionals

It is also important to involve people with expertise in the business life of the community and in the local job market—people who can provide access to employers and to training programs. Such individuals may be sympathetic business leaders and employers, as well as staff members from agencies responsible for employment, training, and vocational rehabilitation services.

Educational Leaders

Educational institutions in the community are often the last to become actively involved in meeting the needs of individuals with psychiatric disabilities. Few colleges, for example, provide special services to assist individuals who are at risk of leaving school because of mental health problems, or those who want to return to school after a hospitalization or other crisis. Furthermore, most academic content in the core mental health disciplines (psychology, social work, nursing, counseling, psychiatry) has not been revised to reflect the new values of empowerment and integration. Nonetheless, there are potential allies among faculty members who are teaching in these areas; among ex-patients or family members who are currently employed in these settings; or in offices of special services for people with disabilities or other special needs. A small but growing number of colleges are beginning supported education programs—a valuable resource.

Community Political Leaders

Finally, it is important to solicit the involvement of at least some of the political leaders in a community—people whose support will eventually be needed to provide funding directly or to apply for funding; to take on potential community opposition; and to advocate for changes in the roles and responsibilities of housers, employers, and service providers. These are the "gatekeepers" to the process of political and structural change in the community, and the group needs to nurture them as such.

It is often the case that such leaders, because of the press of time, will not want to be involved in every activity of the group, so it is important to keep connected to these individuals in ways that respect their time constraints. It is also frequently the case that some of these leaders will not want to be visibly identified with the group in an ongoing way. They can be more effective by periodically providing information, and then strategically supporting the group while maintaining the posture of "objective" nonmembers. Timing is also important; the group should wait to involve community political leaders until it has a clear focus for action.

In similar ways, the group can strategically add other leaders or "gatekeepers," either as people who attend periodically to stay informed or as actual group members. These may include key leaders of the mental health and rehabilitation service systems at the state/provincial and local levels.

FIGURING OUT FINANCING

For those who advocate for community integration, the issue of funding represents the perennial "good news and bad news." The bad news is that money to pursue changes that will make a fundamental difference seems to be only rarely available.

The Center for Community Change through Housing and Support works throughout North America and beyond trying to promote fundamental changes in communities and states that result in increased integration. Our strong values-based philosophy, and our unwillingness to work with people who are not committed to fundamental change (e.g., those who resist full involvement of consumers in their change efforts), have created periodic tensions with government agencies and other organizations that fund us to do our work. The need to develop resources—particularly to work with groups with lots of energy and vision, but with few of their own resources—sometimes seems endless. I remember complaining recently about the chronic lack of stable funding to pursue community integration to Pam Hyde, a very forward-thinking rights attorney and former commissioner of mental health in Ohio. Pam responded: "You know, Paul, if your funding ever becomes stable, that's a sure sign that you're no longer doing what really needs to be done." It is also an axiom in movements for social change that one can always find money to do the wrong thing. When a group wants to do the "right" thing, however, it is typically confronted with the daunting and ongoing task of piecing together multiple sources of money, contributed time, and other resources to accomplish its goals.

The good news, however, is that once a group really knows what it wants to do, the resources somehow seem to organize themselves—although, to be certain, there is a lot of hard work along the way. Thus, a group that has a clear mission is already much further ahead of the game than many others. The group's plans are directed by, and will directly benefit, the people on whose behalf it is working. Through its planning, the group has already involved an extensive network of potential supporters in the local community, and perhaps at county and state levels of government as well. The group knows the "lay of the land," and has gathered all of the critical information it needs to develop an agenda for change. And the group has clear action strategies—ones that, over time, will potentially increase consumers' self-sufficiency, increase their productivity as workers and contributing members of the community, decrease the need for costly hospital and jail expenditures, decrease homelessness, and decrease the need for intensive community services. These are outcomes that are very important to a variety of funders. Thus, it is important to keep these outcomes clearly in mind throughout the process of seeking funding.

The group will need to decide early, and continually redecide, what kinds of funds it will and will not accept. Obviously, the group should be skeptical about funds for segregated settings or for many transitional programs. Another rule of thumb is to be extremely careful about money that is targeted for establishing structures or programs that are intended to remain in place, in the same form, for a long time. Groups that pursue this kind of funding often find that it is very difficult to change such a structure or program after it is started. It is far better to take on a different priority, or to keep looking for funding that will allow group members to do what they believe in and to change their approach as they gain more experience with achieving various outcomes.

The Group's Role: To Provide Services or Not?

A critical early step will be to decide whether the group wants to serve principally as an advocacy organization that draws its strength and agenda from its personal relationships between people with and without disabilities, or whether it wants to seek funding to develop housing, create employment opportunities, and provide support service itself. These are very distinct roles, and the decision to choose between them or to combine them should be taken very thoughtfully. Many local mental health associations, associations for retarded citizens, and chapters of the Alliance for the Mentally Ill, for example, have begun to develop services without carefully considering the effects that this will have on their ability to advocate for change. In the process, many have become a part of the status quo in mental health systems, and now focus primarily on maintaining their funding for providing services, rather than on the broad changes needed in how services are provided or in how communities behave. In spite of the organizations' values about integration, many end up defending segregated housing and work approaches, since that is what they are funded to do; in effect, therefore, they succeed in only further compounding the problem they started out to address. So it is critical to continue examining the question of whether the group can both provide services and maintain its core beliefs about integration, and, if it provides services, whether it should accept certain kinds of funding. The following material about fund raising applies to whatever activities the group chooses to pursue, from planning efforts to housing development to the provision of support services.

Grantsmanship

Today, one can pick up any listing of periodicals and books in human services and see scores of manuals on "grantsmanship." To be sure, some specific skills are involved in researching funding opportunities and writing grant proposals, and a group's approach also varies depending on whether funders are federal, state/provincial, or local government agencies or private foundations. What most of these manuals emphasize, however, is that the most important ingredients of successful proposals are as follows: a focus on an issue that is important to the funder; a clear and "do-able" plan of action that is likely to produce specific results (results that also are important to the funder); evidence that the group proposing the project has the capacity to carry it out; and a request for funding that is realistic but reasonable. Usually this means the absolute minimum required to get the project done, combined with lots of extra work and other resources.

Developing an Ongoing Capacity to Seek Funding

The last time I checked, no one was funding "community change projects to promote integration." As a result, groups have to examine the variety of funding opportunities that can be pieced together to promote the broad changes they are interested in. Piecing funding together is essentially a matter of lots of investigative work—both reading and extensive networking. And although seeking funding from a variety of sources can be both time-consuming and frustrating, it is advantageous to diversify the funding of a change effort as much as possible, so as not to place the entire effort at risk if one funding source should become unavailable. (It is also important to retain as much autonomy from funders as possible.) Seeking funding, moreover, is a process of continually checking the degree of overlap between the various characteristics of funders and the goals and resources of the group (see below). Finally, it is a matter of advocating for the development of new, more relevant funding sources that will focus directly on integration.

A number of summaries of the major current funding sources are relevant to community integration; unfortunately, they tend to be outdated almost before they are written, since both government and foundation funding programs undergo rapid change. Therefore, groups will need a systematic method to become aware of all relevant funding possibilities that are currently available, as well as those that will become available in the future. It is usually a good idea to charge the entire group with thinking about resource development, to be sure that each individual sees this as a responsibility, and then to designate specific individuals or small groups to explore funding possibilities in the specific areas in which the group is most interested (e.g., housing development, employment training and support, creation of a citizen advocacy program, development of a supported learning project, etc.). These individuals and subgroups should be expected to make periodic reports to the larger group about what they have found, where they have gotten stuck, whether they need assistance, and so forth.

It is important to be on the mailing lists for *all* relevant funding from federal agencies, state/provincial agencies, county and municipal governments, and foundations. If one group member works in a local college or university, usually the institution's office of research funding support or "sponsored programs" will be able to generate a list for that person, though the office may well be reluctant to do this for the group itself. It is also critical to find out which foundations are potential funders. Local foundations are the best sources, since they have the greatest interest in local outcomes. Often the local United Way, a source of funding itself, will know about relevant local foundations. The United Way often provides free technical assistance to local groups on fund raising, grantsmanship, and even nonprofit organization development. Groups that contribute time to United Way's many planning committees may gain valuable insights that help them pursue funding down the road.

There are also excellent foundation directories available in most local libraries; these are organized by the kinds of projects they fund, the levels of support they provide, geographical breakdown, and key contacts. Generally, foundations prefer to fund short-term (i.e., 1- to 3-year) projects that will accomplish specific goals, especially if the results are generalizable to other communities. Their proposal requirements are usually much less formidable than those of government agencies. It is especially important in seeking foundation funding to establish informal contact with the key program contact for the particular content area, to discuss the group's ideas, to send concept papers, and so forth, before the group actually submits a proposal. Foundations have brochures that list all of their requirements, funding cycles, and priorities, as well as projects they have funded.

Local businesses or even individuals may have funds they wish to invest in an effort that is clearly focused on improving their local community. People who have had family members or friends with psychiatric disabilities, or who have other reasons to be interested in consumers' needs or in broader disability or low-income issues, can be approached for support. Local funding builds local support by the community as well.

Finally, depending on its specific project focus, the group will want to work with other organizations in order to advocate for new funding that is directly targeted to the kind of integration outcomes the group is promoting. These might include low-income housing coalitions, committees for employment of people with disabilities, disability coalitions, business roundtables, chambers of commerce, mental health coalitions, homeless coalitions, associations of cities or counties, and others with which the group has an overlapping agenda. It is especially important to become involved with organizations that are capable of lobbying and legislative action; serving on the committees of such organizations will ensure that the group's agenda is included in the overall advocacy approach. Although this means that the group will sometimes work on behalf of legislation or funding that does not explicitly relate to people with psychiatric disabilities, this work makes the group part of a larger, more powerful, and more integrated movement for change.

Testing the "Fit" between the Group's and the Funder's Goals

The best way to determine the overlap between the goals of a potential funder and those of the group is to identify the specific outcomes that a funder is seeking (e.g., the availability of more permanent affordable housing; reduced use of SSI benefits by consumers; reduced use of hospitals or jails; reduced incidence of homelessness among people with mental illnesses). As can be seen, most of these could be described as "negative goals." They tell a group to solve a problem, but don't tell it how. That is a real advantage when a group wants to try something new. And even though a group may not agree at all with the funder's statement of the problem (group members may say, for example, "The problem is not to reduce hospital use, but to create opportunities for a high quality of life in the community"), the plan, of course, is to use the funding to promote integration at the same time that the group is "solving the system's problem." Through succeeding, the group is also educating the system in the process, and helping policy makers to reframe the issue as one of integration. And the trick is developing a convincing argument that what the group is proposing will actually solve the problem as the system defines it. When a funding source is not explicit about the outcomes it is seeking, it is useful to examine what the source has funded in the past.

A major dilemma many groups encounter is that funding agencies often will allocate far fewer resources than are needed to promote a decent quality of life in the community for people with psychiatric disabilities, precisely because their focus is on these limited definitions of the problem. The result is often an implicit expectation from a funder—for example, "Do anything to keep people from using the hospital, as long as it doesn't cost much." With mandates like this, it's little wonder that many local programs become so controlling of individuals they serve. It is the only way they see to meet the expectations of the systems that are funding them, and therefore the only way to continue receiving funding.

Through networking, it is also important to get a handle on the values of those who may provide funding. Increasingly, there will often be an overlap at a formal policy level between the group's explicit values and those of a potential funder, because of the recent emphasis in mental health policy on "consumer empowerment" and "integration." Unfortunately, the program rules that are intended to implement these policies may have changed much less than the words in the policy statements themselves, imposing constraints on programs that undermine the group's goals. For example, a recently funded "supported housing demonstration program" in one state requires that all program participants receive a minimum of 10 hours of professional services each week, regardless of whether their individual needs change over time.

Often, a group can find government officials at a middle management level who are strongly supportive of its goals. By building strong relationships with them, the group may be able to use some sources of funding much more flexibly than the program announcements might suggest. The most effective strategy here is simply to get these individuals involved and enthusiastic about the group's planning, and, in the process, to begin building relationships between them and individuals with disabilities. Also, groups should always keep a lookout for "flexible pots of money," no matter how small. These discretionary funds, available through government as well as private sources, are often most the useful ones for very innovative, untested approaches. They are ideal for pilot projects that demonstrate effectiveness, then qualify for ongoing funding, and (ideally) change the way similar projects will be funded in the future.

Writing a Grant Proposal

Developing a Concept Paper. One basic building block of a successful grant proposal is a clear idea of the group's activities and of how these will specifically accomplish the group's goals. Usually the group starts by developing a plan that everyone believes will succeed; it then writes up the plan as a brief "concept paper," and circulates it to a few critical thinkers for review. This is also a good time to get informal feedback from the funder about how the idea can be strengthened.

Obtaining Local Support. After reviewing the feedback from the various reviewers, and paying particular attention to the funder's reactions, the group can revise the concept paper and redistribute it to appropriate individuals and agencies within the community, asking for letters of endorsement, offers of matching funds, and other forms of community support. Meanwhile, the group can continue to work on the formal proposal.

Writing the Formal Proposal. If a group has not written a formal proposal before, it is often helpful to get help from someone in the community who has experience in writing successful grant proposals. Often the best candidate is someone who has already received funding from the agency to which the group is sending the proposal. This person's role is not to affect the content of what the group is proposing, but to help the group articulate its proposal and package this in a way that will be successful. Another excellent strategy is to secure copies of successful proposals that have been funded by the agency in the past. Usually the group will have to get these from other local organizations rather than from the funder itself.

All funding agencies have different requirements for a proposal, and it is always best to follow those requirements rigorously. Often, the flexibility that groups experience in discussing their ideas with a middle manager or a "program person" vanishes when the formal review of the proposal is undertaken by people focused on accountability, organizational history, and so forth. Similarly, it is important to stick rigidly to deadlines. A good rule of thumb is to plan how long it will take to write the proposal and then double that estimate. The process may still be hectic, but the proposal will get done on time.

Often formal proposals require a statement of the problem, which may or may not require a review of the literature. There are several excellent sources of summary literature reviews related to community integration, including the following:

The Center for Community Change through Housing and Support
Institute for Program Development
Trinity College of Vermont
208 Colchester Avenue
Burlington, VT 05401
(802) 658-0000

The Research and Training Center on Community Integration
Syracuse University
724 Comstock Avenue
Syracuse, NY 13244-4230
(315) 443-4484

The Center for Psychiatric Rehabilitation
Boston University
750 Commonwealth Avenue
Boston, MA 02165
(617) 353-3549

Thresholds National Research and Training Center on
    Rehabilitation and Mental Illness
2001 N. Claybourn Avenue, Suite 302
Chicago, IL 60614
(312) 348-5522

The National Resource Center on Homelessness and Mental
    Illness Policy Research Associates, Inc.
262 Delaware Avenue
Delmar, NY 12054
(800) 444-7415

After summarizing what is known about the problem, the group will need to specify its plans to address the need; these are usually formulated as long-term goals, short-term objectives, and action steps. A summary chart with overall project deliverables, outcomes, and time lines is often helpful. The group will generally have to provide evidence that it can carry out the project effectively. How long it has been in operation; what other projects it has completed successfully (such as many of the information-gathering projects described above); what resources it currently has, or has been promised by other sources; how stable it seems to be; and whether it is a legal entity (e.g., a not-for-profit corporation); are all relevant here. For a group that is just getting started, it often makes sense to team up with a more established organization and to pursue funding jointly. This can work well if there is a strong overlap in the two organizations' values, and if each group can maintain the level of autonomy it needs. For projects related to housing (particularly housing development), funders tend to be very rigorous about the financial capabilities and "track record" of the group, so it is often essential to team up with an established organization in this case.

The group will need to develop a budget that is low enough to be competitive, but high enough to get the job done. A common reason for projects' either not being funded in the first place, or failing to deliver their intended outcomes after they are funded, is that budgets are unrealistic. They are either so low that the group is essentially promising to pull the world along with a shoestring, or so high that the funder doubts that the group has the inclination or ability to be "lean and mean." The best way to develop a pragmatic budget is to go through the action plan and realistically estimate every cost for every phase of the project. If the group has no experience with certain projects, other groups that have done similar work should be asked about costs. If the group has been given samples of successful proposals, their budgets should be reviewed to be sure that no key costs are left out. Once the budget has been drafted in this way, it should reflect the true cost of the project. Now the group is ready to figure out whether it can become more competitive by completing the project for less money. If the budget is already in the funder's "ball park," there is no point in trying hard to reduce it. If it needs to be reduced, the group should ask questions such as these: "How can we get this step done in a different way that will cost less?" "Can we get anyone to donate things—furniture, space, and so forth?" It is usually to a group's advantage to show multiple sources of funding for a project, as well as "in-kind" contributions from the group itself or others. The latter show that the group is strongly committed to the project; that it is being economical, stretching its resources; and that it enjoys a strong base of community support.

Although some agencies frown on attaching extensive supplementary materials to the proposal, it is often useful to include letters of support from a variety of groups and interests, any documents that the group has produced in the past, resumes of key individuals who will be involved in the project, and so forth. Some agencies require a number of "certifications" (e.g., equal-opportunity statements, audit requirements, review by a human subjects committee for certain research, etc.). The group will want to cap the proposal with an "executive summary" that describes (in no more than one or two pages) what the need is, what the group plans to do to meet the need, and what the expected outcomes are. They should send the proposal off with a succinct cover letter that communicates the group's competence and enthusiasm. Finally, it is important to attend to the "small stuff," such as details about the quality of the typing and the photocopying. In funding competitions, first impressions *do* count.

Low-Cost and No-Cost Resources

Many of the successes that groups achieve in communities involve little or no money, but instead represent the use of human resources and relationships: the employer who decides to create job opportunities for several consumers; the landlord who begins to rent units to consumers, and then convinces other landlords to do the same; or the community member who decides to develop a long-term relationship with a person with a psychiatric disability. Communities represent a plethora of such nonmonetary resources, and we all know that the best relationships and life opportunities are those that are provided freely.

Similarly, small amounts of money can go a long way in creating life opportunities. For example, a small revolving loan fund contributed by a local congregation can make the difference between an unanticipated rent increase's being merely a bother or a precipitant of homelessness. Such funds can also pay for furnishings and deposits for consumers moving into new apartments. Donated memberships to the YMCA/YWCA can make integrated recreation possible on a person-by-person basis. Physicians' or dentists' making their services available to just a few people with little or no income can mean that, for the first time, consumers have personal doctors.

I remember visiting many years ago with a small group of consumers in Princeton, New Jersey that had decided to solicit this kind of cooperation from all of the physicians in this rather wealthy town. The consumers anticipated that only a handful would respond. Instead,

they got so many volunteers that they almost didn't have enough people with disabilities to sign up: Each physician took on just one or two
new patients at no cost, and each person got to have his or her own
doctor.

The moral of all of this is that funding is important, but that using
the resources of the community simply to include people is far more
important. Funds should only be used when they support the building and strengthening of community relationships, or when they physically create the opportunities for such relationships. Integration, after
all, happens one person and one relationship at a time.

ACHIEVING COMMUNITY INTEGRATION

Revamping Established Support Systems: Mental Health Systems and Higher Education

Two sets of key community resources, if properly used, can be of particular help in integrating people with psychiatric disabilities into the community. These are (1) mental health service systems; and (2) higher education programs, particularly those responsible for training mental health professionals. This chapter describes strategies for making these sets of resources more relevant to consumers' needs and more effective in promoting community inclusion.

RESTRUCTURING MENTAL HEALTH SYSTEMS TO FOCUS ON INTEGRATION

Chapter Two has described the current professional model of service delivery in mental health: comprehensive community support systems. Although this model is critically important, as long as its service components are developed with the same negative assumptions about people with psychiatric disabilities, and as long as professionals retain power and control over decision making in these programs, it is unlikely that outcomes for individual consumers will be any more positive than has been the case with more traditional services. Increasingly, communities are re-examining their principles and practices in order to make them consistent with a community integration approach, and then applying these principles and practices to the current professional services model.

Making Principles and Practices Consistent
with an Integration Approach

In order to develop a comprehensive and relevant support system in a particular community, it will be necessary to (1) develop service principles that reflect a community integration mission; (2) examine current service programs in relation to these principles; (3) determine which needed services can be undertaken by consumers/ex-patients and their families; and (4) focus on new roles for professionals. Each of these tasks is presented in detail below.

Developing Service Principles That Reflect
an Integration Mission

Again, Chapter Two has described the shift in values and practices that is sweeping mental health systems. An emerging literature suggests that incorporating community support systems principles into existing programs can produce very different models of support (Goering et al., 1990; Brown & Wheeler, 1990; Witheridge, 1990; Pace & Turkel, 1990; Thompson, Griffith, & Leaf, 1990; Bush, Langford, Rosen, & Gott, 1990). There is a similar literature focused on system wide reform, whether at the county (Fleming & York, 1989) or the state/provincial (Wilson, 1989) level.

NIMH (1987b), in a set of guidelines for planning the development of community support systems in every U.S. state, has provided an excellent summary of the principles guiding this approach. According to NIMH, community support systems' services should be consumer-centered; should empower clients to retain control over their lives; should be racially and culturally appropriate; should be flexible as needs change; should focus on strengths; should be normalized and incorporate natural supports; should meet special individual needs; should be accountable to consumers and their families; and should be coordinated with other agencies and levels of government.

Many service systems, whether at a state/provincial level or within a specific agency or program, are finding it of significant importance to clarify these principles and to articulate them clearly as a step toward implementing their mission (see Chapter Five). Following are examples of how two organizations that are pursuing an integration approach have adapted these principles—one a state mental health system (Vermont Department of Mental Health and Mental Retardation, 1991), and the other a local agency responsible for county-wide services (Kent County Community Mental Health Center, 1987). In each case, consumers, family members, professionals, and policy makers were involved in the development of the principles.

A State-Level Example: Vermont. The following principles and concepts are taken from the Vermont Department of Mental Health and Mental Retardation's (1991) 5-year plan for mental health, *Mental Health Directions for the Future, 1991–1996.* In these principles, emphasis is placed on respect for the individual, opportunities for growth and self-fulfillment, preservation of personal dignity, and provision of high-quality services that enable people to live normal lives. Vermont's service principles focus on the following:

- Expectations for individual growth and change.
- Human needs, such as love, respect, security, and health.
- The individual and his or her unique experience and needs.
- Natural supports and relationships.
- Supports to families.
- Serving people in natural, integrated settings.
- Responsive care.
- Adequate, competent, and timely care.
- Continuity of helpers through long-term relationships.
- Protection of the rights afforded to all citizens.
- Prevention through support to families and communities.
- A high quality of care.
- Protecting the public from dangerous individuals.
- Consumer empowerment and self-determination.

A Local-Level Example: Kent County, Rhode Island. An excellent set of guiding principles for the development of mental health services, and for the behavior of staff members in the community, has been formulated by of the Kent County, Rhode Island mental health system (Kent County Community Mental Health Center, 1987). They represent a particularly strong statement of community responsibility for services and of a "zero reject" policy. Kent County's service principles are as follows:

- Providing community support to clients where they live, work, and play, and making the community more responsive through education and support.
- Creating systems of care for children, adults, and older citizens through identifying service gaps, developing programs, and advocating with state and local health and human service systems.
- Keeping clients at home by providing all services in Kent County in people's natural environments.
- Keeping families together through support.
- Having clients form connections through creating their own social networks.

- Establishing commitment through treating people considered "untreatable," supporting those seen as "unsupportable," and reaching those viewed as "unreachable."
- Showing courage through "trying the untried"—succeeding, failing, and making mistakes.
- "The buck stops here"—remembering that Kent County is the agency of last resort and is never relieved of responsibility.
- "Living beyond our means"—growing by experimenting, and then seeking needed resources.
- "One small step"—helping clients to progress from one step to the next.
- "Don't take no for an answer"—being assertive and reaching out to clients, not giving up.
- Doing hard work and teamwork; being the best; and being a leader—an indispensable part of the community.

Challenges to Implementing Principles. Incorporating such principles into the actual operations of mental health systems can be a daunting task, requiring strong values-driven leadership. There are many challenges as well. One is the common lack of stability in leadership in most systems; for example, according to NASMHPD, the average U.S. state mental health director now serves less than 18 months (Schnibbee, personal communication, September 1992). Implementing these principles also requires stable financial support, yet funding is becoming more complex and unstable. Furthermore, the key elements of successful integration are people and relationships, and the current human resources in mental health need major training and support to make the shift to an integration approach; however, the commitment to retraining at a policy or legislative level appears minimal.

In this context, one particularly effective leader of the New Hampshire mental health system (Shumway, personal communication, September 1991) reminds us that training the real "caretakers" of the system (consumers and families) to take leadership is the critical task of system leaders, and that in this process, vision and principles are the most important tools. Shumway contends that systems need an intense inculcation of values, including an ongoing commitment to becoming "consumer-driven" and "family-driven"; inclusive processes for planning, organizing, and communicating, all of which are focused on consumer choice; inclusive processes for strategizing and making political decisions; the development of a clear agenda for change within the system; and an insistence that the key stakeholders accept increasing responsibility for system decisions.

Not all of the principles described above will apply to all service systems or communities, but they do demonstrate the importance of developing a clear statement—not only of an organization's mission itself, but also of the principles through which the organization can be held accountable for *how* it pursues that mission.

Examining Current Service Programs
in Relation to These Principles

Change agents can examine the extent to which current programs are consistent with these principles through a variety of strategies— principally, by asking consumers of services and their families throughout the system for a frank assessment of the strengths and weaknesses of these programs. It is also helpful to ask other key informants in the community for their assessment, such as the mayor or members of the city council, business leaders, the police, health care professionals, social service agencies, the public housing authority, and so forth. All of these individuals and groups will of course have their own perspectives, influenced at least in part by their own self-interests; nonetheless, this can be a valuable way to identify common problems, common goals, and the potential need for change.

It is also important to visit each local mental health program, vocational rehabilitation program, or other program serving people with psychiatric disabilities, and to see how it actually operates. Anthony (1990a), in a very practical address to a meeting of the National Alliance for the Mentally Ill, described a set of "nonnegotiable" questions that advocates should ask of service programs, and specific ways to assess whether these are present or not:

1. *Do service settings treat people as people, not as cases, diagnostic labels, or illnesses?* Advocates can assess whether they feel welcomed and how they are greeted. They can ask about the dropout rate, the daily attendance rates, and things the program is doing to improve its services.

2. *Do services involve people in setting their own goals?* Advocates can ask agency leaders, professional staff, and consumers, "What are your typical client goals?" They can also ask each of these groups, "What is the mission of this program?"

3. *Do service programs evaluate outcomes, attendance, and participation?* Advocates should ask about outcome data and inquire about whether such information is used to *plan* programs, rather than only to examine them once they are in operation.

4. *Do service programs hire staff members on the basis of skills, and have a hiring procedure that assesses skills instead of simply look-*

ing for a positive attitude? Advocates can ask to see hiring criteria; ask whether the interview process includes a review of audiotapes or videotapes of prior work with clients; and ask whether an applicant is observed talking with and working with clients. This shows how seriously the agency takes the work of professionals being hired. In addition, advocates can ask whether agencies affirmatively hire people with psychiatric disabilities.

5. *Do services appreciate, acknowledge, and celebrate the courage of people with psychiatric disabilities?* Advocates should investigate whether agency staff members have any special recognition for people who accomplish goals or achieve other things. What is the nature of the publicity that the agency disseminates? Do they promote the "courage to hope" among people with disabilities?

6. *Do service programs only advocate for those services that consumers and their families want?* Advocates can ask how programs are planned, and how the views of consumers and families about proposed services (or about the benefits of current services) are solicited.

7. *Do service programs only provide supports that are individually tailored and available on a long-term basis?* Advocates should ask what procedures are in place to ensure that services are individualized, and that supports will be available over the long term.

Determining Which Services Consumers and Their Families Can Offer

In the group's initial planning (see Chapter Five), an effort has been (or should have been) made to identify the current capacity of the community to support people with psychiatric disabilities. In advocating for and developing needed supports, the first question is this: What capacity do consumers/ex-patients and their families have to provide needed services in ways that reflect their own preferences? The change agent also focuses on how current mental health services must change so that they will promote integration outcomes. Two examples mentioned in Chapter Three may be helpful here as well.

In Albany, New York, a community housing study revealed that there was a large need for affordable housing, as well as for services that would help consumers select, move into, and succeed in that housing. Rather than contract with a mental health residential program, the state funded an ex-patient group to create a new organization, Housing Options Made Easy. A local mental health program provided initial office space; after a year the group became a separate corporate entity, providing people with rental housing and a variety of support services.

In Portland, Oregon, when it was decided that a local state hospital would close, the state did not approach a community mental health center to plan an intensive program to help patients relocate into the community. Instead, it contacted a very successful consumer self-help group, Mind Empowered, Inc. This group adapted the professional Program in Assertive Community Treatment model, hiring consumers in all key positions (including ex-patient psychiatrists). The program has been very effective in helping people leave that state hospital and helping them succeed in the community. It is an excellent example of how people with psychiatric disabilities can organize to provide *any* of the basic and clinical supports that are needed.

Finding New Roles for Professionals

The framework for support (see Chapter Two) relies first on the resources of the individual; then on friends, peers, and family; then on community activities and services; and only then on the formal mental health service system. Thus, the role of the professional becomes first to support anyone else in the community who will meet a particular need, rather than initially offering a mental health intervention. In a community support approach, then, the role of the professional becomes that of supporter to the community. Instead of primarily acting as a treatment agent, the professional combines the roles of community organizer and change agent with those of a skilled personal supporter. Individuals may still wish to use counseling and therapy to assist them in achieving increased mastery over their lives. If this is the case, it may be preferable to help such persons find therapists in the community who are skilled in working with people with severe disabilities. Perhaps the clearest and easiest way to avoid seeing these "community support components" as formal services is to remember that the outcome of any service intervention, or even program, should be to help each consumer maintain a home, a job, and a set of friendships and other social connections.

To facilitate this outcome, professional services must become more relationship-based. Relationships between professionals and consumers must begin to reflect an essential equality, and must be reoriented to putting the consumers in the "driver's seat" as far as making decisions is concerned. The citizen advocacy movement has significantly demonstrated the value of long-term peer relationships, based in friendship and support, in promoting more inclusive communities. The growing self-help and peer support movement among people with psychiatric disabilities is likewise demonstrating the value of such relationships (Zinman et al., 1987). Two examples of reshaping the role of the professional so that it is increasingly directed by consumers, drawn from the diverse communities of Kitchener/Waterloo, Ontario, and Nassau County, New York, are described later in this chapter.

There is, in fact, a major element of liberation in giving up the cloak of omniscience or magical powers that many have bestowed on mental health professionals. In fact, it can be argued that most of what professionals need to know about successful community integration they do not yet know, simply because professional training and the activities of service systems have not been clearly directed toward integration and empowerment. Fortunately, the path to discovering successful approaches to integration is one that can only be pursued in partnership with consumers and their families. And a first step along that path is for professionals to acknowledge their lack of knowledge and the fact that they have few guideposts. In an uncharted land, however, allies are frequently more valuable than maps.

Adapting Community Support Services to an Integration Approach

As noted in Chapter Two, the primary strategy for shifting the activities of a mental health program or system into the larger framework for support is to systematically restructure the mission, policies, funding, operations, and evaluation of current services toward goals of integration and consumer self-determination. Movement in this direction can be accomplished through a broad variety of practical steps. These include adopting the community integration approach in all mission and policy statements (see above); training all staff members in the content and implications of this new mission; systematically changing the ways that professionals, agencies, and government bureaucracies relate to people with psychiatric disabilities, by inviting such people to be part of all planning and policy development activities; providing support and training to make this possible; and incorporating real power and decision making into consumers' roles. Agencies or systems can involve consumers in significant numbers as teachers and learners in all training events, and can affirmatively hire qualified individuals with psychiatric disabilities at all levels in policy, service delivery, and research/evaluation positions. They can decide to shift funding from professional services to services that are designed and operated by people with disabilities themselves. Furthermore, they can make the system accountable to the people it serves by asking consumers how they would like a particular service need met (e.g., through conducting consumer preference studies) before starting any service or program; by routinely evaluating the satisfaction of consumers with every service;

and by changing or discontinuing a service if results suggest doing so. Finally, they can routinely evaluate all services in terms of the concrete outcomes that those services are producing for consumers.

Revamping Basic Components of Community Support Systems

Many community programs throughout North America are engaged in exactly this type of fundamental restructuring of their activities. Before specific examples of such efforts are presented, some of the ways in which each of the basic components of a community support system can be modified to promote integration and empowerment should be considered.

The following suggestions for change focus on critical issues to consider within basic community support systems. The description of these key issues is, of course, not exhaustive, since each community is starting from a different stage of development of community support services, and has unique cultural values and historical challenges to deal with. For a review of the basic content of each of these components, the reader may wish to review their definitions in Chapter Two.

Client Identification and Outreach. Services that promote integration seek to engage individuals with psychiatric disabilities on their own terms, and to let them know how services will meet their needs. Staff members work with concrete needs for housing, income, and so forth, since this is often much more effective than attempts to convince individuals directly that they need mental health services.

Unfortunately, some systems confuse the need for assertive outreach with an overly aggressive posture that leaves people with disabilities with no option other than to leave the community if they are determined not to work with the mental health system. This practice is compounded by the belief among many members of the general public that mental health agencies are somehow not doing their job if they do not control unusual or disturbing behavior in the community—a belief that stems from a lack of understanding of the voluntary nature of community mental health services, and of the rights and responsibilities of citizens with psychiatric disabilities for their own behavior in the community. The key watchwords here are to see people with disabilities as responsible for their behavior, and to allow them to experience the natural consequences of their behavior while persistently continuing to offer help to improve their situation.

Effective outreach must balance the need for persistence; a strong respect for the voluntary nature of the services being offered; a commitment to staying in touch with the concerns of the larger community and to responding to those concerns; and a clear respect for the rights of the individual to make choices about whether to participate in services that are offered. Mental health agencies need to provide the public with continuing education about these issues as well, so that everyone will understand service providers' occasional inability to solve problems in the way some community members may want them solved.

Mental Health Treatment. Community service programs that are shifting toward integration struggle with several critical issues related to treatment: medications, the need for counseling, the role of choice, and the role of residential settings. Several facts now seem clear, based on the research literature and the writings of people with psychiatric disabilities. First, many people with psychiatric disabilities benefit from medications. On the other hand, given the powerful and often distressing nature of many drugs, and given the common experience of involuntary medications, many individuals have serious reservations about their use; such individuals often refuse drugs outright. Finally, many individuals want help in moderating their use of drugs so that they can function more effectively at work and in intimate relationships. For these reasons, programs are moving away from a focus on compliance to a focus on choice. They are working with individuals to help them become educated users of medication, achieve their own goals of whether and how often to use medications, and to make decisions about what effect medications are likely to have on goals other than symptom control (e.g., employment).

Although therapy has been de-emphasized, it now seems clear that many people with psychiatric disabilities want and can benefit from psychotherapy or supportive counseling, and it is important to respect this as a right comparable to the right of any other individual seeking mental health services. Furthermore, many of the clients seen in outpatient settings (derogatively termed the "worried well" by some advocates) often face many of the same challenges in living—particularly the persistent effects of unemployment, the lack of affordable housing, and other pressing social needs—as people with diagnosed psychiatric disabilities. Thus, some organizations are restructuring the relationship between outpatient and community support services; services are being shared, and in each case less emphasis is being placed on formal diagnosis and more on specific needs. In addition, choice of counselor is a critical aspect of integration and empowerment in each case, as is the ability to change counselors if the initial choice should not work out.

Finally, as community programs begin to "decongregate" group homes in favor of integrated housing, many are realizing the need for either crisis-oriented residential settings (see below) or residences where people with psychiatric disabilities can pursue rehabilitation and growth goals while not losing their own housing. In this context, such programs as Burch House in New Hampshire, Soteria House in California, or Spruce Mountain Inn in Vermont represent settings in which people can pursue their own life goals for a limited time, with or without medications, before returning to their own housing.

Crisis Response Services. Community programs that are shifting to an integration approach are beginning to develop a variety of crisis responses that are intended to *prevent* crises, through a graduated set of interventions that focus first on "wellness" and only later on emergency response. Figure 6.1 illustrates this new philosophy by showing the various crisis services and the relative resources that are needed for each in the form of a triangle; this suggests that when most of a community's resources are invested in "wellness" services, only the smallest amount needs to be dedicated to hospitalization or other restrictive interventions (Biss & Curtis, 1993). For example, Washington County, Vermont has developed a "Warm Line" staffed by consumers, which provides as much social support as people want on a 24-hour basis; the community mental health center's "Hot Line" is thus reserved for specific psychiatric crises. Another example of crisis prevention is the Center of Attention in Santa Clara County, California—formerly an apartment to which any member of an ex-patient community could go when support was desired, and call a number of other consumers who had volunteered to provide support as needed (see Chapter Three). This service was and still is very effective in preventing hospitalization among community members; it has now become a mobile volunteer support system.

Common ingredients of professional programs that are effective in preventing crises are low enough staff-to-client ratios among case managers or community support workers, and an emphasis on building strong relationships between professionals and the families and friends of individuals with disabilities. Crisis prevention is essentially a matter of developing relationships that are continuous enough and trusting enough that problems can be anticipated or dealt with in the earliest stages.

A second emerging strategy for reducing hospitalizations is to create nonhospital alternative services that work with people in their homes until crises are resolved. The Home Intervention Team in Washington County, Vermont, for example, works with individuals who have refused all other voluntary services and are about to be in-

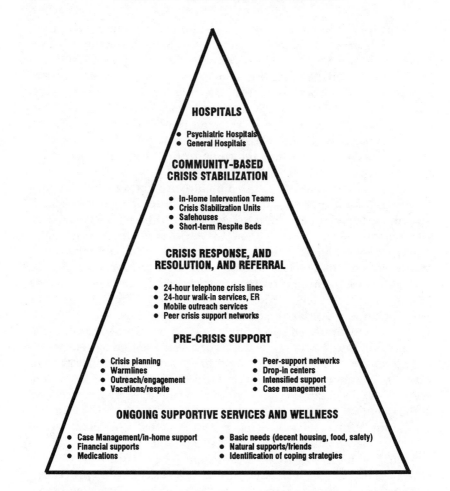

FIGURE 6.1. Comprehensive community crisis response systems. From Biss and Curtis (1993). Copyright 1993 by Center for Community Change. Reprinted by permission.

voluntarily committed to the state hospital. These persons are offered a service in which staff members will stay with them in their homes, or in an agency-operated apartment, for as long as needed until the crisis is resolved. The program serves individuals who are actively suicidal or are experiencing major symptoms of mental illness. As such, the program has been especially effective in avoiding hospitalization among people who, in most other systems in North America, would certainly be involuntarily committed for extended periods.

A final set of strategies involves moving the locus of hospitalization closer to home and blurring the boundaries between hospital and community programming and staffing. I have visited the Schenectady Shared Services Program in New York, and met staff members who spent part of their time working in community programs and the rest working with consumers in the local hospital—a very effective example of continuous support within the home community.

At a service system level, there are many emerging examples of integrated admissions and discharge planning in which hospital stays are shortened and community and hospital staffs work jointly on specific parts of a coordinated treatment plan. Table 6.1 describes elements of such integrated hospital–community work.

Finally, integration-oriented agencies are rethinking the kinds of residential programs they provide, particularly as they stop using group residences for long-term housing; many of these facilities are being converted to short-term treatment settings that serve as alternatives to hospitalization. We are seeing the expansion of crisis apartment programs, such as in Maine; the use of families to provide short-term crisis support, such as in the Northeast Kingdom section of the state of Vermont; and consumer-operated "safe houses," such as in San Diego, California.

TABLE 6.1. Core Elements of a "Seamless" Admission and Discharge Process: Integration of Efforts by Community and Hospital Staffs

Prescreening by community treatment team
- Consideration of alternatives to hospitalization
- Local hospital as first inpatient option considered
- State/provincial hospital role in screening admissions
- System-level monitoring of appropriateness of admissions

Joint discharge planning (within 24 hours of admission)
- Purpose/outcome of admission
- Reasons why other alternatives not used
- What specifically will change as a result of hospitalization? When will this happen? Who is responsible for its happening?
- What specifically will change in the community during hospitalization? When will this happen? Who will be responsible?
- What are the critical review points and accountability mechanisms?

Joint hospital treatment
- Continuity of relationships
- Community staff on treatment team
- Staff privileges for community physicians

Joint community treatment/programming
- Regularly shared information
- Visits, shared staffing
- Some community services by hospital staff

Health and Dental Care. Helping people with psychiatric disabilities gain access to high-quality health and dental care is a priority for many programs. Too often consumers lack the resources to purchase the care they need; moreover, many health care providers ignore or discount consumers' physical health concerns, assuming that these are emotionally based. One interesting example of the goal of helping people with psychiatric disabilities to have their own personal physicians, involving a program in Princeton, New Jersey, has been described at the end of Chapter Five.

In locations where adequate health care is available, it is often necessary for mental health professionals and advocates to educate physicians, nurses, and others about the need to serve people with psychiatric disabilities on an equal basis. Finally, in many areas with inadequate mental health services, general medical practitioners are often the major service providers for people with psychiatric disabilities; it is important that they be provided with adequate information as well.

Housing. Programs pursuing an integration approach, as noted in the discussions of supported housing in earlier chapters, are emphasizing choice, regular housing, and flexible supports. Specific strategies include the development of a support plan that relates to the new living environment; concrete and emotional support during the transition into housing; and attending to any special needs, such as those of single parents with psychiatric disabilities seeking housing. A series of national surveys (Yoe, Carling, & Smith, 1991) describe the development of over 700 supported housing programs in the last several years. Examples of such programs are provided in Chapter Seven.

Work. Organizations pursuing integration in the workplace are focused on the critical issues of individuals' career aspirations and of figuring out ways to provide supports that are not stigmatizing, both on and off the job site. Often an after-hours peer support group is helpful in this regard. Programs are also working with employers in the United States to help them understand and respond to the new requirements of the 1990 Americans with Disabilities Act, and specifically to design the reasonable accommodations that people request. Finally, programs are helping individuals to pursue their rights under this legislation. Examples of such programs are presented in Chapter Eight.

Income Support and Entitlements. Many local service programs now work directly with public benefits agencies, such as the local welfare office, the local housing authority, vocational rehabilitation services, and the Social Security office. These agencies help consumers get the benefits to which they are entitled, and also advocate for changes that will enhance respect for consumers and the timely delivery of benefits. The state of Ohio, for example, through the leadership of the state mental health department, developed a highly effective program to help people with psychiatric disabilities to receive their SSI benefits much more quickly than was the case in other states. This program involved working with the Social Security staff, training mental health care providers, and providing information directly to consumers. Recently, the federal Social Security Administration announced plans to restructure the disability determination and appeals process in very similar ways.

Programs are also placing much greater emphasis on work, and on coordinating the entry into employment with the receipt or termination of benefits. This is a critical issue: SSI, for example, also provides eligibility for Medicaid, which is the major source of health insurance for many consumers in the United States.

Peer Support. Funding for a variety of peer support options is expanding, both through federal funding for a series of demonstration programs that offer a wide range of community support services provided by consumers, and through state- or provincial-level funding for such options as self-help groups, drop-in centers, rights protection and advocacy services, and so forth. New Jersey, for example, has funded a variety of consumer-operated housing options, and Tennessee recently funded a statewide network of consumer-operated drop-in centers. Unfortunately, such funding still represents only a miniscule portion of overall mental health funding.

Family and Community Support. Programs interested in expanding services to families and in working with families as partners are pursuing a variety of approaches, including helping to develop family support and education projects, which are then maintained by the family groups themselves. This pattern was successfully used in Vermont, where an initial family support and education group was begun in Burlington, Vermont, through Howard Mental Health Services. The program was then expanded statewide and taken over by the Vermont chapter of the Alliance for the Mentally Ill, which grew out of the initial group. The chapter now provides family education, support, and organizing services throughout the state, as well as training programs for professionals.

Programs are also seeking family members to serve on boards of directors, developing procedures to involve families in treatment and offering respite services to families. Many local programs have developed effective strategies for working with other key community members, such as employers, landlords, and others to provide a variety of supports. These strategies are described in detail in subsequent chapters.

Rehabilitation Services. A rehabilitation approach is being adopted in most programs serving people with psychiatric disabilities, both vocational and social rehabilitation programs are increasingly focused on individuals' goals as the driving force behind services, as well as on integration outcomes. As with any set of changes, however, it is important to investigate the extent to which such programs have merely changed their language rather than their practices. Anthony, Cohen, and Farkas (1982) provide excellent guidance about whether programs are truly rehabilitative in nature.

Protection and Advocacy. Protection and advocacy are services that are expanding in the United States, primarily because of federal funding through the Protection and Advocacy for Mentally Ill Individuals Act, as well as funding from some state and local governments. The aims of many advocacy programs are to expand access by advocates to all parts of the professional mental health system; to help consumers become organized so that they can better advocate for their own needs; and to provide information to consumers about their rights and about various service options that are available.

According to Anthony and Blanch (1989), ex-patient advocates are focusing their attention on a number of major civil rights issues, including issues of involuntary interventions; limiting the expansion of outpatient commitment; the increasing number of people inappropriately or involuntarily maintained on medication; the practice of seclusion and restraint in community hospital settings; and common discriminatory practices, such as denying parents with mental illness custody of their children.

Case Management. To be effective, case management must be outreach-oriented and available when and where it is needed. It is also critical that caseload sizes be realistic. Programs with years of experience in effective case management, such as the Program for Assertive Community Treatment in Madison, Wisconsin, contend that an average caseload of 20 for routine work with individuals, or 10 for work with people whose needs are very great, is essential to community success.

Other critical issues with which progressive case management programs are struggling include creating sufficient authority among case managers to give them the "clout" they need in the system to help individuals gain access to services, and keeping policy makers informed about parts of the service system that simply aren't working well on behalf of consumers (See Downs, 1990). Local programs are increasingly hiring consumers themselves as case managers. Finally, as I have noted in Chapter Three, the term "case manager" is one that many consumers find offensive: They neither see themselves as cases, nor desire to be managed. In response to this concern, terms such as "client services coordinator," "community support worker," "community resource coordinator," "community support worker," or "individual life planner" are being increasingly used.

At an agency-wide or even community-wide level, an increasing number of mental health systems are using case management as a core service to replace many of the specialized facility-based programs that have been used in the past. Table 6.2 presents a strategy for how case management teams with low caseloads, typically referred to as "assertive community treatment teams," can incorporate staff members who previously worked within specialized programs in a fragmented and uncoordinated fashion. For example, staff members who used to teach skills classes in a day treatment center can be assigned to an *in vivo* skills training team to work with consumers who are being served by that team. Other teams include staff members with special skills

TABLE 6.2. Assertive Community Treatment Teams:
A Strategy for Converting Facilities to "Wrap-Around" Services

Facility-based program	→	Team-based services (specialists)
Day treatment program	→	*In vivo* skills teaching (rehabilitation specialists)
Clubhouse program	→	Social network building and integration
Vocational program	→	Helping consumers choose, get, keep employment (work specialists)
Residential program	→	Helping consumers choose, get and keep housing (housing specialists)
Substance abuse program	→	Integrated mental health/substance abuse service (substance abuse specialists)
Medication clinic	→	(psychiatrist/psychiatric nursing specialists)

in employment, housing, substance abuse, nursing, and so forth. Incorporating staff members into these teams has several benefits: Team-
based services are typically outreach-oriented in nature, and thus
replace services in which consumers have to go to specific sites to
receive assistance; staff members with specialized skills can teach these
to other staff members on the team; and services provided to individuals with a variety of needs are much more easily coordinated within
a team than they would be across multiple programs or agencies (this
is especially important during times of high need, when services are
"wrapped around" an individual). Finally, having such expertise in
teams allows agencies to phase out facility-based programs and divert
those resources to more outreach-oriented community services.

A Local Community Example:
Kitchener/Waterloo, Ontario

The cities of Kitchener and Waterloo, Ontario, had a very traditional
set of mental health programs, until recently; a number of these were
operated by the local branch of the Canadian Mental Health Association. Several years ago, a new executive director was hired who had
a strong background in community integration of people with developmental disabilities. He decided to completely redesign the agency's programs and organizational structure, in order to promote integration
and self-determination. Management changes included eliminating middle management positions, and setting up mechanisms so that the executive director and new program directors were directly accountable
to the direct-service staff and to consumers. Consumers were invited
in significant numbers onto the board of directors. Traditional day
treatment programs were restructured, and resources were provided
instead for individual life planning staff, who were expected to establish continuing relationships with consumers and to offer goal-oriented
services. Consumers were hired to fill staff positions, including one
of the program manager positions. The organization then began working with other service providers and agencies in the community (such
as a local network of group home programs)—both to influence those
with more traditional values to move toward greater integration and
empowerment, and to ensure that consumers would receive the services they wanted and needed.

   The process used in this change was a lengthy one, in which all
members of the agency community were first involved in careful
deliberation about a new mission and in the articulation of a new set
of values. These values included the following: social justice; individual
and collective responsibility; access to appropriate and adequate
resources and supports; self-determination; community integration;

integrity; partnership; excellence; accountability; and creativity. The planning process also focused on the development of a new language, communication style, and organizational culture. Expected outcomes were defined, and basic operations within the organization were redesigned. Programs were restructured to shift power to consumers. Throughout the process, a clear goal was on empowerment for *all* participants, and on creating a healthy and accountable organization. It was recognized from the outset that staff members would have to make the greatest shifts in power. Furthermore, it was recognized that the agency needed to redirect its current resources, since no new funds were anticipated.

The agency created a new menu of services that reflected what consumers said they would find helpful:

- Services to the general public (a 24-hour help line staffed by volunteers; a self-help resource center; a stress management service; a support service for elementary school children with emotional problems).
- Services related to public education and community development (family education; a resource library; a speakers' bureau; a newsletter, brochures, and displays; a mental health week; a mental health curriculum for school-age children; and advocacy).
- Community support services for people with psychiatric disabilities (life planning; support coordination; individualized support; volunteer development; and self-support groups).

Outcomes of the planning process included creating a single point of entry to the agency's services; reducing middle management positions (as noted above), and giving staff members the authority and responsibilities necessary to empower themselves and to promote empowerment among the people they support; making staff members responsible to the service needs of people rather than for a single service (i.e., making them generalists instead of specialists); decentralizing management to each local community, and giving communities more input and influence over services; introducing a department to ensure quality of the services provided; individualizing services and making them holistic, flexible, and portable by reducing the barriers between services, and by amalgamating the management of services; and establishing an administration that focuses on being a resource to staff members rather than on exercising control over them.

In this process, described by the agency (Jones, 1993) as a "movement toward empowerment—living our words," key consumer concerns were realized: clarification of the agency's dual responsibility for service provision and for advocacy; creation of an individualized planning process, where the person supported is in control; deprofessionalizing services to maximize the involvement of people who have used services, community volunteers, and family members in all aspects of planning, policy development, management, and service provision; accountability to individuals for all activities on their behalf; recognition of the benefits of mutual support; and establishment of a determination to move from control to support, as well as from hierarchical to collective organization.

Only after this restructuring was completed did the organization approach its funding sources to ask for permission to reorganize existing funding, and to seek new funding for expanded integration services. The agency then began the process of developing new relationships with other service providers in the community, based on its new mission and its new sense of clarity about its responsibility to serve as an agent of community change.

At an individual client level, the agency is now developing resource materials on the "Discovery" process through which local facilitators (e.g., paid staff or advocates) can convene key members of consumers' social networks to engage in futures planning focused on recovery and integration goals (Joyce, 1994a, 1994b).

Interestingly, such a major change process invariably creates further opportunities for change. Shortly after the agency planning process was complete, the Ontario provincial mental health authority began emphasizing the need for community-wide service systems. The agency was in an excellent position to respond, because it had such a clear sense of what people with psychiatric disabilities wanted. On the other hand, the service system was dominated by agencies that did not share its values of integration and empowerment. The agency was also in the position of primarily providing nonclinical support services, and was not offering treatment, crisis services, or other clinical interventions. Therefore, it had not had to consider its position on issues involving medications, involuntary treatment, and other such dilemmas with which mental health clinicians are frequently concerned.

In spite of these differences, the agency continues to assume a position of leadership in the Kitchener/Waterloo community, and has begun convening community-wide meetings of service providers, consumers, and family members to design a comprehensive system of services. In the process, it has taken elements of successful case management programs across North America and incorporated them into its individual life planning approach. The agency's staff members are negotiating (both among themselves and with other service providers) which clinical functions they are comfortable in taking on, and how they will work with other service providers involved in those they choose not to offer. Although the service system has not yet been fully planned or implemented in the Kitchener/Waterloo area, this set of developments represents an excellent example of local leadership based on values of integration and empowerment, and shows how such leadership can create significant change in a community.

A Local Community Example: Nassau County, New York

A second example of community-wide change involves a demonstration project designed to transfer decision making to consumers in a case management program in Nassau County, New York, partly in response to the New York State mental health system's articulation of principles that services should be "consumer-selected," "consumer-directed," "flexible," and "individualized" (Bertsch & Dolan, 1990). Local planners quickly recognized that these principles were antithetical both to the traditional value of professional control and to the characteristics of the current local service delivery system. Consumers in the local area were typically offered only one service provider, as contrasted with an open marketplace in which consumers choose from among several options. At a more fundamental level, planners recognized that the current system offered no opportunity for consumers to determine what programs would be established to serve them. They were asked to select from the services designed for them; if they refused, they were seen as "treatment-resistant." Providers, on the other hand, placed a premium on serving more and more people for longer and longer periods, based on the rewards of the system. Furthermore, services were sufficiently underfunded that providers could serve the maximum number for whom they contracted with the state to provide services, and could still avoid serving consumers who were seen as "difficult" or who demanded highly individualized services. Because only services within a narrow range were reimbursed by the state, providers were discouraged from spending any time planning with consumers or advocates for services that might actually respond to what they wanted, rather than services that were reimbursable. In short, the rules and regulations of the system consistently thwarted the service principles. An aphorism comes to mind: "Idealists can build castles in the heavens, but the devil is in the details."

An opportunity presented itself to make the actual mechanics of service delivery more consistent with these principles when the New York State Office of Mental Health developed a flexible pool of funds for its new intensive case management program, and each community received an allocation of these funds. Funds were to be spent at the discretion of the case managers. In Nassau County, mental health policy makers, professionals, and consumers designed a proposal to pool these funds with other new funding available for innovative initiatives, creating an initial fund of $660,000. The pool was used to create a credit card system, managed by the Mental Health Association of Nassau County. As each consumer is assigned to a case manager, an account is opened in that consumer's name. Over 900 such accounts were opened in the first year. Case managers have access to the funds only for emergencies, whereas the consumer controls the portion of the funds to be used for nonemergency purposes (i.e., for purchasing services). The consumer gains the ability to direct the use of the funds by signing an agreement to do so, to direct the work of the case manager in the process, to meet at least quarterly with the case manager, and to evaluate the services of the case manager.

With the assistance of the case manager, the consumer then develops a service plan focused on enhancing his or her natural support system, and selects resources and services that will make the plan a reality. These resources and services need not be related to mental health treatment and need not be provided by a mental health agency. Expenditures to meet the goals of the plan are decided by the consumer, but must be approved by either the case manager or another agency representative, but not both; thus, the consumer needs to obtain the agreement of only one person with whom he or she is involved in order to use the funds. An appeals process is available in cases in which there is conflict over how the funds should be spent.

Although clearly these funds are not completely under the control of consumers, the effect of even this limited shift in buying power in the system has been dramatic, changing the culture of service delivery. After the credit cards became available, service providers began to organize "service provider fairs" in which they sought to attract consumers to their services. In essence, they had to prove to consumers that what they were offering was worthwhile and effective.

In addition, consumers were given the opportunity to identify shared interests and then to pool funds, thereby creating consumer-operated service alternatives. Such pooled funding arrangements faced initial difficulties in having sufficient numbers of consumers opt for any specific service; over time, however, they have resulted in the creation of peer support and advocacy groups, social clubs, a consumer rock band, a weekly "dining out" experience through a consumer-run kitchen, and a number of drop-in centers. Consumers must commit to ongoing funding of such services, and if sufficient numbers do not, the service is discontinued. This experiment is seen by local advocates as an important intervention in the community, the effects of which go beyond the new opportunities and resources that have been created. A larger effect may well be a renewed, ongoing dialogue about choice and empowerment throughout the Nassau County service system.

Many similar developments are occurring throughout North America. The Center for Community Change through Housing and Support has a great deal of material relating to improving state/provincial and local support systems, which is available upon request.

MAKING CHANGES
IN HIGHER EDUCATION PROGRAMS

As higher education prepares to meet the challenge of community integration, it starts at a substantial disadvantage. Traditionally, professional training programs in mental health (psychiatry, psychology, social work, nursing) have focused principally on pathology and on the treatment needs of individuals, rather than on the whole person. They have not incorporated into their training curricula much of the knowledge that has been exploding in the field in the last decade and a half (Carling, 1990c, 1990d). Thus, change in these programs is critically needed. This section describes an agenda for change within higher education. It includes two distinct approaches: (1) reforming the curricula through which mental health professionals are trained; and (2) using higher education programs as resources for people with psychiatric disabilities and their families.

Reforming Professional Training Programs

The Need for Change

Halter, Bond, and Graaf-Kaser (1992), in a review of the most popular introductory college psychology texts, recently found that coverage of the issue of lobotomies far outweighed any mention of people's needs for housing, work, and supports; that families were still consistently blamed for "causing" psychiatric disabilities; that virtually no mention was made of community support systems; and that the consumer and family movements were ignored. In summary, virtually all of the developments that have transformed the mental health field in recent years have not yet found their way into the textbooks from which the next generation of mental health professionals is learning. Because higher education has been in many ways the last bastion of tradition, policy makers and planners in public mental health appear to have assumed (at least until recently) that major service system reform could be accomplished without a fundamental transformation of university curricula. In the 1990s, we can count on the fingers of two hands the number of training programs in the United States that have a specific focus on psychiatric disabilities.

The emergence of the community support systems model, and the growing interest in consumers' operating their own services, raise profound questions for each of the academic disciplines involved in mental health; they suggest the need for a fundamental rethinking of the role of higher education and of clinical training. Some of these questions include the following:

1. Is the concept of separate disciplinary training an outmoded one in preparing professionals to work in a community support and rehabilitation approach?

2. In a services approach that focuses on the whole person, and on the simultaneous need to assist the individual and to transform social institutions, how relevant are the traditional distinctions between clinical skills and skills related to policy development, planning, community organizing, and advocacy?

3. How prepared are higher education settings to promote the development among their faculty of knowledge and skills related to psychiatric disabilities, to shift their research focus toward community integration, to develop programs that promote their own integration (such as supported education services), and to become partners with public mental health systems in retraining staff members in those systems?

Successful Strategies for Change

As communities seek to make higher education more relevant to the needs of people with psychiatric disabilities, several successful strategies have been used: (1) developing some initial successful projects in order to generate broad interest in this area; (2) helping higher education leaders to develop a better understanding of what is helpful to consumers and their families in achieving community integration, and to review their own responsibilities in achieving this goal; and (3) helping higher education programs to restructure (in some cases dramatically) the training programs they offer in this content area, including reconsidering the kinds of students they wish to recruit, and beginning to see themselves as direct resources for people with psychiatric disabilities.

It is also central to consider the issue of "markets." Marketing is a predominant concern in the higher education industry today, since it is increasingly subject to competition for fewer students and to budget cuts. Higher education programs are most responsive to becoming involved when they see, in addition to a clear community need, a major opportunity to develop a new training market (e.g., community mental health workers, or people with psychiatric disabilities and their families) or a research market (e.g., evaluation of mental health services); or when there are some resources available (even if limited), so that they can "share the risk" of such new ventures with other partners (e.g., a state/provincial or county mental health department). Some successful examples are described below.

Beginning with Small Successes. It is helpful to start with a particular project that represents an initial goal on which educators and students can focus their energies, as opposed to jumping in and initiating a broad planning process. Building on such small successes in a strategic way can stimulate much broader interest throughout a college or university, and can pave the way for larger change efforts. Some initial projects that were undertaken at the University of Vermont included the following:

1. Having consumers and family members provide guest lectures in relevant courses within the core mental health disciplines.

2. Initiating a course in one department that focused on psychiatric disabilities and community integration. This course was then cross-listed in other departments, so that students in any of the core disciplines could take it.

3. Developing a set of field experiences through which students could begin to have positive contact with people with psychiatric disabilities and their families, ranging from individual projects that were taken on as part of a class to formal field-based training experiences. Examples of such field experiences included interviewing a group of consumers about their preferences for housing and work; volunteering in professional and consumer-operated community support programs, or in family support efforts; pursuing formal internships or practicum experiences within high-quality community programs; and providing personal assistance to people with psychiatric disabilities and their families over the course of a semester or a year.

Rapp (1990), in a presentation on higher education change strategies at the annual National Alliance for the Mentally Ill conference, described a similar set of successful strategies used at the University of Kansas to develop what has become a widely acclaimed M.S.W. program specifically designed for training case managers to work with people with psychiatric disabilities. On the basis of this experience, he recommended the following strategies to change agents:

1. Finding a "champion" within the faculty.
2. Finding the best social worker in the state who is working in community mental health—a person who is excited and exciting—and asking this person to teach a course, perhaps without pay.
3. If this person is not used to organizing a course, getting copies of the curricula used in some other excellent programs.
4. Securing some student stipends for field work.
5. Advertising these stipends before they are actually secured, in order to stimulate broad interest among students; the result is that a larger number of students will sign up for them and ultimately will be willing to work without stipends, and the stipends can then be given to the most needy.
6. Giving free Alliance for the Mentally Ill memberships to students.
7. Getting consumers and family members into the curriculum in any way possible (as speakers in classes, as subjects of dissertations, as students, etc.).
8. *Not* using anything but the most excellent community support agencies.
9. Being sure to monitor the content of classes, as well as the experience of students in the field.

Each of these approaches helps to begin building a "critical mass" of faculty and students interested in this area. These small successes also increase the commitment of individual faculty members and students, as well as practitioners and other collaborators. Finally, they lend an air of reality to subsequent discussions of larger change efforts, particularly those that involve multiple departments.

Planning for Change within Higher Education Settings. Planning for change in higher education settings requires first an understanding of some of the major barriers to change. Davis (1990), in a recent presentation on the process of collaboration with higher education, provided an excellent summary of some of the larger systemic barriers to achieving a competent work force in mental health systems. He pointed out that the mental health field is in a crisis as far as human resource development is concerned; that knowledge of what to do with regard to services is limited; that few resources are allocated to research on effective approaches; that interest in human resource development among public mental health agencies is variable and generally *laissez-faire;* that faculty and students in academia have little interest in psychiatric disabilities; that there is little information on effective linkages between public mental health and academia; and that there is a poor fit between public mental health needs and college curricula. Public mental health agencies, on the other hand, are labor-intensive, with 80–90% of their resources allocated to staff. Whereas the priorities of mental health tend to be first service, then research, and only then training, the priorities of academia are often exactly the opposite.

Rapp (1990) has summarized a number of specific barriers to collaboration that must be considered in the change process. These include low initial interest among faculty and students; a generally held view that a focus on public mental health is inconsistent with the mission and values of the academic program; a lack of faculty expertise and commitment; an already cramped curriculum; cumbersome organizational structures; a lack of knowledge about the benefits of collaboration; and a lack of resources on the part of both parties. So, although the involvement of higher education is critical for the long-term goals of a skilled work force, of effective research, and of higher education as a resource in the lives of people with psychiatric disabilities, there are very substantial barriers to this involvement.

The Vermont mental health system has engaged in a successful higher education planning effort with the state's only university, the University of Vermont, over the last several years. The following strategy was used (Carling, 1990c, 1990d):

1. *Involving key leaders in the effort.* A multidisciplinary task force, consisting of department chairs of each of the relevant disciplines, was asked to plan a variety of higher education initiatives.

2. *Securing some initial funding for planning.* Funds were secured from NIMH to develop a higher education plan; these were used to have faculty members travel to conferences, visit excellent programs, and the like. Limited state funds were also found to pay for internships in high-quality community programs, and then to offer these internships competitively to the different academic departments.

3. *Gathering critical information.* The task force heard testimony from consumers, families, service providers, and policy makers on the need for higher education programs, and examined the characteristics of the current work force, along with its educational aspirations. Information was also gathered on the extent to which current college programs offered relevant training in community support systems and in community integration.

4. *Providing individual support to the faculty.* Technical assistance was provided to individual faculty members who wished to develop or modify courses to make them more relevant to the needs of people with psychiatric disabilities.

5. *Disseminating information on successes.* In cases in which new programs were developed, new courses offered, or new internships created, information on these successes was disseminated to the larger mental health system and throughout the university.

The outcomes of this planning effort were the creation of a new specialization within the M.S.W. program, focused on community health and mental health; the creation of a new course in the M.A. program in counseling, focused on community mental health; the development of a number of courses in the Department of Psychology, focused on public policy related to psychiatric disabilities and to children and adolescents with serious emotional problems; plans for a master's program in psychiatric nursing; and the creation of a new community and hospital residency program in the Department of Psychiatry, focused on public mental health. In addition, other colleges in the state have developed a strong interest in public mental health programs.

Through funding from NIMH, Boston University's Center for Psychiatric Rehabilitation has developed and nurtured a sizeable network of higher education settings throughout the United States that wish to modify their curricula to incorporate a psychiatric rehabilitation approach. This project has involved sharing of curricula, technical assistance to develop new curricula, and "seed" funding for trying out new training approaches on each of the campuses. The effort has resulted in a significant increase in the number of higher education programs focused, at least in part, on the needs of people with psychiatric disabilities.

Restructuring Training Programs. A number of academic programs have been specifically developed to focus on the community integration of people with psychiatric disabilities. One excellent example of a multidisciplinary master's-level training program already in operation is the program at the University of Cincinnati (Hellkamp, 1993), which represents a collaboration among the social work, psychology, nursing, and psychiatry departments of the University of Cincinnati and Loyola University, and includes participation and funding from the Ohio Department of Mental Health. This program trains students in multidisciplinary seminars and team field placements, and has successfully recruited both consumers and family members as students. Its graduates are in high demand both within the Ohio system and elsewhere.

Other excellent comprehensive programs—in this case, organized within one academic department—are the master's-level and doctoral-level programs in rehabilitation counseling, with a specialization in psychiatric rehabilitation, at Boston University. These programs are offered by the staff of the Center for Psychiatric Rehabilitation, a national research and training center, through the university's Department of Rehabilitation Counseling. The center offers two master's-level programs, one on campus and one off campus, for practitioners in the field. The on-campus option consists of intensive competency-based classroom training and field experiences in the psychiatric rehabilitation approach. The off-campus program offers equally intensive training; students send in audiotapes and videotapes for faculty review, and also spend a period of residency on campus. The doctoral-level program offers a Sc.D. degree in rehabilitation counseling. All programs stress the need not only to demonstrate awareness of knowledge and skills, but also to acquire these skills and to demonstrate effective use of them over time. Students completing the program show very positive attitudes toward working in the area of psychiatric disabilities, and tend to stay in the field. This focus on skills development provides evidence, according to Anthony, Cohen, and Farkas (1990), that "burnout" in this field may principally be a function of inadequate training.

Another program that has been widely recognized is the M.S.W. program at the University of Kansas. This program, described above (Rapp, 1990), has developed a new approach to case management that has been replicated in a large number of communities; this approach is referred to as the "strengths model" of case management.

A final example is found in the Program in Community Mental Health, offered by Trinity College of Vermont and the Center for Community Change through Housing and Support, in which students throughout North America can receive either a certificate, a master's degree, or continuing education credits. This program focuses on working more effectively both with adults with psychiatric disabilities, and with children and adolescents with serious emotional disturbance and their families. The program offers training in clinical and management skills; it serves an integrated student body that includes current mental health professional staff, as well as individuals with psychiatric disabilities and their families who wish to become service providers.

The Trinity College program is unique in that it provides instruction in a variety of ways including having their faculty travel to local areas, using local experts, internships, video instruction, and the teaching of courses through a variety of communication technologies. Groups of students in each local area form integrated "learning communities" to discuss content and to complete projects together, typically using the facilities of a local community mental health program. Students and faculty throughout North America communicate by electronic bulletin board discussion groups, as well as by telephone and facsimile machines. All students complete intensive internships designed to develop needed skills. Finally, the program plans to work with other colleges and universities to help them update their curricula.

Using Higher Education Programs as Resources for Consumers and Their Families

In spite of the challenges facing change agents as they attempt to move higher education programs toward becoming real partners in the process of community integration, the reality is that colleges and universities represent significant and largely untapped resources for consumers and their families, beyond their responsibility for training students. Colleges can play an important role in community integration in a variety of ways.

Having Colleges Become Supported Learning Sites

Colleges can arrange to welcome back consumers whose education has been interrupted by the onset of a psychiatric disability, and arrange to support them so that they will succeed. Several successful models have emerged, pioneered by the Continuing Education Program at Boston University's Center for Psychiatric Rehabilitation. These include programs at the University of Massachusetts (Boston) and at Adelphi University in New York, and an initiative throughout the community college system in California. These initiatives are described in Unger et al. (1987).

Organizing a Pool of Educators, Researchers, Consultants, and Advocates

Faculty members in colleges often represent a pool of very talented individuals who can conduct research for a system on effective community support and community integration strategies. As educators, they also have the potential ability to train new mental health professionals in ways that will advance community integration, to train researchers who will make a commitment to developing new knowledge, and to retrain current staff members in the mental health system. Moreover, as advocates, they can bring credible testimony to public hearings and legislative sessions about the need for community integration. Faculty memberrs in Vermont, for example, have conducted a variety of studies for the state mental health system, including a feasibility study of phasing down and closing the only state hospital (Carling, Miller et al., 1987); a task force on crisis options for consumers (Blanch, 1988); a task force to design a consumer-operated advocacy system in the state (Carling, 1987); a study of the community needs of patients remaining in the state hospital (Tanzman et al., 1990); and a statewide study of consumer preferences for housing and supports (Tanzman et al., 1992).

Having Colleges Become Resources for Citizen Involvement in Community Integration

Colleges and universities can become contexts in which community-wide meetings can be held to explore integration issues, and in which faculty, students, and citizens in the community can become involved in a critical community issue, such as housing. As an example, faculty members in Vermont convened a colloquium series for other members of the university community, state officials, local service providers, and the general public, in which experts on community integration were brought in from across North America to give their perspectives on how Vermont could operate a state mental health system without a state hospital. Following each presentation, the faculty convened groups of interested citizens who wished to work on particular issues. One such group organized a consumer preference study, and started a process through which several consumers were able to purchase their own housing in a limited-equity cooperative (Cioffari, Blanch, Wilson, Carling, & Pierce, 1988).

Integrating Higher Education Planning into the Larger Work Force Agenda in Mental Health

As mental health systems face more pressure to be accountable and to demonstrate tangible outcomes in consumers' lives, there is a growing interest within these systems in the competence of the mental health work force. This interest represents an obvious opportunity for partnerships with higher education. Over the last several years the Vermont Department of Mental Health and Mental Retardation, with assistance from NIMH, has funded a major planning effort designed to create a competent work force for the 21st century. This effort, staffed by the Center for Community Change, has built on some of the successful higher education strategies described above. It has focused on this key question: "What mechanisms, funding, and programs need to be in place to ensure that all staff who work with adults with psychiatric disabilities, and with children and adolescents with serious emotional problems, are competent to provide state-of-the-art services and to promote tangible outcomes?'' The task force, consisting of consumers, family members, professionals, policy makers from several state departments, and a variety of higher education representatives, has developed a comprehensive set of recommendations to improve the competence of the entire mental health work force over time (Cioffari, Burchard, Carling, & Copeland, 1993):

1. Developing a Vermont Mental Health Training Institute responsible for designing and offering comprehensive training, and for approving higher education programs targeted to mental health workers.
2. Developing a set of comprehensive standards describing the specific knowledge and skills needed by all staff members working in public mental health, either with adults with psychiatric disabilities, or with children and adolescents with serious emotional problems.
3. Establishing individual staff development plans for all staff members in the system, developed and implemented by local staff supervisors in mental health programs, who themselves participate in a statewide "training of trainers" program to ensure their competence.
4. Developing a comprehensive set of training programs targeted to three levels of training—basic staff skills, advanced staff skills, and management skills—to be offered both through the institute and through higher education settings.
5. Developing a specific set of strategies to upgrade the salaries and benefits of mental health workers, and to improve the organizational culture in mental health programs.

This comprehensive set of recommendations is being used to pursue a number of legislative initiatives that will (it is hoped) ensure long-term state funding to meet these goals. Several work groups drawn from the original task dorce, have designed the institute, and the salary and benefits improvements, both of which are awaiting approval from the state legislature as this book is being written. Competency standards and individual staff development plans for all staff in the system have been piloted and are about to be implemented statewide. These processes include feedback from consumers and familes regarding what staff skills are necessary. Comprehensive training programs based on the competency standards are in the final stages and should begin in 1995. These are ambitious goals, particularly within a highly constrained fiscal environment for publicly funded programs; however, the energy of the group has been sustained through the commitment to a clear vision of consumer outcomes, as well as through having a comprehensive plan to pursue, one piece at a time. Thus, even if some parts of the plan are not immediately funded, or will take longer to implement, a strong, ongoing coalition working toward improving work force competence over time has been established.

Similar efforts are taking place in many locations in North America. The Center for Community Change though Housing and Support has a variety of materials available on change in higher education and professional training programs.

In summary, then, colleges and universities throughout North America represent significant potential partners for promoting community integration by taking on a leadership role in organizing state-of-the-art training for current and future mental health professionals, as well as by becoming valuable resources to consumers and families, who become students, teachers, and joint participants in a variety of community activities and projects that can be initiated within these academic settings.

CHAPTER 7

Improving Access to, Preserving, and Developing Housing

> Housing is the number one need of ex-patients. . . . When I speak about the housing needs of those who have been classified mentally ill, I do not mean shelters, group homes, supervised apartments, and other so-called solutions. Most ex-patients . . . want real homes, rooms or apartments in which they can live permanently, either alone or with someone of their choice.
>
> —JUDI CHAMBERLIN (quoted in Ridgway, 1988a, p. 6)

In many communities today, efforts to assist people with a label of "mental illness" to obtain decent housing occur primarily on an individual basis: One person at a time is helped to find a place to live, which is generally an existing housing unit in a community. This chapter, on the other hand, is intended to provide information about how the overall capacity of an organization or a community to provide affordable housing for people with psychiatric disabilities can be increased through efforts to secure significant numbers of housing units. Obtaining sufficient amounts of decent, affordable housing in communities is a result of three separate but often related strategies: (1) improving assess to existing housing, (2) preserving affordable housing, and (3) developing affordable housing.

Improving consumers' access to existing housing involves deciding who will be responsible for routinely helping consumers to find decent housing, who will work with landlords and others to locate units, and what resources will be needed to make this happen. It also involves identifying properties (available through public housing authorities, through individual landlords, or through currently planned housing development) that offer better opportunities both for integration and for higher-quality housing than consumers' current residences do.

Preserving affordable housing typically requires a well-organized approach to identifying properties that have affordable units, but that are at risk for "gentrification" or conversion to more expensive housing. Groups wanting to preserve these properties must generate various purchase, ownership, and financing alternatives, usually in concert with other groups concerned about affordable housing in the community. For example, an affordable housing coalition can purchase a rooming house that is threatened by "gentrification," or can arrange for the tenants of a low-income housing development to purchase the development after the 20-year U.S. federal commitment to rent subsidies has expired.

Finally, housing development involves the purchase and rehabilitation of existing housing that needs repair, the construction of new housing, or the acquisition of existing housing for immediate occupancy. It can involve rental units, single-family homes, or cooperatively owned units; Toledo, Ohio, for example, has pursued all three of these approaches. Housing development is the most complicated of the three types of efforts, and requires advocates to draw upon the unique expertise of the housing field.

Deciding which of these three approaches to take on—and some communities take on all three—must depend upon the available housing stock in the community, the preferences of consumers, and the interests and resources of the group involved. Completing a housing planning process, as described in Chapter Five, will provide an excellent basis for decisions about how much effort to put into each housing approach.

IMPROVING ACCESS TO EXISTING HOUSING

Strategies for improving access to existing housing include: (1) deciding who will help individuals to locate and select housing; (2) working with public housing authorities; (3) working with landlords; and (4) becoming involved in currently planned housing development.

Deciding Who Will Help Individuals with Housing

In order for people to be able to gain access routinely to available housing, it is important to decide who will be responsible for this service on a neighborhood- or community-wide basis. Mental health agencies throughout North America have begun to hire "housing coordinators" to work with the real estate community to gain access to housing, and have made housing access a specific responsibility of many case managers as well. In some cases local mental health systems are organizing housing development corporations, separate from mental health service providers, to assume this responsibility. Several examples of this kind of initiative are described at the end of this chapter. Other communities are using organizations that are concerned with disability issues but are not part of the mental health system (e.g., independent living centers) to help with housing. Oakland, California, provides a good example of this approach. In still other communities, such as in Albany, New York, ex-patient groups are taking on this responsibility. There are advantages and disadvantages to each approach.

Some of the advantages of mental health professionals' assuming greater responsibility for housing are that they often have access to funding and to the other supports people with psychiatric disabilities need, and can coordinate the availability of supports with whatever living situation a person selects. Often the assurance of such supports from the mental health agency makes landlords much more open to renting to people with disabilities. And if a crisis occurs, the mental health agency is often in a position to continue paying rent so that the unit is not lost. Some of the disadvantages, however, involve balancing roles that many service providers have come to see as incompatible: providing and managing the housing, providing the mental health supports, and "policing" the housing. Many landlords, along with the general public, expect mental health agencies to control their clients' behavior. To retain access to the housing, many mental health agencies in turn will impose program requirements on tenants as conditions of living there—required use of medications, required attendance at day treatment programs, required participation in case management services, and so forth. Often special clauses in leases impose requirements and responsibilities on tenants with psychiatric disabilities that are not imposed on any other tenants. And often these conditions, even though they are generally illegal, will allow people with disabilities to be evicted and lose their housing without the due process required for all other tenants. Finally, to the extent that mental health agencies continue to be seen by the community as directly responsible for housing provision, there may be a tendency for housing professionals to remain uninvolved, and not to assume their responsibility to arrange housing for all community members.

Independent living centers, because of their commitment to people with a range of disabling conditions, are often in a position to have a broader knowledge of community housing, the network of landlords, and so forth. They are typically strongly oriented toward integration and consumer empowerment. On the other hand, until recently, most of these centers have not served people with psychiatric disabilities, and they are often not aware of the special needs that relate to these disabilities. They are also often not involved with mental health centers in coordinating housing and supports, so these relationships need to be built. There are of course notable exceptions, such as the independent living center in Boston, Massachusetts.

Providing housing through ex-patient organizations often has significant advantages in terms of knowledge of the needs of the group, a strong focus on empowerment and integration, a strong respect for the preferences of consumers, and the availability of peer support. This is not to say that some consumer groups do not replicate restrictive professional programs. In fact, I have visited several that do—but they appear to be very much the exceptions. One problem is that many ex-patient organizations are poorly funded, and are often in jeopardy when systems are faced with funding problems; this undermines the availability of a stable source of housing assistance. Their relationships with formal mental health services vary greatly, so often these relationships need some development as well if consumers are to have easy access to the mental health supports they want. Successful examples of such an approach are increasing; they can be found in Philadelphia, Pennsylvania, St. Louis, Missouri, as well as in Albany and Oakland (see above).

Finally, it should be emphasized that it is not necessary to have only one organization assist consumers with their housing needs. What is necessary is a system of opportunities that enables *anyone* with a psychiatric disability to receive housing assistance from the kind of organization that he or she thinks will best meet his or her housing needs. Examples of such networks are given at the end of this chapter.

Working with Public Housing Authorities

There are over 70,000 local public housing authorities in the United States. These agencies are responsible for providing affordable housing to people with low incomes, those with disabilities, and those who are homeless. In working with these organizations, it is necessary to understand the context in which they operate and the constraints they face in meeting the housing needs of communities. Until the 1960s, these agencies were typically funded to create large housing projects for low-income families or for elders; although they provided affordable housing, they became increasingly plagued with crime, drug use, and other problems. In the late 1960s, the predominant approach to housing shifted to rent subsidies and then to rent vouchers: The federal government approved units in the regular rental stock in the community as "decent, safe, and affordable," and then issued subsidies or vouchers to low-income and disabled tenants so they could select among those units. Although this is a much more integrated approach, the program (HUD's Section 8 Rent Subsidy Program) has been terribly underfunded since its inception, never reaching more than about one-third of U.S. residents who qualify. In Canada "rent-geared-to-income housing" or "social housing" represents a more broadly available and more stable source of affordable housing, representing Canada's stronger commitment to housing as a *right*.

Furthermore, there has been an increasing controversy within elderly housing projects, which fewer and fewer elders are seeking out; as a result, increasing numbers of people with disabilities are choosing these units, often as a last resort. Although some communities have managed these projects in ways that have enhanced the lives both of elders and of individuals with disabilities, others are engaged in substantial conflict over the needs and rights of each group, with attempts being made to exclude the people with disabilities or segregate them into specific buildings. Until recently all of these attempts have failed, due in part to the use of the U.S Federal Fair Housing Act. In 1992, however, new federal legislation (Fair Housing Amendments Act, 1993) was passed that allows public housing authorities to offer separate housing sites to people with disabilities, and to organize services only in those sites. Although people are not required to live there, they may then be refused tenancy elsewhere if they need services that are only available in the segregated setting.

Local housing authorities administer a number of housing programs such as the rent subsidies and vouchers mentioned above, which can be used for regular community rental units; they also manage the waiting lists for rent subsidies in their communities, which can be several years long. They have new mandates, however, to give priority to people who are homeless or at risk of homelessness, including people with psychiatric disabilities. Typically, residing in a mental institution qualifies a person as being "at risk" of homelessness, and therefore a high priority for a housing subsidy. Public housing authorities also manage a number of other federal (HUD), state, and local housing programs used to purchase, rehabilitate, and construct affordable housing. Local groups should participate in the priority setting for these agencies through the Comprehensive Housing Affordability Strategy planning process (see Chapter Five), and should work closely with their local housing authority on a variety of strategies to gain access to or create affordable housing. In Columbus, Ohio, for example, the local mental health housing corporation, Community Housing Network, installed a special telephone in the housing authority office and used this phone to let the authority know when a mental health client needed housing. The authority responded quickly to these calls, since they knew that recipients, in contrast to many other potential tenants, would be well supported. Thus, this group greatly improved the housing authority's service to people with psychiatric disabilities, all for the price of a monthly phone bill.

Other communities, such as Waterbury, Connecticut, have found it very effective to offer mental health and related support services to *all* tenants in public housing settings, in return for the housing authority's allocating more housing resources to people with psychiatric disabilities, and becoming involved in housing development that includes these individuals.

Working with Landlords

Working with landlords is an essential aspect of assisting consumers/ex-patients with their housing needs. Communities as diverse as Burlington, Vermont, Salem, Oregon, Ottawa, Ontario, and Winnipeg, Manitoba, are finding the following strategies helpful. First, it is critical to get to know landlords personally and to find a mutual agenda. Building relationships with a small number of landlords, and making sure those relationships result in successful experiences in providing housing for people with psychiatric disabilities are key elements. Most landlords are primarily concerned about such issues as timely rent payments, upkeep of housing units, and avoiding behavior that will disturb other tenants or make adjacent housing units difficult to rent. Some landlords are also motivated by a desire to help others and to contribute to the community. By getting to know landlords as individuals, advocates can develop strategies that will meet landlords' needs and expand housing opportunities at the same time; they can also begin to determine the specific "environmental demands" that people will face who live in units managed by these landlords. A consumer may well lose his or her housing because of a poor fit between the expectations and style of a particular landlord and the behavior or expectations of the particular tenant.

Second, it is important to understand and respect both tenants' and landlords' rights. A major role of advocates, and of those wishing to provide housing assistance, is to be aware of the rights of individuals in community housing, and to insist that no special tenant responsibilities be imposed on an individual simply because that person has a history of involvement with the mental health system. People have a right to occupy rental units if they continue to pay their rent and follow all of the other rules of tenancy described in their leases. People have a right not to be discriminated against or given any special treatment insofar as their housing is concerned, solely on the basis of a psychiatric disability. And people are entitled to the same due process, if there is a challenge to their tenancy, as any other tenants. Therefore, a major responsibility of those involved in housing is to advocate that people with psychiatric disabilities use the same lease forms as any other tenants. With the passage of the Federal Fair Housing Act Amendments (1989), problems in this area should decline to the extent that individuals hold the leases to their own housing. Similar provincial legislation in Ontario granting all tenants, including those living in group homes, full rights as tenants. The protections under these laws are, in fact, another reason why programs or service agencies should avoid signing leases on behalf of people with disabilities.

Ensuring that people have their own leases and that they are standard leases, however, does not guarantee that the tenants understand their leases or that the expectations of landlords (e.g., concerning "reasonable behavior") are clear. Therefore, an important responsibility is to make sure that each lease is "translated" into clear expectations for both a tenant and a landlord.

Landlords also have rights. They have a right to expect that rents will be paid, that their tenants will take reasonable care of the housing units, and that the tenants will conform to reasonable standards of behavior so that other tenants' rights are not violated. In supporting the rights of tenants and landlords, it is usually helpful to promote an active dialogue and direct negotiation about these issues between the parties involved.

Third, it is important to provide ongoing support and problem-solving assistance both to tenants and to landlords. A major responsibility of the service provider, whether this is a professional or a peer support group, is to provide ongoing support to each tenant so that the housing situation remains satisfactory and available. Of particular importance are providing assistance to consumers in taking responsibility for their housing units, including paying rent; providing assistance in adjusting to the demands of the environment, including helping to build positive relationships with neighbors; and making on-site crisis assistance available. Another important aspect of support is advocating for landlords to keep their properties well managed. Often people with low incomes live in situations in which landlords are relatively inattentive to repairs. Supporters may also be called upon to mediate tenant–landlord conflicts, and also to support landlords on issues such as violation of the conditions of tenancy or eviction. The basic principles of working with landlords are being available and operating in a professional, businesslike manner.

There are four key ways to attract landlords. First, many communities have established ways to help assure continuous rental income, such as a "housing contingency fund" that allows rent to be maintained for a unit if there are problems (e.g., if the tenant is rehospitalized). A growing number of states, including Minnesota, Vermont, Tennessee, Ohio, and New York, provide such funds to local communities. These funds are also useful for rent deposits and for a variety of initial expenses that tenants incur. This fund can be set up as a grant program or as a revolving loan fund. Second, some mental health programs offer "free consultation" to landlords about tenants with whom the landlords are having difficulties. Landlords who have problems with tenants are often quite isolated and unsure of what to do; therefore, they may take the only course that they see open—eviction. Providing problem-solving support of this type is very valuable to landlords.

Third, it is important to "back the landlords up" in cases where tenants are consistently failing to take responsibility for paying rent, not keeping their units in proper condition, or refusing to change behaviors that are very problematic for other tenants. In such a case, although an advocate may be supporting a tenant in moving on to a situation that he or she can manage more effectively, it is also important to support the landlord's actions in insisting that the person continue to follow lease requirements, and to take care of the unit, and (when the landlord decides to exercise the right) in evicting the tenant. In such cases, if the relationship with the landlord has remained positive, someone else can then be referred to that unit, at the same time that the evicted person is being helped to find another home.

Fourth, it is helpful to express appreciation and even public recognition for those landlords who have become most involved with integration efforts. At the same time, this publicizes the successes of people with disabilities in the community, and attracts other landlords to become involved.

As a final note, my consistent experience in communities throughout North America is that when landlords who rent to low-income persons are provided with the types of supports described above, people with psychiatric disabilities become the *most* desired tenants among these landlords. Although this may strain belief among some readers, the reasons for this phenomenon are simple: Such landlords typically rent to individuals with many challenges, such as substance abuse, lack of after-school supervision for young children, inconsistent incomes, and so forth. When the landlords are approached by a service agency that offers strong supports to tenants of a particular type, such tenants stand out as comparatively very desirable.

Becoming Involved in Currently Planned Housing Development

An excellent way to gain access particularly to high-quality housing units is to become aware of all affordable housing in the community that either is being planned or is currently under development. The way to do this is simply to become involved with the various housing organizations in the community: neighborhood development corporations, community land trusts, housing coalitions, public housing authority planning processes, and so forth. Housing coordinators, as mentioned above, often develop such relationships as a key part of their job. Often the state housing finance or community development agency has a list of these organizations in the community. The local housing authority or community development office may also have such a list, and certainly a well-connected local nonprofit housing developer knows the "road map" of the area's housing community. Meeting with these groups, identifying mutual concerns, and becoming involved in their work (even joining their boards of directors) allow advocates to become fully informed about potential opportunities for affordable housing. These activities also set the stage for integration-oriented groups to participate financially in such development activities (see "Developing Affordable Housing," below).

In Burlington, Vermont, for example, there is a very active community land trust movement, which makes housing affordable by having a nonprofit group (a land trust) purchase properties and then sell the buildings on them as housing, while keeping the land (which tends to increase in cost over time much more quickly than the buildings) in a perpetual trust. Purchasers also agree to limit their profit when they sell the property. The local mental health program has begun working with the Burlington Community Land Trust on several fronts: planning housing development for people who are homeless, in concert with the local homeless coalition; and encouraging people with psychiatric disabilities to become members of the land trust, and therefore to be eligible for their housing when it became available. One outcome of this collaboration has been the development of a number of new housing options, including several limited-equity cooperatives in which people with psychiatric disabilities, using their SSI, now own their own housing.

PRESERVING AFFORDABLE HOUSING

As noted in Chapter One, an increasing problem in recent years has been the sharp decline of the affordable housing stock in most communities. This has resulted from many factors, including trends in the housing industry, which has become increasingly speculative and oriented toward short-term profit. These tendencies have fueled the "gentrification" of neighborhoods where affordable housing used to predominate; such housing has been replaced with "upscale" condominiums or luxury housing. Large numbers of units are lost to arson and neglect as well. Finally, many of these buildings in the United States formerly received HUD Section 8 rent subsidies from the federal government; these 20-year subsidies, and their related responsibility to use the property for low-income tenants, are now expiring. This leaves the owners with the option of converting these properties to some other use. Meanwhile, during the same period, U.S. federal funding for affordable housing has declined so sharply that only about 10% of the affordable housing stock lost to these trends has been replaced. Each time an affordable housing property is lost, people are displaced, and the competition for housing among those with limited incomes is intensified. Therefore, it makes sense to become involved in efforts to preserve affordable housing. There are three basic strategies for becoming involved in this issue.

First, it is important to find out early through community networks about properties at risk. If advocates have built an effective working relationship with landlords, low-income housing groups, development organizations, and the public housing authority, it is likely that they will hear early enough about at-risk properties to be able to take action. Often significant numbers of people with psychiatric disabilities will already be living in such properties. Second, advocates can participate in or even organize coalitions to take action, securing a temporary restraining order from a court if necessary; such an order prevents the property owner from engaging in eviction, demolition, conversion, or other action while preservation efforts are proceeding. Third, advocates can work with these coalitions to obtain local, state, and federal funds for the purchase and renovation of housing (and, if needed, the provision of services to people there); they can also help the tenants themselves purchase the property and reorganize it into some form of cooperative or joint ownership, such as a limited-equity cooperative.

Getting involved in preserving affordable housing presents a number of unique opportunities for further community integration. Large numbers of individuals get "stuck" in such settings after an initial "placement" by a service agency many years before. Each current resident, for example, can be offered assistance to move on to a more desirable housing situation. Often such properties, because of the threat of conversion or eviction, also have a number of vacancies. Depending on the current composition of tenants, this provides an opportunity either to obtain additional units for people with psychiatric disabilities, or to promote integration through achieving a better mix of low- and middle-income groups in the building.

DEVELOPING AFFORDABLE HOUSING

If an organization has thoughtfully explored ways of improving access to existing housing, is well connected to housing preservation efforts, and finds that there is still not enough affordable housing in the community of the types that people with psychiatric disabilities prefer, it may consider becoming involved in housing development. There are several important considerations here. First, developing integrated housing makes sense not only from the perspective of community integration principles, but from a real estate perspective as well. Robert Laux, of Creative Management Associates in Portsmouth, New Hampshire, assists groups throughout the country in developing integrated housing. In addition to the obvious benefit of increasing integration potential, Laux (personal communication, May 1991) points out that regular housing builds financial stability; that is, since regular housing increases in value, the owners can take income out over time and reinvest it in more housing. In addition, regular housing costs less (e.g., housing developed under the HUD Section 202 program, which is typically segregated by disability group, can cost up to three times as much and take twice as long to produce as regular housing). Moreover, regular housing creates long-term uses as *housing,* rather than as facilities. Finally, regular housing is easier to obtain, since it is available through multiple-listing services.

Second, through the process of identifying funding options and formulating a plan for the property, advocates will need to investigate options for ownership, property management, and service provision, to ensure that the housing remains a desirable living situation over time. Generally speaking, the "ideal" situation would be for many consumers to own their own housing, on either an individual or a cooperative basis. Alternatively, when it is dictated by individual circumstances, family members may own the housing. An increasingly popular option is for local nonprofit housing development corporations, whose mission focuses on affordable housing for *all* community members, to own and manage properties. Examples of this approach are described at the end of this chapter. These ownership strategies avoid many of the role conflicts described above in which human service or mental health agencies can become entangled, and frees up these agencies to do what they should do best—provide supports to people living in their own homes. Thus, in this "ideal" approach, the "framework for support" (self-help; family, neighbors, and friends; generic community services; and formal mental health services) provides necessary supports. Clearly, depending on local circumstances, other arrangements are possible. Private investors may become involved in ownership; this can be a valuable source of additional funding, as long as measures can be built in to ensure the long-term availability of the housing for the group's intended purposes.

Similarly, mental health agencies can stimulate the development of a housing development corporation, which will work with a variety of other housing groups in the community to develop affordable integrated housing. Karoff and McCabe (1992) provide an excellent analysis of the pros and cons of establishing such a corporation. They note that before making a decision, it is important to consider what kind of housing is needed; whether other entities exist that could be persuaded to provide affordable housing for people with psychiatric disabilities; what types of financing are available for housing production; and how such a corporation will be organized. Similarly, before development begins, the authors encourage groups to define the field of operations for the new entity (the local, regional, or state/provincial level); to decide how the housing units will actually be produced; and to decide on the ideal tenancy structure for the consumers who want to live in the housing (rental housing, cooperative ownership, sublease, etc.). Many such housing development corporations have now been organized across North America for the express purpose of increasing access to housing for people with psychiatric disabilities. Two very different examples of such housing development corporations are described below: a local entity in Franklin County, Ohio, and a statewide effort in Rhode Island.

Another strategy that is especially helpful is the creation of a housing development fund—a pool of money that can be drawn upon quickly to "buy into" development efforts that are already underway in a community. The reader should understand that because of the absence of adequate or easily accessible funding, most affordable housing development efforts by community groups are very tenuous and fragile enterprises, requiring multiple sources of funding and high levels of uncertainty. The majority of such "deals," in fact, fall apart before they ever produce housing, often for the lack of only a very small amount of money, when viewed in the context of the overall project budget. Although this is discouraging, it is also a very opportune climate for a prospective new partner to become involved in such a "deal" and literally save the entire plan by contributing a relatively small amount of funding. In such situations, the new partner may well gain far more units in the project than the actual dollar contribution would indicate, simply because the partner has made it possible for the overall project to survive. There are multiple examples in which, for funding of as little as $10,000, mental health groups have been able to gain access to a significant number of units in this way.

In any of these arrangements, it is most critical to continue thinking clearly about the ultimate goal of creating homes for people with psychiatric disabilities; of making a clear distinction between those homes and the services people receive; and of providing assistance to people within the framework for support. And it is frequently very helpful to formalize the relationships among these diverse partners, so that each knows what to expect of the others.

It is not realistic, in a book of this scope, to provide sufficient information about the highly complex process of housing development for the reader to go out and begin developing housing. Fortunately, there are a number of excellent resources available for those groups that wish to consider playing a role in housing development in their communities. These include: Molinaro (1988); National Association of Home Builders, National Research Center (1989); and Ohio Department of Mental Health, Office of Housing and Service Environments (1989). For those who are interested in this subject, however, it cannot be stressed enough that groups will need the expertise of housing professionals, to whom what may seem a complex process is actually a matter of doing day-to-day business.

Housing development can be thought of as occurring in three distinct phases: (1) preliminary steps, in which the group organizes itself to become involved in development; (2) the predevelopment phase, in which the group's plans are finalized; and (3) the development phase, in which the group either rehabilitates or builds housing, or acquires housing for immediate occupancy. Each of these phases is summarized below as a way of acquainting the reader with the overall flow of the development process. It should also be stressed that the description below, drawn largely from Molinaro (1988), is focused on community-wide efforts to develop housing. In cases in which a group is interested in focusing more narrowly—for example, on a single building—the process can be much simpler, especially if an existing local housing organization is taking leadership responsibility for all housing aspects of the effort.

Preliminary Steps in Housing Development

According to Molinaro (1988), preliminary steps typically include (1) hiring a housing staff person who is knowledgeable about real estate and who can "translate" the needs of the group to the housing community; (2) organizing a local planning effort, often a "housing task force," responsible for gathering some essential information to guide development (see below) and for formulating a housing plan, necessary to secure funding; (3) orienting the staff person and the task force to the group's goals, to current housing options, and to other key groups that will need to be involved in the effort; and (4) organizing the work of the staff person and the task force, including beginning to collect necessary information (a data base), beginning to develop the housing plan, beginning community relations activities, contacting state and local housing development officials and organizations, beginning a public information campaign if necessary, and initiating communication with local lenders.

The Predevelopment Phase

The predevelopment phase (Molinaro, 1988) typically includes completing three distinct activities: assembling a data base, completing a housing plan, and establishing a housing development corporation. Although the first two activities need to be completed in sequence, the third can begin while the group is still finalizing its housing plans.

A number of specific steps are associated with assembling the data base: (1) analyzing the existing housing inventory, including housing owned by the mental health system, and determining needs on the basis of consumer preferences and demographics; (2) analyzing overall market conditions; (3) analyzing the impact of existing housing programs for people with low incomes or with disability labels on decisions to locate future housing development; (4) formulating site selection criteria; (5) identifying future housing opportunities and financial resources, including determining the need for subsidies to the housing, whether these are cash payments to tenants (called "external subsidies") or subsidies to the cost of the development itself (called "internal subsidies"); and (6) preparing the data base so that it can be understood by nontechnical readers.

On the basis of the suggestions in Chapter Five, the advocacy group may already have gathered the most central information that will determine its housing strategy—information on where and how mental health consumers want to live. The group may also have collected some information on the housing characteristics of the community, as well as the economic situation of people with psychiatric disabilities. Now it is ready to gather any additional information it will need, as noted above, to create a data base that will specifically guide future housing development efforts.

The housing plan should specify (1) the number and types of units to be produced; (2) how the units will be produced; (3) who will produce the units; (4) the location of the housing units; (5) who will occupy the units; and (6) what supports will be available to the tenants. Many communities have now produced such housing plans. Notable examples include Philadelphia; Toledo and Cincinnati, Ohio; Seattle, Washington; and Columbus, Ohio (described below).

According to Molinaro (1988), housing plans are usually organized into the following sections: (1) a general overview; (2) a summary of the data base; (3) demographic information on people with psychiatric disabilities; (4) a summary of general market conditions; (5) ownership strategies; (6) financing strategies; (7) financing prototype; (8) issues, opportunities, and constraints; (9) community relations strategies; (10) criteria for selection of occupants; (11) public documents; and (12) a general summary.

The Development Phase

The development phase can involve either construction or rehabilitation of housing, or simply the acquisition of housing. The primary purpose of the development phase is to determine the financial feasibility of the housing project being considered (i.e., whether the net income will be sufficient to pay off the debt incurred in development).

Construction/Rehabilitation

The specific activities included in development that involves either rehabilitation or construction are (1) hiring a project manager; (2) organizing preliminary financial assistance; (3) revising financial projections; (4) completing financing arrangements; and (5) preconstruction activities.

The project manager is typically responsible for organizing the development team, which should include an architect, an engineer, legal counsel, a financial specialist, a community relations specialist, a management specialist, and representatives of those who will provide supports to tenants (consumers, family members, and service providers). The team meets regularly as the project unfolds.

The preliminary financial plan involves several elements: the acquisition costs of the property; information from the architect, from the builder, and from other technical specialists; and information from local government officials. Information from the data base will also be needed for the preliminary financial plan, including information about the maximum rent that tenants can pay; expected vacancy rates; estimated annual operating expenses; and the methods the group plans to use for financing.

After it is clear that the plan is financially feasible, the architect and the engineer are hired to design development documents. The housing management specialist then supplies more refined management figures. One or more general contractors examine the development documents and submit cost estimates, and the group submits the plans to local government agencies for project approval and permits. Finally, the housing development team finalizes permanent financing; closes on construction loans; and obtains all required governmental permits, zoning, and licenses.

Acquisition and Occupancy

Acquiring housing for immediate occupancy on a broad scale is substantially simpler than either constructing or rehabilitating housing. In many communities in the United States, significant amounts of property are often available through such sources as regional and area HUD offices (which can direct a group to vacant or abandoned housing); auctions or distress sales; foreclosures, such as those available now in many areas in connection with the savings and loan crisis; and other sources. As in other development, however, the group needs to determine the financial feasibility of the project by calculating whether the net projected income is sufficient to repay the debt incurred in actually making the housing available.

As with the construction/rehabilitation process described above, it is important to install a project manager, who will (1) assemble the members of the housing development team; (2) convene the team; (3) collect any needed information; and (4) keep the project on time and on budget.

The first step in financial planning is to prepare a physical plan and calculate preliminary costs. These include acquisition costs; any site alterations needed; "soft" costs, such as insurance, taxes, financing fees, legal counsel, and consulting fees; and costs involved in zoning variances, public utilities, making allowances for traffic or other public requirements, and so forth. In preparing the preliminary financial plan, the group will need similar information to that discussed above under construction and rehabilitation: the maximum rent that all tenants can pay; vacancy rates; annual estimated operating expenses; operating costs; off-site maintenance; replacement fund; and potential methods of financing. Using this initial information, the group can complete a preliminary calculation of the financial feasibility of the project.

If this analysis indicates that the project is feasible, the group is ready to finalize its financial plans by reviewing more detailed project costs and confirming the purchase price, closing costs, escrow balances, and estimates of initial costs. This will provide the information needed to obtain preliminary commitments for financing. If these figures still indicate that the project is financially feasible, the group is ready to proceed with a final financial plan; this involves negotiating with the lender to secure the financial commitment, and making any adjustments or changes required by those negotiations. The group is now ready to close on the property, to complete necessary renovations, to rent the property, and to begin managing the housing.

"DECONGREGATING" CURRENT RESIDENTIAL FACILITIES

As part of a community-wide effort to improve access to, preserve, and develop housing, many groups across North America are confronting the issue of the future uses of group homes, boarding homes, and other residential facilities that have been used in the past as a form of semi-institutional permanent housing for people with psychiatric disabilities. Often mental health systems that are emphasizing supported housing will convert these facilities to other treatment settings, such as crisis residences or "step-down" facilities for people leaving long-term institutions (Fields, 1990). In those cases, it is very important to be involved in the planned reuse of those settings, in order to be sure that they are promoting the kinds of services that are consistent with empowerment and integration.

In other cases, however, these properties represent valuable resources that can be put up for sale, in order to raise funds for more integrated housing approaches. Alternatively, such facilities can themselves be converted to regular housing, and may even represent a home ownership opportunity for some consumers.

Aside from the issue of the housing itself, various other important issues must be dealt with in "decongregating" residential programs. Nagy and Gates (1992) have produced an excellent summary of the experience of one program as it proceeded with "decongregation." They describe the shift to a new set of operating principles that consumers and staff members needed to develop as they began working with each other in regular housing: an expectation of permanence and exit from the housing by choice; control by the tenants over access by others; control by the tenants over the physical features of appearance and responsibility for maintenance; and the promotion of a "territorial attitude" among consumers. In order to accomplish this change, supervisors needed to model new behaviors, and to support staff members as their jobs changed in fundamental ways—from supervising clients in a group home to providing supports to individuals anywhere in the community that support was needed. The staff members had to adjust to loss of control in the face-to-face situation; an increase in the chances of personal embarrassment; others' perceptions of staff roles vis-a-vis clients; the blurring of personal and professional roles; an increase in perceived personal responsibility for the clients; and anxiety about social integration.

In order for all parties concerned to make the shift effectively, staff members needed help in developing and promoting freely given relationships; the organizational structure itself needed to be "deinstitutionalized"; and outreach and communication with the broader service provider network and with the community at large were critical. Staff members needed to be retrained in new roles and interventions, and new recruitment strategies needed to be developed. With this thoughtful approach, the shift from a group home program to integrated housing with flexible supports was accomplished smoothly.

Similar housing efforts are occurring in many communities. The Center for Community Change through Housing and Support has a broad range of materials available related to supported housing, housing access, preservation and development, and decongregating residential programs.

EXAMPLES AT LOCAL AND STATE LEVELS

A Local Community Example: Western Massachusetts

Through a coordinated effort undertaken by the Western Massachusetts Regional Office of the Massachusetts Department of Mental Health, a number of communities were helped to take on the housing needs of people with psychiatric disabilities in a systematic way that produced significant housing opportunities. This effort involved several distinct strategies:

1. Raising the consciousness of key constituencies in mental health and housing, through a regional conference focused on innovative housing and integration strategies and on consumer self-determination.

2. Establishing clear policy directions based on consumers' perspectives, through conducting a series of consumer preference studies.
3. Making technical assistance available to local communities in integration-oriented approaches, provided by the Center for Community Change through Housing and Support.
4. Encouraging local programs, through clarifying policies and through making funding more flexible, to "decongregate" their group homes and to shift to a service approach emphasizing integrated housing and flexible, outreach-oriented supports.
5. Funding the development of innovative new projects, including those focused on home ownership for people with psychiatric disabilities.

The results of this multipronged effort have been broad and dramatic. They include a major shift in programs across the region to an integration approach, and extensive organizing among people with psychiatric disabilities to assert their rights and to begin developing their own services. In addition, several group homes have undertaken successful "decongregation" efforts, in which consumers and staff members have gained access to regular housing, and shifted supports to these new housing arrangements (Nagy & Gates, 1992). A number of limited-equity cooperative projects have been initiated, including one in Berkshire County through a local housing authority. In this effort, consumers who are prospective owners have worked as a group over an extended period to plan the housing, develop budgets, and design the rules that will govern the cooperative. This cooperative is designed to be integrated and accessible to a wide range of income groups; to be affordable on a long-term basis to current and future residents; and to represent an investment in consumers' future security.

I had the opportunity to meet with the members of this group shortly before the housing cooperative was developed, after they had engaged in considerable planning. It was extremely impressive to see people with psychiatric disabilities, who had never believed that home ownership (or in some cases even housing stability) was possible for them, struggling with all of the issues that homeowners today are challenged by. It was obvious to me that incredible power and strength can come from operating in such a valued role.

Similar cooperatives have been extensively developed in Madison, Wisconsin, through the Madison Mutual Housing Association, to improve access to integrated housing for people with a broad range of disabling conditions. Racino (1993) provides an excellent description of the actual operations of this relatively mature effort.

A Local Community Example: Franklin County, Ohio

Franklin County (Columbus), Ohio, is another community that has pursued a systematic strategy (involving many individual initiatives) to increase affordable housing and to shift the locus of decision making to people with psychiatric disabilities. As one of the Robert Wood Johnson Foundation's Demonstration Program Mental Illness sites, the county mental health board initiated an ambitious process of creating a central mental health authority, establishing case management through community treatment teams throughout the county, and restructuring each of the community mental health programs to emphasize a community support approach.

With regard to housing, the county developed a housing plan (Franklin County Mental Health Board, 1987), using the strategy described above (Molinaro, 1988). This comprehensive plan is an excellent resource for those interested in county-wide or regional housing planning. In addition, the county sought outside consultation from the Center for Community Change through Housing and Support, assessing its entire stock of residential programs, and solicited recommendations for shifting those resources to a more integrated housing approach. Based on an assessment of consumer preferences, the housing plan specified the types of housing and the neighborhoods that were of greatest interest to consumers. Case management teams were created and made responsible for helping people find decent housing. The housing plan also made it clear that a number of areas in which individuals wanted to live lacked sufficient affordable housing to meet this need.

In order to increase access to housing, and to develop new housing, the county created a housing development corporation called the Community Housing Network, which took on the roles of landlord, property manager, and development coordinator; essentially, it serves as a real estate agency for people with psychiatric disabilities. This corporation operates quite distinctly from service-providing agencies. Although consumers are referred to the Community Housing Network by their case managers, once they receive their housing they are no longer under any obligation to continue services as a condition of keeping their housing. The county was also able to secure funding from the state for rent subsidies, and from federal, state, and local government, along with private lenders, for housing access and development activities.

Results of these efforts have included a much stronger emphasis on housing among the community treatment teams; a significantly increased affordable housing stock available to people with psychiatric disabilities, based on their preferences; much greater choice among decent housing alternatives for consumers; and a stable organization responsible for assisting consumers with their housing throughout the county.

A Statewide Housing Strategy: Rhode Island

A third example, in this case on a statewide basis, comes from Rhode Island. The state mental health department, working closely with consumers, families, and local service providers, conducted a study of consumer preferences for housing; it then initiated a statewide housing development corporation responsible for gaining access to and developing housing for people with psychiatric disabilities. This corporation, Thresholds, Inc., enjoys corporate autonomy from the state, which used traditional funds for capital improvements for mental health group homes and institutions to fund the effort. The corporation has a majority of people with psychiatric disabilities and their families on the board of directors, and has focused exclusively on integrated housing (both rental and ownership options).

Forming a separate nonprofit agency to develop housing has had several advantages for the Rhode Island mental health system, including an ability to respond quickly to market conditions, and an ability to create a structural separation between housing and services. It has also provided a consistent entity with the opportunity to develop effective relations with the housing community, and to acquire needed expertise in the creation of housing. The core development strategy that Thresholds uses is to work with local housing nonprofit organizations. Unlike for-profit groups, these nonprofits have a natural affinity for working with disadvantaged people. They are committed to long-term affordability and to providing people with opportunities for permanent housing. They also have a long-range commitment to their communities, and are skilled at developing multiple subsidies and financing arrangements to help keep housing affordable over time. Thresholds finds that often with very limited investments, and given the complexity of financing community housing, it is able to make financially marginal projects developed by others successful; it therefore gains access in greater proportion than its specific contribution to a project might represent.

The results of this initiative are the development of a stable organization responsible for meeting housing needs; strong partnerships between community mental health providers interested in developing integrated housing and the local housing community; a greatly expanded stock of affordable housing accessible to people with psychiatric disabilities; and a clear shift among service providers toward a supported housing approach.

CHAPTER 8

Creating Employment Opportunities

We need full-time employment. If they just keep getting part-time jobs and workshops, they're just putting off what they're eventually going to have to face—that we should be working the same as everyone else.
—A consumer (quoted in Hutchison, Lord, Savage, & Schnarr, 1985, p. 21)

In many communities, the majority of people with psychiatric disabilities have only two options: to be unemployed, or to work in entry-level positions with low pay and little chance of advancement. Work represents a core value in Western society; it is an essential element of the way we define our worth as individuals, as well as the way society appraises our value. Work is also essential to having the financial resources that make housing, education, and social participation possible. Recent research (Downs, 1989) indicates that people with psychiatric disabilities look to employment to meet a broad range of psychological, financial, and social needs. Therefore, increasing consumers' access to the full range of employment opportunities in a community needs to become a major priority of advocates and service providers.

Strategies for helping people with psychiatric disabilities to obtain meaningful work have changed significantly in recent years with the decline of sheltered and segregated work approaches; with the emergence of "transitional employment programs" in integrated work settings; and with the adoption of a "supported employment" approach, focused on long-term integrated work options. Traditionally, employment efforts have been based on helping one person at a time.

Those who received help were typically seen as ready or nearly ready for competitive employment; even then, they were typically offered a "train, then place" approach. Even recent attempts to implement supported employment, which emphasize the "place, then train" approach, often focus only on certain individuals who are seen as most ready to work.

In contrast, employment approaches that are based on integration and empowerment principles emphasize work assistance to a much broader range of individuals with psychiatric disabilities. Instead of offering help only to those individuals who are judged to be ready or nearly ready to work in competitive employment, this approach recognizes that *all* citizens have a right to meaningful employment or to other productive activities in the community, such as volunteering, and thus is focused on people who have never worked; people whose work or vocational progress has been disrupted; people who are currently working, but whose work is at risk of disruption because of a psychiatric disability; and people who simply want to explore new work options. The overall goal of these approaches, then, is to assist all such individuals to reach their vocational goals. This chapter describes strategies that have been successfully used to increase a community's employment opportunities for *all* of its members, including mental health consumers/ex-patients.

CHARACTERISTICS OF SUCCESSFUL EMPLOYMENT ASSISTANCE APPROACHES

Although strategies for increasing employment vary greatly from community to community—reflecting differences in the communities themselves, the specific preferences of individuals, and the service capacities of the areas—successful work assistance approaches appear to have a number of common characteristics. These include individualized career planning, help with job access, and aid in job retention; peer support; coordination with services and benefits; and assurances of confidentiality. Each of these characteristics is discussed briefly below.

Individualized Career Planning

Each person's work identity and career path is unique, and the meaning of work is highly individual. Furthermore, people who have never worked or who have not worked in some time may need to engage in substantial planning, in order to identify career goals to be resumed or new career directions to be taken. Some individuals, in addition to planning, may want to try out a number of work situations as part of this planning process. Some individuals will want full-time work; others will want to start with part-time or volunteer work, either because of the significant change that work represents for them, or because they are still quite undecided with regard to a career. Therefore, it is critical that any work assistance approach start with a posture of basic openness to meeting each person exactly where he or she is in the process of thinking about work, and to helping each individual discover his or her own vocational interests, preferences, successful past experiences, and future goals.

Effective career planning involves such diverse activities as the identification of both skills and interests; an ability to assess the needs and demands of specific work environments or career choices; the identification of specific vocational goals; and help with concrete activities, such as resumé development.

Individualized Help with Job Access

Effective work assistance does not just require planning. It may also involve, depending on the individual, the identification of potential jobs or other experiences that match an individual's goals, or that are natural "stepping stones" to the realization of those goals; training in job interview skills; help with arranging interviews; assistance with practical details, such as clothing and transportation; and assistance with references.

Individualized Aid in Job Retention

Once an individual has secured a job, effective work assistance becomes focused on such issues as job retention, performance improvement, and advancement. This may include help with "learning the ropes" of a particular job; clarifying job expectations; providing emotional support; providing or facilitating skills training; and offering support to the employer through being available "on call," or through planning and arranging reasonable accommodations as discussed later in this chapter.

Peer Support

Peer support is a critical factor in employment success, and effective work assistance approaches help to link individuals with peers—particularly other individuals who are facing the challenge of re-entering the work force, as well as individuals who have successfully made this transition. Peer support groups focused on employment that meet after working hours are a particularly effective ways of meeting this need.

Coordination with Services and Benefits

Even when an individual returns to work a full-time basis, there is often a continuing need for various entitlements and benefits (e.g., medical insurance, or supplementary income programs that represent a "safety net" if the individual's work situation should change). Although recent changes in U.S. Social Security legislation and related Medicaid rules have removed some of the disincentives in those programs to return to work, very careful coordination between entitlements and benefits, and the pacing of returning to work, are critical to employment success. This is especially the case since many individuals have come to rely on these benefit programs for basic subsistence, and may be reluctant to return to work because they fear the loss of these benefits. Thus, encouragement to return to work must be coupled with a high level of familiarity with benefits programs, and with their opportunities and pitfalls related to employment.

Similarly, it is critical to coordinate employment assistance with other aspects of treatment and support. Medications can have a major negative or positive impact on an individual's ability to perform on a job. Similarly, appointments with a case manager, rehabilitation worker, or therapist can be scheduled in a way that supports re-entry into employment (e.g., in the evening), or in ways that disrupt this goal. Thus, it is critical to rearrange and replan any services that are needed on an ongoing basis, so that they will support and enhance employment success rather than undermining it.

Assurances of Confidentiality

Stigma, as noted throughout this book (see especially Chapter Four), is a major factor in the social integration of workers with psychiatric disabilities. Therefore, it is paramount that each individual be in charge of decisions about whether or how much to disclose to the employer and to coworkers about his or her psychiatric history. Disclosing this history may result in benefits, such as protection under the antidiscrimination provisions of the 1990 Americans with Disabilities Act, entitlement to reasonable accommodations in the workplace, and arrangement of supports that may be needed at the work site. However, such disclosure also opens the door to an individual's being treated very differently and perhaps being greatly disadvantaged in the workplace. Thus, this decision is inherently personal, and people should be offered assistance in making it thoughtfully. Once this decision is made, it affects the nature of all contacts with the employer, as well as nearly every aspect of the roles of both the individual and the person who is assisting in the employment process.

USING A SUPPORTED EMPLOYMENT APPROACH

As noted in Chapter One, the supported employment approach was first developed as a model for people with developmental disabilities. Its original components included (1) personal choice; (2) individual employer-paid jobs; (3) substantial work (usually at least 20 hours per week); (4) availability of a support worker/job coach to train the person on the job, to support the person's employment, or both; (5) integration with nondisabled coworkers on the job; and (6) ongoing supports after the worker has mastered the job. Wehman and Kregel (1985) have concluded from their experience with people with developmental disabilities that the four critical activities for implementing supported employment are job placement, job site training and advocacy, ongoing monitoring, and follow-up.

As the supported employment approach has taken hold in mental health, concerns have been raised about how the original approach needs to be modified to meet the specific needs of people with psychiatric disabilities. Among these concerns is a desire for more flexibility in the definition of "substantial work" in order to allow participation of people who want to work fewer hours, especially since many individuals are reluctant to jeopardize their benefits at the start of their employment experience. A second concern has to do with whether a job coach is necessary at the job site. Many people with psychiatric disabilities do not need to be taught a job any differently than any other worker needs to be, and the presence of a coach can potentially increase stigma and social isolation by emphasizing differences between an individual and coworkers. A final concern has to do with the need for a strong emphasis on making long-term supports available after the initial period of success on the job; a person with a psychiatric disability may require more ongoing services than a person with a developmental disability may. U.S. federal regulations that encompass the definition of supported employment given above have been rewritten to accommodate many of these differences in needs. Also, as Anthony and Blanch (1987) point out, there are many possible "routes" to supported employment: directly from a mental health treatment setting (such as a hospital), from a psychosocial clubhouse program, from a transitional employment setting, through a self-referral, through an individual's family, or through a vocational rehabilitation program.

THE BUILDING BLOCKS
OF A SUCCESSFUL EMPLOYMENT INITIATIVE

In order for an integration-oriented employment initiative to be effective, various components or "building blocks" need to be put in place. These include (1) an effective network of support services; (2) access to a variety of career development and training opportunities; and (3) access to employers. Each of these three components is described briefly below.

A Network of Supports and Services

In order to ensure that people with psychiatric disabilities can obtain the help they may need at any point in the process of returning to work, it is important that a network of relevant supports be available. These include peer supports, supports for families, and services directly focused on rehabilitation. Thus, what is needed is a network of people to help an individual figure out what kind of work he or she wants, including longer-term career interests; to help the individual do what needs to be done to prepare for getting a job; and then to help him or her with actually getting, keeping, and advancing in the job. In addition to people, supports include tangible items such as clothing, transportation, funding for training programs, and so forth.

A rehabilitation-oriented organization that is knowledgeable about psychiatric disabilities (e.g., a psychosocial rehabilitation clubhouse or supported employment program) can be an especially important resource, as long as it operates according to integration and empowerment principles. The rehabilitation approach, as it has been adapted to psychiatric disabilities, demystifies the process of employment by describing it as a matter of "choosing, getting, and keeping" a job (Anthony, 1990b). A person's ability to complete this process successfully depends on the congruence of the job with the individual's goals, as well as on the individual's skills and personal supports that are directly relevant to the demands of the job. Therefore, the process of rehabilitation emphasizes (1) an exploration of the individual's employment goals; (2) an assessment of the person's current skills and supports that are relevant to that goal; (3) an identification of the skills and supports that will be needed for the person to achieve his or her goal; and (4) the development of those skills and supports. Many excellent materials are beginning to become available that focus on successful rehabilitation practices, as well as on effective strategies for securing employment in integrated work settings (e.g., Anthony, 1990b; Hasazi & Collins, 1988; Danley & Mellen, 1987).

Access to Career Development and Training Opportunities

Instead of having individuals with psychiatric disabilities focus immediately on getting jobs, it is often much more useful to engage in a career planning process focused on individuals progressing toward and realizing their longer-term work goals. Obviously, this process can take place while a person is working as well. In order to work toward their goals, people need access to a broad range of career development and training opportunities, as well as a variety of work experiences. The best way to help people gain access to the kinds of jobs that reflect their career goals, and that offer them chances for significant mobility and advancement, is to make full use of any career development and training opportunities that may exist in the community (and to create new opportunities as they are needed). This involves exploring the kinds of training available through vocational rehabilitation and employment training agencies, as well as through the various trade schools and academic programs in the community. Transitional employment programs may offer time-limited work experiences in integrated settings that help an individual to develop basic work skills and to explore different types of employment. It is then necessary to work with these groups to ensure full access for people with psychiatric disabilities. Making use of community opportunities also involves learning which private organizations or government programs have grants to assist people in obtaining equipment for various job options (computer equipment, tools, uniforms, etc.). Finally, gaining access to these training options may well require the development of specialized pools of funding to be made available to individuals who wish to return to work.

Access to Employers

Helping consumers to obtain employment requires developing good working relationships with employers throughout the community. Thus, the most effective advocates in this area are often individuals or agencies that are themselves employers, including service-providing agencies that have become part of the business community in their area, and perhaps are involved with the local chamber of commerce or business roundtable. Being perceived first as a person with common concerns among business leaders, and only secondarily as someone who also employs people with disabilities, can be an advantage in building peer business relationships. Other effective advocates are those who can offer a service to business: a ready source of capable workers; a source of support to those workers; or a source of information on reasonable accommodations and other aspects of creating a more inclusive work force, in response, for example, to the requirements of the Americans with Disabilities Act (see below).

SPECIFIC COMMUNITY STRATEGIES FOR RESPONDING TO EMPLOYMENT NEEDS

In order for all community members, including those with psychiatric disabilities, to have the opportunity for meaningful work, it is critically important to involve employers and others in the effort to take advantage of existing employment opportunities; to overcome barriers to employment; and, when necessary, to create new employment opportunities. Communities that have begun to achieve greater success in employment have used strategies in the following key areas: (1) creating or refocusing services related to employment, training, and career development, and retraining service providers in relevant skills; (2) developing community resources, including training opportunities; (3) working with employers; (4) creating employment opportunities within mental health systems; and (5) creating employment through consumer-operated services alternatives. Each of these strategies is discussed briefly below, with examples.

As in the case of housing strategies, certain fundamental information is needed to guide employment strategies; this includes information on the kinds of work that people with psychiatric disabilities want, and the needs that they are expecting to meet through employment. Chapter Five, has provided a considerable amount of information about how to conduct a community-wide employment preference study. This information can be used to inform a group's strategies about the types of jobs and training opportunities it will try to gain access to or develop; the ways in which it chooses to structure the relationships among workers, service providers, and employers; and the specific supports it will develop as well.

Creating or Refocusing Services Related to Employment, Training, and Career Development; Retraining Service Providers in Relevant Skills

The policies of mental health and vocational rehabilitation agencies are shifting toward integrated employment strategies. A recent policy statement of the National Association of State Mental Health Program Directors (NASMHPD, 1990) is a useful tool for advocating that these shifts be translated into more widespread support of such strategies in local communities. This policy statement, for example, "recognizes the fundamental importance of integrated, paid, and meaningful employment to the quality of life of persons with severe psychiatric disabilities," and asserts that "mental health authorities should assume a leadership role in significantly increasing the rate of employment among individuals with psychiatric disabilities" (p. 1). The statement provides guidelines as to what constitutes effective employment support, including the following:

> career planning, job goal selection, job placement, self-presentation in writing and in person during pre-employment screening, negotiating reasonable accommodations, acquiring specific job skills, obtaining transportation and clothing appropriate to the work setting, estimating how earnings will impact entitlements, such as SSI, SSDI [Social Security Disability Insurance], Medicaid and Medicare, education in using Social Security Administration work incentive programs to greatest advantage, establishing positive relationships with coworker and supervisors, and assistance in changing jobs. (p. 1)

In spite of these policy advances, many staff members in mental health and even in vocational rehabilitation agencies are relatively unfamiliar with the specific skills required to help integrate people with psychiatric disabilities into jobs with career potential in normal employment settings. Therefore, a major effort needs to be placed on helping staff members acquire these skills, and on promoting the involvement of other organizations that may have skilled staffs, even if these agencies are oriented primarily toward other disadvantaged groups. Such organizations include supported employment projects focused on people with developmental disabilities; local or state commissions on the employment of people with disabilities; and groups that have been successful in working with other disadvantaged groups to become employed (single parents making the transition from welfare, displaced homemakers, etc.).

Within service programs, the first critical steps are to adopt a rehabilitation-oriented mission focused on tangible employment outcomes for consumers; to restructure policies, funding, and programs to be consistent with this approach (see Anthony et al., 1982, for specific guidelines); and then to systematically retrain the staff and supervisors of the organization in the new approach.

What do staff members of mental health or vocational rehabilitation programs specifically need to do in order to work effectively on employment issues? Basically, they need to be guided by rehabilitation, integration, and empowerment values; to keep focused on employment as an outcome; and to possess the specific knowledge and skills to help people achieve these outcomes. A comprehensive competency-based approach to these staff skills has been developed by the graduate training program in supported employment at the University of Vermont (Hasazi & Collins, 1988). Competencies have been developed by this program in the following areas: (1) vocational assessment; (2) individual program planning; (3) direct vocational services; (4) coordination of community resources; (5) consultation and in-service training; and (6) program administration.

One excellent short-range strategy for training or retraining current staff members is to have them visit successful employment projects in other communities. Another is to "import" trainers from successful communities to critique current efforts to provide employment, make recommendations for change, and train staff and advocates in some of the skills needed to implement those changes. Finally, there is a growing literature on supported employment both within mental health and in the larger disability community; in additon, a new national organization of advocates and service providers—the Association for Persons in Supported Employment (P.O. Box 27523, Richmond, VA 23261-7523)—has been formed. The association sponsors annual national conferences on supported employment. Other relevant conferences are those of the International Association of Psychosocial Rehabilitation Services, state and national community support conferences, and the national "clubhouse" conferences convened by Fountain House in New York. Subscribing to the *Psychosocial Rehabilitation Journal* (available from the Center for Psychiatric Rehabilitation, Boston University, 730 Commonwealth Avenue, Boston, MA 02215; [617] 353-3549) is also very helpful. The Center for Community Change through Housing and Support has resources available about employment strategies, reasonable accommodations, and related issues.

It should also be emphasized here that many nonprofessional groups, such as peer support groups and independent living centers, also work effectively to help consumers/ex-patients secure employment, and typically do so through a much less formal process.

Developing Community Resources, Including Training Opportunities

In order to gain access to or create an adequate network of opportunities for employment in the community, advocates need to know the following about the labor market in the community: job growth trends, readiness of employers for hiring, the nature of unemployment, the ways people typically find jobs in the community, and both the "visible" and the "hidden" job markets in the community. Then advocates will need a specific set of strategies to take advantage of the local job market and to maximize work opportunities.

One formal way to proceed is to complete an analysis of the local labor market, and then to develop a specific marketing strategy (Hasazi & Collins, 1988). According to Hasazi and Collins, a labor market analysis is intended (1) to determine local labor needs and trends, and (2) to develop strategies for matching the labor needs of the community and the employment needs of the individuals advocates are focused upon. It seeks to identify employers in a specific geographical area; to obtain information about appropriate employers, rather than simply locating specific job openings; and to compile information on these potential employers that will facilitate individuals' getting jobs there. There are many potential sources of information for this analysis, including the chamber of commerce (listing of major companies); the state employment agency and job service (current trends in vacancies); vocational rehabilitation (jobs commonly available to people with psychiatric disabilities); employers (direct and indirect contacts); mail and telephone surveys to identify high-turnover positions; and classified ads (trends, requirements).

It is important to identify job growth trends in the community. Typically, most job growth occurs either in small businesses or in the public sector (city, county, state/provincial, and federal governments, or private nonprofit service agencies). Employers identified can be separated by degree of readiness to hire individuals, and strategies for approaching them can be based on this readiness. For example, are employers not hiring, and therefore ready for awareness-level intervention? Are they formally looking for potential future job openings because of increased awareness of the need? Do they know that openings are going to occur in the near future? Or do they need employees now? It is also important to understand unemployment trends in the local area. How much unemployment is "frictional" (resulting from time spent in looking for existing but unfilled jobs), how much is "cyclical" (resulting from a downturn in the business cycle), and how much is "structural" (resulting from a mismatch between the skill demands of unfilled jobs and the qualifications of job seekers)?

How do people find jobs in a particular community? Most people find jobs through friends, relatives, or acquaintances. Only a small minority find work through the "visible" job market, such as by directly filing applications, responding to want ads, or using public employment services. The most difficult source is want ads, since at least half of those who read them are already employed, and the job seeker is competing against anyone who can read. Few employers use want ads, and they tend to do so primarily for low-level or "no-future" jobs.

The "hidden" job market, on the other hand, is often the best source of positions. These are best identified through telephone directories, chambers of commerce, friends, relatives, and acquaintances. The best strategies for actually securing these jobs are telephone contacts and "informational" or "networking" interviews.

Working with Employers

Depending on the relationships that individuals want to maintain with their employers, various approaches to working with employers are potentially helpful. Often employers simply need basic information to overcome their misunderstandings about psychiatric disabilities. They may need help in understanding the provisions of various laws related to employment rights (such as the Americans with Disabilities Act), or of laws that provide incentives for them to hire people with disabilities. Employers will also typically not be familiar with the reasonable accommodations that are relevant to many people with psychiatric disabilities, and thus may need help with aspects of the workplace that are specific foci of antidiscrimination legislation, such as interview procedures, health care benefits, and job descriptions (including essential tasks of a job and required qualifications). They may need some assistance in learning to negotiate reasonable accommodations respectfully with individuals.

Employers may also need help in figuring out how to keep the employer role separate from that of service provider, particularly when employment is in a service-providing agency; in setting clear and consistent expectations for performance and for appropriate behavior on the work site; and in developing effective strategies for communicating with service providers, if individuals desire this. In addition, employers may need help in planning for extra supervision or support, planning for backup coverage in the event of absences, creating policies that respect both confidentiality and accountability, and developing grievance mechanisms that will keep any problems from turning into major disputes. Finally, employers may need help in anticipating potential interpersonal problems and designing awareness programs for coworkers of individuals with disabilities. They may also need support if and when there are problems on the job, and especially appreciate the quick availability of such support.

Job Development

"Job development" is any activity intended to locate multiple employment opportunities that may then be offered to individuals with psychiatric disabilities, based on their interests. Job development, as contrasted with helping individuals find specific positions, is particularly appropriate in a very tight job market. It is also appropriate for creating transitional employment opportunities, or for developing positions for individuals who have particular difficulty with the job search and interview process. In order for job development to be effective, it must take into account the characteristics of the geographical location and the individuals being served; it must be systematic; and it relies heavily on the job developer's interpersonal skills. In addition, it may involve strategies that are very similar to those used by individual job seekers.

A number of personal and professional attributes of the job developer (Hasazi & Collins, 1988) seem to be critical. These include (1) good communication and interpersonal skills; (2) good public relations and sales skills; (3) reliability and dependability; (4) good organizational skills; (5) persistence and perseverance; (6) genuine interest in and knowledge about persons with disabilities; (7) knowledge of and interest in the business community; (8) ability to build credibility with employers; and (9) ability to identify businesses most likely to have appropriate job openings.

Traditionally, there have been four distinct approaches to job development: the charity approach (appealing to an employer's "conscience"); the legal approach (using laws and regulations as leverage); the personal approach (using personal acquaintances as contacts); and the business approach (demonstrating why it's good business to hire people with disabilities). Each of the first three approaches often has an adverse effect—whether it is leaving employers with low expectations (charity), developing adverse and suspicious relationships (legal), or introducing limitations based on who is involved (personal). The most effective approach is the business approach, particularly when combined with the best features of the personal approach.

It is also helpful to distinguish between generic and specific job development. In generic job development, the focus is on the overall job market in the community. This may involve conducting detailed labor market analyses (see above); identifying businesses most likely

to have openings; focusing efforts on executive or upper-level personnel; concentrating on employers with a large labor force; making
presentations to these employers and to others in the business community to raise their awareness; and, through all of these activities,
creating job opportunities for people with psychiatric disabilities in
a given geographical area to choose among. Specific job development,
on the other hand, is focused on obtaining a specific job on behalf of
someone who has limited skills in finding employment. A job developer
approaches this type of job development in the same manner as any
individual seeking employment; in addition, he or she emphasizes
proven successes involving people with psychiatric disabilities, and
provides specific information about the abilities and interests of specific
individuals with such disabilities.

The Americans with Disabilities Act;
Reasonable Accommodations

The Mental Health Law Project (1992) has produced an excellent summary of the provisions of the 1990 Americans with Disabilities Act,
as well as an explantion of how this important legislation applies to
people with psychiatric disabilities. The American with Disabilities Act
specifically makes it illegal for employers to ask job applicants about
psychiatric treatment, past or present; to deny a job to someone with
the necessary experience and skills because of the person's past or current psychiatric treatment or possible future treatment; to deny a job
or promotion because of a belief that a person with a psychiatric disability won't be able to "handle" the job; to refuse to make reasonable modifications in workplace rules, schedules, policies, or procedures
that would help a person with a psychiatric disability perform the job;
to force an employee with a psychiatric disability to accept a workplace modification; to contract with other organizations and individuals
that discriminate against people with psychiatric disabilities; or to retali-
ate against people with psychiatric disabilities for asserting their rights
(Mental Health Law Project, 1992).

   With regard to who is covered, the act prohibits discrimination
against any person with a disability who is "qualified" for a job,
whether he or she currently has a disability, has a history of disability,
or is even perceived to have a disability. Psychiatric disabilities are specifically included in this legislation, if they are extensive enough that
they may interfere with working. People who are friends or relatives
of those with disabilities are also protected if they are seen as potentially missing work because of these relationships.

   Employers are required to provide reasonable accommodations
to people with disabilities, as long as such a person identifies himself

or herself as having a disability and as needing such accommodations, and as long as this does not represent an "undue hardship" to an employer. An employer may not fire, punish, or threaten a person who tries to use the provisions of the Americans with Disabilities Act. "Reasonable accommodations" are defined as modifications in job expectations, the work environment, personnel policies, training, or other aspects of the employment setting and its operations, intended to increase access to the workplace and to increase successful job performance by people with disabilities.

Making reasonable accommodations for people with psychiatric disabilities is still a matter of experimentation, exploration, and learning in the workplace. A recent summary (Carling, 1993) provides a comprehensive review of the literature in this area. Typical examples of recommended accommodations (Mental Health Law Project, 1992), are as follows:

- Flexible scheduling, such as allowing an employee to take a certain number of hours off every week, or changing his or her working hours to accommodate visits to a therapist or clinic.
- Providing extra unpaid leave for short-term medical or psychiatric treatment.
- Offering an employee a private work space to eliminate the stress of working with large numbers of people, or arranging for an employee to work off site, such as at home.
- Restructuring job duties by changing when or how a task is accomplished, or switching assignments with another employee.
- Providing job coaches or other individualized on-the-job assistance.
- Changing an employee's supervisor if another supervisor would be more patient and flexible.
- Educating coworkers to improve their attitudes toward people with disabilities.
- Reassigning an employee to a vacant position.

Mancuso (1990) describes a number of specific examples of accommodations that have actually been provided:

1. *Changes in interpersonal communication.* These include arranging for all work requests to be put in writing for a library assistant who becomes anxious and confused when given spoken instructions; training a supervisor to provide positive feedback along with criticisms of performance for an employee re-entering the work force who needs reassurance about his or her abilities after a long psychiatric hospitali-

zation; allowing a worker who personalizes negative comments about his or her work performance to provide a self-appraisal before receiving feedback from a supervisor; and scheduling daily planning sessions with a coworker at the start of each day, developing hourly goals for an employee who functions best with added time structure.

2. *Modifications to the physical environment.* These include purchasing room dividers for a data entry operator who has difficulty maintaining concentration (and thus accuracy) in an open work area; and arranging for an entry-level worker to have an enclosed office, to reduce noise and interruptions that provoke disabling anxiety.

3. *Job modifications.* These include arranging for someone who cannot drive or use public transportation to work at home; restructuring a receptionist job by eliminating lunchtime switchboard duty normally handled by someone in this position; and exchanging problematic secondary tasks for part of another employee's job description.

4. *Schedule modifications.* These include allowing a worker with poor physical stamina to extend his or her schedule to allow for additional breaks or rest periods during the day; and allowing a worker to shift his or her schedule by 90 minutes twice per month in order to attend psychotherapy appointments.

Creating Employment Opportunities within Mental Health Systems

Until recently, mental health systems have been one of the most consistent sources of employment discrimination against people with psychiatric disabilities. Many mental health agencies, in fact, still have policies against hiring ex-patients; they may also discourage professional staff members from disclosing any personal experiences they have had with receiving mental health services. These practices perpetuate a "we–they" mentality that promotes a sense of incompetence and inferiority among consumers. As consumer groups grow in strength, however, mental health agencies are coming to recognize the unique knowledge and skills that consumers have acquired from their experience with psychiatric disabilities and with the mental health system.

Mental health systems, in fact, represent a very significant resource for employment of consumers who have an interest in the "helping professions." Programs, agencies, and systems that are interested in using this resource fully can systematically begin to make jobs available to consumers in these ways:

1. Examining and changing existing policies, hiring practices or requirements, and other potential barriers to employment.
2. Identifying needs of clients of the agency that are not being met, or that could better be met by consumer staff.
3. Reviewing current full-time jobs and restructuring them to make a number of part-time roles available to peer helpers.
4. Identifying clients who are interested in roles as service providers, and offering them training and support.
5. Pursuing strategies for reasonable accommodation in the workplace, including providing support to current employees who wish to acknowledge their history of involvement with mental health systems.

An agency or program that wants to take on such an effort might designate a group of individuals to work on opening up employment opportunities within the agency. The group should consist of a majority of consumers, and should include staff members and managers committed to this effort, as well as family members. The group should initially develop a mission statement that focuses on maximizing opportunities for integrated employment in the agency. This should include not only hiring consumers on a long-term basis to provide services, but also exploring the variety of ways in which consumers can do short-term work in the agency to gain valuable job experience. An important point for the group to bear in mind is that for many ex-patients (W. J. Montague, personal communication, September 1990), returning to work in the mental health system, particularly after some success in more integrated settings, can be a source of restimulation and distress, since it was within mental health systems that they once experienced the extreme sense of powerlessness inherent in the patient role. Furthermore, some individuals may fear that mental health professional "peers" will continue to retain significant power over them, and may continue to see them as people with the potential for serious work difficulties and/or eventual failure. Thus, providing peer support for these returning workers is essential. Finally, beginning to hire people with psychiatric disabilities in a mental health agency typically results in current professional or support workers' feeling more open about "coming out" about their own past experiences in the mental health system. Acknowledging the value of this experience, and of the role modeling that "coming out" represents, is important.

As noted above, agencies often have explicit policies that prevent hiring consumers. They may specifically exclude current service users, or they may require specific degrees or prior experience for certain jobs that are actually not necessary. Similarly, many positions are defined as needing to be full-time, although many consumers may only want to work part-time. A careful examination of policies, hiring practices, and job requirements may often lead to plans for major change in these areas. An excellent first change is to develop a strong affirmative hiring policy for people with a history of psychiatric disability. Another is to consider membership on the agency board of directors for a significant number of consumers.

Through surveying clients of the agency, the group can begin to identify service needs that consumers feel are not being met at this point, or that they would prefer to be met by consumer staff members. Often people will want more social support, or will prefer that a consumer staff person be involved when a crisis occurs. Others may prefer that mutual support groups be organized by consumers on the staff. Many of these identified needs can be met with part-time staff. For many consumers, the availability of positions with a limited number of hours has great appeal, since such positions allow a higher quality of life and some re-entry into the work force while not jeopardizing benefits.

Similarly, it is helpful to talk with consumers about the specific ways they feel they can be helpful to one another, such as providing companionship or assistance with material needs (e.g., shopping or transportation). Some agencies begin by creating "case manager aide" "crisis aide," or "support worker" positions, in which consumers work alongside professionals to provide support and to learn various professional roles. Such an approach should not, of course, serve as an alternative to an aggressive effort to hire people with psychiatric disabilities at all levels, including management positions. Those involved in a variety of efforts to hire such people in mental health agencies stress that it is important to avoid creating "consumer jobs," but rather to hire affirmatively in current positions, and to create positions that a variety of community members might fill (including consumers).

Through full involvement of as many consumers as possible in this planning effort, as well as through focus groups and other methods, the organization can develop a pool of consumers who are interested in service provision. It can then use the newly created opportunities within the agency, as well as the broader employment development efforts described above, to respond to these needs. Consumers may also want to form one or more support groups to help one another continue to explore these work interests; to identify training needs; and to brainstorm ways for the mental health agency to continue to promote additional job opportunities, both within the agency and in the larger mental health system.

Mental health agencies can sometimes secure state/provincial or federal funding to establish, in cooperation with local colleges, a mental health training program that provides certificates or degrees to people interested in working in the field. It is far better to initiate such a service through a regular educational institution than in a mental health setting. Examples of such efforts can be found in California, Massachusetts, New York, Maine, Connecticut, Vermont, Ontario, and elsewhere.

Mental health agencies throughout the United States have begun hiring people with psychiatric disabilities. A recent national survey of mental health programs offering housing and community supports, conducted by the Center for Community Change through Housing and Support (Yoe et al., 1991), and funded by the National Institute on Disability and Rehabilitation Research, found that programs emphasizing the new integration paradigm were more likely to hire people with psychiatric disabilities in a wide range of positions. An important finding of this survey was that people with psychiatric disabilities were being hired in virtually all job categories and at all levels of these organizations—from senior management to entry-level roles, and from full-time to part-time positions. This finding indicates the range of positions that consumers can hold, as well as the potential variety of accommodations needed. Even psychiatrists hired by an agency can be consumers/ex-patients, as Mind Empowered, Inc., of Portland, Oregon, discovered (see Chapter Three).

Creating Employment through Consumer-Operated Service Alternatives

The final strategy for mental health systems to help expand employment opportunities is to foster the development of consumer-operated services, and to assist in the development of consumer-run businesses. Although consumer-operated services are discussed in more detail in Chapters Three and Ten, it is important to emphasize that, as mental health systems move to becoming more "consumer-driven," they simply must increase funding for services that are controlled by and provided directly by consumers. Advocacy, mutual support groups, hot lines, assistance with crises, help with housing and employment, the creation of drop-in centers and "safe houses"—all these provide opportunities for additional employment, as well as ways to experiment with services approaches that are more acceptable and more responsive to consumers than more traditional, professionally provided mental health services may be.

A number of communities have recently begun to provide "seed money" and business advice to groups of consumers who wish to operate their own businesses. Typically, this involves creating a service organization in the community (a retail bakery, a clerical services agency, etc.). Such businesses not only require some capital to start with, but often need subsidies for several years as well. However, they can be valuable sources of full- and part-time employment; they can also serve as training sites for consumers not yet interested in regular competitive work. Finally, they can be a significant step toward empowerment of consumers, as community members see another "success" story involving people with psychiatric disabilities.

LOCAL COMMUNITY EXAMPLES

Institute for Community Enterprise
(Northampton, Massachusetts)

The Institute for Community Enterprise had been operating a number of mental health and rehabilitation programs for many years. Several years ago, it undertook an organization-wide process to examine the extent to which it was operating with a focus on integration and empowerment. As a result of this planning effort, the agency took a number of steps, including expanding its board of directors so that a majority of members would be people with psychiatric disabilities. The agency also began hiring consumers as staff members in a variety of positions. As a result of this new climate of openness, the strong historical rehabilitation focus of the agency, and initial experience in hiring consumers, clients and management staff decided to shift decision making in the agency's employment program to the consumers of that program.

As a result of this decision, the program shifted toward an exclusive focus on integrated employment settings. The organization expanded its mission from being only a service-providing agency to becoming an economic development partner, and helped to create several consumer-operated businesses. Peer support groups for consumers returning to work were organized, as were various services geared toward helping people plan for careers, obtain jobs, and negotiate reasonable accommodations. The fact that the program itself was aggressively committed to hiring consumers was a major asset in this process, since staff members were discovering the kinds of accommodations that were needed at the same time as they were helping other employers to make the same efforts. Recently, this agency started an Institute for Consumer Empowerment, through which consumers provide technical assistance and consultation to mental health agencies.

The changes that this agency undertook had a strong effect on increasing employment among consumers, as well as making the services available much more reflective of those that consumers found helpful. In addition, these changes had a strong "ripple" effect on other mental health and rehabilitation agencies in the area, which had been struggling with similar issues and appeared to benefit greatly from the leadership and role modeling of the Institute for Community Enterprise. As a result, a number of agencies in western Massachusetts now include people with psychiatric disabilities on their boards, have begun hiring consumers, and have undertaken a broad range of initiatives related to integration and empowerment.

Oakland Independence Support Center (Oakland, California)

The Oakland Independence Support Center is a consumer-operated drop-in and service center for individuals with psychiatric disabilities, particularly people who are homeless and are not interested in the services of traditional mental health agencies. The agency is staffed entirely by ex-patients, and provides a broad range of services related to housing, work, and entitlements. The service model combines a strong orientation to peer support and self-help with skills training and individual planning.

The center makes services available that address all of the practical barriers to employment, such as having a fixed address, decent clothing, and funds for meals, transportation, and job searching. Through a profound sense of respect for the individuality of each person who approaches the center for service, staff members are able to assist individuals effectively in making work-related decisions, and then in finding and keeping jobs. People are also helped to access other training opportunities or to return to school, if that is consistent with their vocational goals.

Staff members also work closely with government agencies to coordinate access to benefits, and then to help people move off those benefits as they return to work. Because this is a multiservice organization, people can also receive help related to housing, education, substance abuse, or other needs.

Laurel Hill Center (Salem, Oregon)

The Laurel Hill Center is a multiservice agency focused on community integration and support for people with psychiatric disabilities. The agency has a particular focus on working with individuals with the most severe disabilities, using integrated housing, work, and social environments; it has been successful in helping people who have been chronically homeless, as well as people with serious substance abuse problems, to find and succeed in regular housing over an extended period of time (Brown, Ridgway, & Anthony, 1991).

The center operates a comprehensive employment program that works closely with the local vocational rehabilitation service to help people plan employment goals, and to learn the skills and organize the resources necessary to achieve their goals. With a strong commitment to a rehabilitation approach and to integration and empowerment, the agency has included people with psychiatric disabilities on its board of directors, and is active in hiring consumers in its service programs. Employment programs include a consumer-operated business that performs a variety of services in the local area, and has recently received a contract to provide eyeglasses to all welfare recipients in Oregon. The center also operates an extensive supported employment program, which focuses on helping consumers obtain jobs, developing jobs, organizing reasonable accommodations, and providing support on and off the job.

Programs such as these demonstrate that, with a strong commitment to rehabilitation, and to the guiding values of integration and empowerment, service providers can help people with even the most significant psychiatric disabilities to get and keep satisfying and meaningful work.

CHAPTER 9

Promoting Social Integration

It would be good [to have a couple of friends]. . . . And people my own age too. . . . You can't always spot the loneliness. There are so many ways of covering it up.

—A young woman in Toronto
(quoted in Hutchison et al., 1985, p. 23)

In the life and fabric of a community, relationships are our basic support. This chapter focuses on a most critical challenge in the struggle for integration and empowerment: social integration. The chapter begins by briefly defining social integration, describing the social experience of a psychiatric disability, and detailing a number of the key barriers to social integration that advocates and staff face. Next, the chapter describes the timeliness and the critical nature of promoting social integration, and proposes several goals for such an effort. The chapter then reviews the major implications of a social integration approach for mental health workers, summarizes the key strategies that are being used to promote social integration throughout North America, and concludes with three local examples of efforts to promote social integration.

WHAT IS SOCIAL INTEGRATION?

Social integration, according to Reidy (1992), can be simply defined as affording people with psychiatric disabilities the opportunity to participate in all aspects of community life. This means, as much as possible, that such people live in typical housing within the community;

have acquaintances, friends, and intimates among a wide range of people; work in regular employment settings; be educated in community schools; and participate in worship, recreation, shopping, and other pursuits alongside other community members.

To promote social integration, it makes sense to direct the efforts of formal services toward maximizing contact between people with psychiatric disabilities and potential friends or other supporters. The simplest strategy is to ensure that virtually all such efforts take place in regular work, housing, and educational settings, in ways that lessen or remove any distinction between persons with and without a label of "mental illness." Services of this sort focus increasingly on supporting the natural supports in an individual's life, such as friends, family members, employers, coworkers, landlords, neighbors, teachers, and so forth. When crises occur, efforts are directed not only toward assisting the individual but toward mending and strengthening the natural support network, so that it becomes more and more capable of resolving crises with little or no professional help. In this way, service providers can overcome the typical impact of hospitalization or other crises, which is to *increase* social isolation (Holmes-Ebert & Riger, 1990).

Social networks are perhaps the critical component of well-being. Relationships serve multiple functions in everyone's life (Strauss, 1989), including ventilation ("talking things out" and expressing emotions); reality testing; material support; social approval and acceptance (belonging, being accepted as one is); constancy (sharing a history with others); modeling and social learning; motivation (giving and receiving encouragement, sharing positive expectations, being believed in by others); symptom monitoring (giving and receiving feedback on impending problems, becoming aware of how one is behaving); problem solving (serving as a sounding board for others and vice versa, planning for alternative courses of action); empathic understanding (feeling understood); reciprocal relating (being a partner, sharing and giving to others); insight (gaining a better understanding of oneself); and loving and being loved.

In addition, "typical" community members use various professionals and services (doctors, dentists, counselors, laundries, restaurants, etc.) to meet various needs in life. Formal services working toward a goal of community integration for people with psychiatric disabilities carefully avoid developing "specialized" programs that replace the obligation of these professionals and services to meet the needs of *all* community members. Instead, mental health workers and advocates often become directly involved with the providers of community services, in order to increase access for consumers/ex-patients. In other words, the focus shifts to working with and changing communities themselves, rather than just individuals with disabilities. Reidy (1992) goes on to stress that the real emphasis of social integration must be placed on the *quality* of actual participation by consumers/ex-patients in the community, and that true social integration involves three essential elements: access to valued roles, chances to participate in life-enriching activities, and opportunities to develop a wide range of voluntary relationships.

For all of us as human beings, social satisfaction lies in the extent to which we belong, or how each of us answers these questions: Where do we belong? To whom do we belong? Obviously, we all struggle with this set of issues over the lifespan. For people with disabilities, the issue is often whether they will have the opportunity even to struggle with these questions in the same ways that "typical" citizens do.

THE SOCIAL EXPERIENCE
OF PSYCHIATRIC DISABILITY

Lutfiyya (1988) has written a moving document on social relationships among people with disabilities including those with psychiatric disabilities, in which she summarizes the experience of social integration. She describes two critical components of this experience that are important to understand, if we are to promote true social integration: separation and clienthood. It is important for change agents to understand these issues if they are to overcome the variety of obstacles or barriers to social integration.

Separation

Lutfiyya describes a recent training session with the staff of a residential program, in which staff members pointed out that none of the residents with whom they worked had "best friends," that only a few could claim one or two "close friends," and that all had a limited number of acquaintances. The majority of these relationships were with staff members, with other residents, or with other professionals with whom the residents conducted business. Lutfiyya goes on to describe how most human service programs effectively set up barriers between people with disabilities and most other members of the community by surrounding the consumers with paid staff members and with others receiving the same services. In the process, family connections may be ignored or broken, friends may be discouraged from keeping in touch; and, in effect, a person's social history becomes lost. This is engendered by, and in turn promotes, a profound sense of "different-ness" between people with and without disabilities.

In short, according to Lutfiyya, people with disabilities are sepa-rated from their families and communities, and cast into roles of de-pendency. Even when they are physically present in the community, they are kept at a social distance from other community members. Housing people with disabilities in segregated environments, or hav-ing them work in segregated settings, only compounds the problem: Communities are reinforced in the belief that consumers are different and can neither successfully fit into nor contribute to society. "Typi-cal" community members lose the chance to meet and get to know people with disabilities, and thus opportunities for people to grow together and to build attachments are lost.

Clienthood

When they enter formal health or mental health programs, most peo-ple with disabilities are turned into "clients," which often implies a dependent and passive relationship with staff members and other caregivers. When the client role becomes life-defining, a person's uniqueness is lost, and the emphasis is placed on the person's service needs or problems; professionals are then brought in to "solve the client's problems." Clients, in turn, learn a narrow range of accept-able behaviors through which they can get their basic needs met. Such rigid and distant roles promote resentment and a deep sense of aliena-tion among people with disabilities, who struggle to maintain some sense of control over their lives. These roles also contribute to "burn-out" among staff members, who are expected to control all aspects of the lives of clients, including their social connections. In such con-texts, people with disabilities often become desperate for relationships; they then behave in ways that are described as "attention-seeking," "withdrawn," "difficult to engage," "promiscuous," or other labels that imply social inappropriateness.

OBSTACLES TO SOCIAL INTEGRATION

In my own experience of knowing many people with psychiatric dis-abilities as clients, as friends, and as colleagues, it is clear that isola-tion and loneliness are among their central concerns. When people are still involved in the formal mental health service system, their iso-lation is what makes service providers reluctant to promote more in-dependent housing or work arrangements. Similarly, the fear of loneliness is what prompts many individuals with psychiatric disabilities to resist leaving segregated or congregate environments—in short, to remain isolated within the world of mental health. And the belief in the inevitability of social rejection is what explicitly guides many mental health programs, with the best of intentions, to organize themselves so as to provide sheltered social environments for clients. This is not to say that consumers do not have much to offer to one another (see below), but they also need much more expanded social networks if they are to get on with their lives. Even in a U.S. national demonstration project of progressive supported housing programs, staff and tenants cited, as a major problem, the continuing social isolation of tenants (Livingston & Srebnick, 1991).

The psychological impact of this sense of clienthood and isolation is vividly described by Reidy and Shea (1990), who quote several friends: "Am I so unlovable that only paid professionals are willing to talk with me?" "Am I so poor and disabled that I will never be able to find a spouse?" Reidy and Shea point out that consumers have often developed a sense that they are aliens, and expect routine rejection. They conclude that social integration will only be advanced if change agents are willing to acknowledge and attempt to alleviate this profound sense of alienation.

Aside from beliefs and practices within mental health systems, advocates must consider a number of other practical barriers to social integration. These include personal characteristics of consumers (such as shyness, limited scope of interests, or lack of awareness of interests); logistics (such as lack of money for social activities, lack of transportation, or lack of support from others to socialize); inexperience (such as negative attitudes about consumers' social potential on the part of others, whether these be community members or staff); and fear (whether on the consumers' part or on the part of others).

I remember once talking with a "citizen advocate" whose role was to help people with severe disabilities make social connections in the community. She described her efforts with one individual who had multiple problems and a very long history of living in an institution. After considerable discussion, she found that he was very interested in country music, and she began accompanying him to a variety of concerts and local gathering places. The one he liked best was a bar in a less desirable part of the county. So, somewhat reluctantly, she began going there with him. Each week the bar had an "open mike" night when anyone who wanted to could sing. She watched in terror as this gentleman got up to sing. True to her greatest fears, she saw the experience as terrible: He barely knew the words, couldn't carry a tune, and hardly got through the song, while she sat there experiencing great amounts of social embarrassment and fearing that he would be ridiculed. But she literally held on to the table and kept herself from intervening. At the end of the song, she felt a terrific sense of relief —that is, until he called out, "Let's do another one!" At that point, she couldn't bear it any longer and rose from her seat, asking her friend to come back and sit down. And then something marvelous happened: Two or three other people in the audience called out, "Let him sing," and "Give him a chance." And she sat back down, realizing that he was indeed on his way to developing a richer social network.

WHY IS A FOCUS ON SOCIAL INTEGRATION CRITICAL NOW?

Reidy (1992) describes why a social integration focus is especially timely now, given current trends in mental health systems. First, people with psychiatric disabilities, as part of their growing civil rights movement, are challenging current mental health treatment practices and demanding that they be treated like any other citizens. Second, shrinking public resources make it impossible to sustain a system that tolerates or even fosters dependency. Local resources, such as YMCAs/ YWCAs, churches, and civic organizations, simply must become part of the support picture. Third, a growing concern for consumer satisfaction has highlighted the sense of isolation and loneliness that people with psychiatric disabilities feel, and has identified these issues as central to their quality of life.

KEY GOALS OF A SOCIAL INTEGRATION EFFORT

In order to promote social integration, advocates must move beyond vague notions of mental health consumers' becoming more socially connected, and begin to pursue specific goals that will result in stronger social support systems. According to Lutfiyya (1988), these goals include increasing consumers' opportunities for social relationships; increasing community support for social integration; increasing the diversity of consumers' social connections; increasing the continuity in their relationships; increasing the actual number of freely given relationships; and increasing intimacy in relationships. Each of these goals is discussed below.

Increasing Consumers' Opportunities for Social Relationships

As noted above, a basic strategy is simply to provide all supportive and collaborative services for people with psychiatric disabilities within integrated community settings. Beyond that general principle, it is important to recognize that all of us meet potential friends through our families and neighbors; in schools and workplaces; at cultural, civic, and recreational events; and through our churches or synagogues. We also come into contact with people through our daily activities, such as shopping, getting the car fixed, going to professional appointments, and so forth. In each case, it requires effort to meet new people. Therefore, consumers need to be provided with as many opportunities as possible to engage in these "normal" sets of social interactions. If necessary, this should include changing any program rules or professional practices that directly interfere with the opportunity for consumers to discover such connections in the regular course of their lives.

Increasing Support for Social Integration

Hand in hand with providing opportunities is providing support for building new relationships. Lutfiyya (1988) gives one powerful example:

> One woman, Helen, wanted to go to church, as she had not attended since she was a child. A church of the right denomination was located, the priest [was] contacted, and a parishioner agreed to sit with Helen during Mass and accompany her to the coffee hour afterwards. For Helen, this effort was not enough. She did not know how to behave in church, and smoked cigarettes, talked, and swore during the service. Not surprisingly, the parishioner became uncomfortable sitting next to Helen, and soon stopped coming to pick her up. Helen needed someone comfortable enough to direct her actions quietly while in church—suggest going out for a smoke, or waiting, being quiet. Initially, a staff person sensitive to Helen's need to attend church and to the limits of appropriate behaviors might have made the difference, by minimizing disruptions, allowing Helen to attend church and meet others in the congregation. This staff person could then encourage a member of the congregation to support Helen, in the hope that a friendship would develop. Enhancing relationships between people with disabilities and typical citizens is not accomplished by throwing unprepared and unsupported individuals together. (p. 5)

Increasing the Diversity of Social Connections

A typical social network may be thought of as a "pie" in which different kinds of relationships form different sized pieces. The kinds of relationships may include those with professional service providers, coworkers, friends, neighbors, family members, and acquaintances. Because professional service relationships often constitute the largest piece of a consumer's "pie," an important goal is thus to increase the size of other pieces. Obviously, when a consumer develops a greater diversity of connections with coworkers, neighbors, and acquaintances, he or she has an increased potential for more intimate friendships; family relationships may also improve as a result (see below). Therefore, it is helpful in working with any individual who is socially isolated to keep in mind a picture of this person's social network, and to consider the ways in which this network might best be expanded and diversified at any given time.

Increasing the Continuity of Relationships

Many of us thrive on meeting new and interesting people, but we are all sustained by those with whom we have had relationships for a long period of time. This continuity is an important source of security, comfort, and self-worth. For individuals who rely principally on mental health workers for connection, even those relationships typically lack continuity, given the high rate of turnover of direct-service staff. Hasazi, Burchard, Gordon, Vecchione, and Rosen (1992), in a research study on the effects of this rapid staff turnover, have concluded that staff departures have an impact on clients that is as great as the stress of divorce or even death. Unfortunately, staff members tend to be unaware of the depth of this impact. For people whose primary relationships are with mental health professionals, this pattern of continued loss has a great effect on their willingness to open themselves to new connections over time. Thus, a major strategy for building consumers' capacity for trusting relationships is to enhance the continuity of professional relationships, and to increase the power of consumers to choose their own professional relationships (e.g., from among a group of case managers).

The experience of staff members in programs that have worked with individuals over a very extended period, such as the Program in Assertive Community Treatment in Madison, Wisconsin, is quite different from that in more typical programs. Staff members are supported to work for a long time in the program, and are encouraged to maintain long-term but changing relationships with consumers over that time. Thus, it is not unusual for a staff member who served as a case manager for an individual a number of years ago to continue a social connection for many years, in which the individual comes to the staff members's house for dinner and vice versa. In the absence of the opportunity for such continuing relationships, it is at least critical to be clear about the nature, purpose, and time limits of the relationship, rather than insisting that a consumer develop a trusting connection with a professional with whom a longer-term relationship is unlikely, simply because the professional wants to "help."

Another important source of continuity is a consumer's family. It is axiomatic, of course, that for family relationships to remain healthy, they must change over time. Within the context of what the individuals want, it is important for people who have been disconnected from their families to be offered help in building healthier relationships with their families—not only because this is an important developmental task for any adult, but also because a caring family represents a critically important source of social support over time. The task of reuniting individuals in relationships with their families takes time and careful attention, but is made much easier within a context in which the individuals are also developing other adult connections that will sustain them in other areas of life. Having these other social connections provides multiple opportunities for ventilation and problem solving, as the process of rebuilding healthy family relationships progresses.

For many individuals (primarily women) with psychiatric disabilities, a major goal is reunion with their children, who may have been lost to foster care, to adoption, or to the custody of others during a psychiatric crisis (Wallace, 1992). A statewide study of housing needs in Ohio, for example (Ohio Department of Mental Health, Mental Health Housing Task Force, 1986), concluded that among people with psychiatric disabilities, 38% of the housing need was represented by single parents who wanted housing in which they could live with their children. In some cases the children were living with these parents in inadequate shelter, but in most cases the children had long since been taken away by social service agencies and placed in foster care. In many cases, service providers were not even aware that these individuals had children, much less that a different housing situation was critical to pursuing the goal of reuniting the families. Individuals need concrete assistance with this issue, help with parenting skills, and emotional support to reconnect and rebuild these centrally important relationships.

Increasing the Number
of Freely Given Relationships

Increasing choice among service providers is helpful as a first step, but the larger goal is to decrease the proportion of people in a consumer's life who are paid to relate to the consumer. Thus, any relationships that a consumer forms must be potentially viewed with respect, since they are freely chosen. Obviously, staff members and peers need to be sensitive to the issue of exploitation in any relationship, but they must also be clear about the variety of social purposes that all relationships meet. When opportunities and support for increasing the number of freely given relationships are provided, an individual's network is strengthened. Volunteer or citizen advocacy programs are an excellent resource for expanding social relationships among people who are especially isolated. Through such efforts, typical citizens make a commitment to become involved in consumers' lives over an extended period of time as friends, and then use these relationships along with their own social contacts to promote a richer social network for the consumer.

Increasing Intimacy in Relationships

Intimacy in General

Intimacy is a challenge for all people, and is only built over time in the context of a trusting set of relationships. Intimacy is also a key element of an individual's recovery process, in which the person rediscovers (or discovers for the first time) his or her own worth, attractiveness, and power. Providing opportunities and support for relationships; focusing on the diversity of connections and their voluntariness; and adhering to a clear sense of honesty, integrity, and directness in relationships all provide the context for deepening trust and intimacy.

All people strive for intimacy, and some individuals are less experienced and less skilled at navigating these waters than others. Often, citizens who befriend consumers who have been socially isolated may initially feel overwhelmed by the consumers' need for attention or desire for intimacy. Similarly, there is ample room for significant misunderstandings about the nature of a relationship when two people have very different levels of intimacy in their lives at a particular time. The basic need in these situations is for compassionate candor. A number of the social integration strategies discussed below also focus on expanding the range of people involved in promoting social integration, so that this need for attention and intimacy can be shared with a number of individuals. In the longer term, it is certainly the case that as an individual's social network expands and deepens, such issues become much less problematic.

Sexual Intimacy and Long-Term Relationships

People with disabilities in general, and individuals with psychiatric disabilities in particular, have typically been perceived as nonsexual or as incapable of developing either healthy sexual relationships or long-term committed relationships with partners. In fact, the early literature on disability is replete with examples of such barbaric practices as forced sterilization. By preventing the development of healthy, developmentally important sexual experiences, mental health programs have inadvertently promoted consumers' seeing themselves either as nonsexual beings or as people who "act out" inappropriate sexual behaviors.

The reality is that too often, people with psychiatric disabilities have simply been denied appropriate developmental experiences, and the information they need about their own sexuality and about responsible sexual behavior. In particular, women with psychiatric disabilities often do not receive adequate medical care related to their bodies and to sexuality. And the needs and rights of individuals who are gay, lesbian, or bisexual have been virtually ignored within mental health programs.

As noted in Chapter Three, there is growing evidence that many people with psychiatric disabilities have experienced some form of sexual exploitation or abuse, whether as children, in institutional settings, or in the marginal neighborhoods where many of them live. Such people need active help in engaging in a process of recovery from this abuse, and in learning strategies to decrease their vulnerability or the risk of exploitation in the community. Some mental health agencies, such as the one in Burlington, Vermont, have developed films, print materials, and support groups to help consumers in this area.

Issues of sexuality within mental health programs are also an important focus for change. Advocates for change can form a planning effort within an agency that focuses on the extent to which programs support the recognition of clients' sexual identity and needs, and promote healthy expressions of sexuality. Such a planning process can identify the specific issues related to sexuality that clients want to have addressed; it can also examine program practices with regard to the common and differing needs of men and women, and the specific needs of individuals who are gay, lesbian, or bisexual. They can propose a variety of changes in programs or the development of new programs. A series of public forums exploring sexuality issues that are important to different subgroups of consumers can be developed. Support groups that encourage younger people to explore their emerging sexual identity can be formed. Separate groups for gay, lesbian, or bisexual youths are critically important. Broad staff training related to sexuality may emerge from such planning. Organized efforts to link people with other community resources related to sexuality are critical as well, whether these be women's health centers; shelters for women experiencing abuse; Planned Parenthood centers; gay, lesbian, and bisexual support groups or resource organizations; resource centers for men; or other groups or services. Helping people connect with such information and allies is a way of helping people find their communities. And planning like this can help to "break the silence" that often surrounds these fundamentally human issues; it can free consumers to ask for the help they need.

Responding to consumers' needs in this area requires first and foremost individuals who are comfortable with their own sexuality, and who are able to be sensitive and respectful. Individuals with psychiatric disabilities often need help in exploring their own sexuality, in accepting and appreciating their bodies, and in learning or relearning the social skills associated with developing healthy sexual relationships. People who have been institutionalized often need help in learning alternatives to what they learned in those settings, such as public displays of sexual behavior, or no sexual behavior at all. Of critical importance is the provision of accurate information about sexuality; physical self-care; contraception; and safe, responsible, and respectful sexual behavior.

The desire for a partner with whom to share one's life is as basic to a person with a psychiatric disability as to any other person. Because of the lack of experience in forming such relationships, or because such relationships may not have been supported by professionals in the past, consumers often need help in negotiating and nurturing the development of long-term committed relationships. After beginning such relationships, consumers may need help in conflict resolution, as well as in making important and far-reaching decisions about marriage and about bearing, adopting, and raising children. Given the profound potential social support in such long-term relationships, promoting change in this area can provide some of the most far-reaching improvements in consumers' lives.

IMPLICATIONS OF A SOCIAL INTEGRATION
FOCUS FOR MENTAL HEALTH WORKERS

Promoting social integration among mental health and rehabilitation workers starts with a belief not only that such relationships are centrally important, but also that they are possible for people with even the most significant psychiatric disabilities. It is only within the context of this fundamental belief that mental health professionals will begin to do whatever needs to be done to promote healthy social networks. This belief is necessary in order to overcome the barriers within programs, and to make relationships with professionals more meaningful to consumers.

Reidy (1992) points out that once mental health workers grasp the meaning of social integration, their first question is often "What's my role?" They also quickly come to understand that the traditional mandate for professional distance, that is, "boundaries" that are expected between helper and client, create a number of barriers to expanding their roles. Finally, they may have legitimate concerns about ethical issues in shifting their roles, such as about the power differences in relationships.

Boundaries and Relationships

Curtis (1992), who provides extensive training for mental health staffs on issues of boundaries and ethics in relationships, mentions that unless staff members are actively and continually struggling with such issues, they are not really engaged in integration and empowerment. The traditional sense of boundaries in clinical relationships was based in the psychoanalytical notion that the task of a therapist was to focus exclusively on the world view of the client, and never to allow his or her own personality, experience, values, and so forth to intrude on the person's unfolding sense of his or her own experience. As the concept of boundaries evolved in practice, it became a way to "understand" the very unique and often unnatural relationship between a paid helper and a client; in the process, it became a normative system in which virtually no reciprocity in relationships was tolerable. In this context, it is not unusual for some agencies to define the greeting of a client by a therapist on a street corner as a violation of confidentiality. Unfortunately, such unnatural constraints on what are often very intimate relationships have served to perpetuate the great inequities in power in these relationships. This fact was pointed out by early feminist theorists (e.g., Friedan, 1963), who saw much of therapy as an exercise in which male "culture bearers" treated women for problems such as depression by defining these problems as internal and personal, rather than as results of political and social oppression. Out of this consciousness came the slogans "No intimacy without reciprocity," and "The personal is political"—slogans that in turn gave birth to consciousness-raising groups among women.

Another rationale for strict boundaries between clients and professionals arises from legitimate concerns about exploitation in such relationships—in part based on differential power, and in part on the fact that professionals often control access to resources that are basic and literally life-sustaining for people with psychiatric disabilities. Therefore, clear attention to roles is critical; however, it should not serve as a barrier to creating relationships that are more genuine and reciprocal, and that include a wider array of activities and connections over time.

Curtis (1992) suggests a number of important questions that staff members can ask themselves as they navigate changing boundaries:

> What is the justification for my behavior or choice in this situation? Can I explain it clearly to the consumer and to other professionals? What are the benefits of this behavior or choice to the consumer? Are there other less problematic ways to achieve the same outcome? Why am I choosing not to use them? What are the benefits to me? Am I getting something out of doing things this way, that I can clearly explain to the consumer and to other professionals? What are the possible problems that could occur for the consumer, other community members, or myself? How could my behavior or choice be misconstrued by the consumer or others? How will I deal with that? (p. 5)

In short, staff members need to become increasingly flexible about boundaries; in the process, they need to be very thoughtful and willing to communicate openly with everyone involved.

Although traditional boundaries have had some value, they lose their utility, according to Reidy (1992), when they become an excuse to maintain attitudes that people with psychiatric disabilities are somehow a "breed apart." In such cases, professionals may use boundaries as a way of avoiding dealing with individuals as valued, respected human beings. The prospect of opening their social networks, their homes, and their lives to persons with psychiatric disabilities may be very threatening to some staff members; if so this requires an honest personal examination of which boundaries need to be preserved and which need to be changed. At a more fundamental level, staff members who are socially uncomfortable with people with psychiatric disabilities are inappropriate as service providers for these individuals.

Shifting Roles

Reidy (1992) points out that staff members need to expand their roles when they focus on social integration, and that the most critical role shift is that of becoming an "ambassador" to the community, or a "community connector." This involves helping consumers gain the skills they need, helping consumers make actual social contacts, and then supporting them in sustaining those relationships.

New Skills

These new roles, according to Reidy (1992) also imply a specific set of skills on the part of mental health workers. Staff members need to be able to do research on a person's interests; they also need to be effective at motivating consumers, providing emotional support, creating opportunities over and over without giving up, and encouraging consumers without pressuring them. Finally, they need to be socially competent, able to follow through and attend to details, but able at the same time to stay in the background.

New Core Attitudes

Reidy (1992) concludes that the most important change required of staff members is the development of four core attitudes: possibility (seeing the capabilities of consumers and the possibility of connecting them with others); necessity (being wholeheartedly convinced that social integration is crucial for everyone involved); equality (seeing people with psychiatric disabilities as equal to themselves and to others, regardless of their current level of functioning); and equanimity (taking things in stride without being pulled off course by setbacks). These attitudes form an excellent set of criteria for recruiting staff and volunteers in social integration efforts.

SUCCESSFUL SOCIAL
INTEGRATION STRATEGIES

Communities interested in furthering social integration between people with psychiatric disabilities and "typical" citizens have a wealth of experience to draw upon from other communities that have begun to take on this critical challenge. Following are eight successful strategies, drawn from the work of a variety of groups that are trying to promote social integration throughout North America.

Promoting Peer Support Networks

Although much of the emphasis in this chapter has been on integrated relationships between people with and without obvious psychiatric disabilities, an important strategy for promoting social integration is to help individuals begin to identify with others with the same disabilities, but in a different and more powerful way than has traditionally been the case within mental health programs. The paradox here is that in spite of the fact that people with psychiatric disabilities have been separated from communities and grouped with others with the same label, the effect of this grouping has been to place them in essentially devalued roles. Peer support and self-help groups are now coming together on a very different basis: with an understanding of the commonality of mental health consumers' experience, and with a clear sense of consumers' abilities to help one another understand what has happened to them and, in the process, to get on with their lives.

According to Deegan (1992), peer support and self-help, in which consumers develop a ''consciousness'' of what has happened, an understanding of how people with psychiatric disabilities are oppressed, and perhaps even the development of a common language through which they can start to talk about their own recovery, is an essential first step in the process of consumers' taking charge of their lives. This positive and powerful affiliation with peers helps many individuals to move beyond the stigmatizing assumption that people with psychiatric disabilities have internalized—that is, the assumption that people with this label are inferior and have little potential. This set of beliefs in itself serves to disconnect consumers from others who have had the same experiences.

In some cases, promoting self-help and peer support results in consumers' wanting to share significant parts of their lives—for example, residing together or even starting an alternative university (F. Friese, personal communication, August 1991). At times, it may seem to advocates that these directions are contrary to integration values; in fact, they are attempts to build community and to build a distinct culture, and therefore can be tremendously empowering to individuals as they choose to move into more integrated relationships in the future. Chamberlin (1987), for example, makes a strong case for such ''separatism.'' The difference between these efforts and traditional segregated services is that consumers are fundamentally making choices and decisions about their own lifestyles; the consumers themselves are in charge; and the bases of coming together are a sense of the oppression of segregated services; and a sense of capability in helping one another.

Developing a Network of Nondisabled Allies in the Community

Advocates and professionals who accept social integration as a critical goal become a core group of allies that can organize a wider network of citizens, staff members, and others to become involved in the lives of people with disabilities, on the basis of freely given relationships rooted in common interests. These individuals, with their sense of individual commitment, can serve as a cadre of "community connectors." As such, they can help to build richer social networks over time. Although citizen advocacy programs and other volunteer efforts in some communities have successfully achieved these goals, it is important not to think automatically in terms of organizing such an effort as a program or service; this often implies a lack of reciprocity, unequal power relationships, and a lack of common interests that bind people together.

Making a Personal Commitment to Building Relationships

Promoting social integration comes from a genuine desire to change the nature of one's own relationships; it is not something that one person does to or for another. Therefore, those who are most effective at promoting social networks are those who have a genuine personal commitment to building relationships and connections with those with whom they are involved. Whether working with, guiding, or teaching someone about specific skills involved in relationship building, or directly accompanying someone to one's own church or synagogue, the quality of the individual relationship is critical.

Creating Access to the "Affiliational Life" of the Community

Relationships are ultimately built on the basis of common interests. Therefore, a major strategy is to shift the "common interest" in a relationship from the person's disability or difference (the focus of a professional–client relationship) to one that has nothing to do with the disability, but instead represents a valued role. McKnight (1987) asserts that the affiliational life of a community represents the central resource for social integration, and is the only long-term supportive alternative to human service "systems of care." According to McKnight, any community, even the smallest one, has a plethora of clubs, social groups, and activities that meet/are carried on every day and night; these are based on common interests as diverse as bridge, horseback riding, macrame, and volunteer fire prevention.

Reidy (1992), in directing a major social integration effort (see below), has developed a set of practical guidelines for creating access to the affiliational life of a community. She advises staff members and advocates to do the following:

- *Get connected themselves.* Staff members or advocates who live in different communities, and who are not closely connected with the social life of the communities in which people with psychiatric disabilities live, are not particularly effective.
- *Involve connected people.* In forming new contacts, professionals/advocates should seek to connect consumers with others who are strategically connected socially.
- *Know the person.* All connections must be based on an in-depth knowledge of the individual consumer.
- *Learn about the group or setting beforehand.* This kind of research is essential to avoid situations such as the one with Helen, described above (Lutfiyya, 1988).
- *Keep it simple and informal.* Staff members/advocates should talk about life for consumers in the way citizens talk about their own lives, avoiding the use of "networking" language, or the mental health mystique of using fancy language for everyday events.
- *Be flexible.* Professionals/advocates should keep an eye on how the supports need to change as the situation and the needs change; they should avoid thinking about connections as "placements" that they can control.
- *Put their best foot forward and help consumers do the same.* "Ordinary" people often have misconceptions about mental health staff or about people with disabilities; thus, it's critical for all parties to present themselves as positively as possible.
- *Pay attention to the match between a consumer and a group.* The quality of the match is much more important than the level of disability over time.
- *Pay attention to details.* Are dues getting paid? Is transportation arranged? Since details can be overwhelming, it's often better to do this with one person, not with five.
- *Follow through.*
- *Work behind the scenes.* Professionals/advocates should not come rushing in to solve problems; they should respect natural consequences, while supporting change.

Working with Consumers One Person at a Time

As noted throughout this book, integration, in any of its myriad forms, cannot be packaged and must involve work with one person at a time. This is especially critical in social integration, since so much of what any person brings to a social situation and set of connections consists of his or her internal goals, needs, preferences, and vulnerabilities. The potential for further social rejection of consumers in the absence of a thoughtful approach, is high. Therefore, it is essential to promote social integration only within the context of real, in-depth relationships with other people, and to do so one person at a time. One practical implication is that when a consumer is being accompanied to a social activity, it is usually better to have just one person do the accompanying, not more. The implication of this is that effective work on social integration occurs within unique, one-on-one relationships. Trying to promote social integration simply through adding this function to a variety of other staff or clinical responsibilities is unlikely to be successful.

Arranging the Involvement of Others

In taking on the responsibility to connect consumers with others in the community, it is easy to become overwhelmed, particularly when a consumer is socially isolated and desperate for connection. Thus, it is critical to involve others in supporting the development of social opportunities, and to provide meaningful connections with each individual consumer, so that clear expectations and limits can be mutually agreed upon. Involving others, such as volunteers, in promoting a consumer's social integration, of course, expands the consumer's access to social networks, activities, and potential social relationships.

Opening Up One's Own Social Network

In a recent workshop on integration for a group of clinicians in Maine, I was struck by the story of a clinical supervisor who reported that until recently she had held a very traditional view of clinical boundaries, and that this had served her well in her work. Unfortunately, she was hospitalized several months before the workshop for surgery. No single room was available, and, to her great dismay, she found herself sharing a room with a former client who was seen by other clinicians as perhaps the most troublesome client in the agency—an attitude she shared to some extent. Over the course of several weeks of hospitalization, she found that her relationship with this person was completely transformed. Pressed by the hospital staff to be compliant and dependent, she began to learn important survival skills from her former client about dealing with an institutional environment. Gradually, she began to understand who this person was at a very different level, and found herself sharing her own experiences and vulnerabilities. After a while, they began to talk truthfully, and somewhat painfully, about each of their very different perceptions of their former clinical relationship. In the process, they became friends. The clinician ended her story by saying that this experience had caused her to significantly rethink her posture with all of her clients.

As powerful as the impact of this story was, even more powerful was the reaction of other workshop participants, several of whom then chose to reveal for the first time that they had experienced a psychiatric hospitalization in the past, but had never felt safe enough in the agency to share this experience they held in common with their clients.

If social integration is not to be pursued as a program or service, then it is critical that professionals or advocates involved in this effort consider opening up their own social networks to those individuals with psychiatric disabilities with whom they want to develop friendly relationships.

Creating Circles of Support

The goal of many social integration efforts is not only to increase the number, diversity, and intimacy of consumers' social connections, but to help create "circles of support" through which friends, neighbors, and coworkers can help to sustain consumers socially and emotionally, including during crises. A major threat to social relationships, particularly those in their early stages, is that when a crisis occurs professionals tend to move in to help, and members of natural support systems tend to back off and let the professionals take charge. Building a strong circle of support with people who are connected to an individual's day-to-day life in the community is the best safeguard against the danger that the person will be extruded once again from the community during a crisis.

LOCAL COMMUNITY EXAMPLES

Social Integration Project (Amherst, Massachusetts)

The Social Integration Project (Reidy, 1992) is a consumer-operated service initiative through which people with psychiatric disabilities and "typical" citizens are encouraged to make social connections; the guidelines listed above are used. In addition to building an experience of social connections that has provided valuable guidance to other communities, this project has also been helpful in training mental health workers in the area to take on a number of the challenges related to boundaries, relationships, roles, skills, and attitudes. The project has been successful in significantly expanding the social networks of members with psychiatric disabilities.

Clustered Apartment Project
(Santa Clara County, California)

Originally funded as a consumer-directed supported housing program, the focus of the Clustered Apartment Project (Mandiberg & Telles, 1990) has been on building a community of ex-patients who will develop an increased sense of consciousness about their experience in the mental health system, and who will then have the capacity to support one another over time. The structures used to accomplish these goals include frequent meetings of the community in which norms, rules, and needs are discussed. Originally, the housing component of this project was organized so that units were scattered throughout the community; over time, however, the members wanted a higher level of support and social connection with one another, and thus began to move closer together. Eventually, this evolved into a "clustered apartment" arrangement of "fourplexes."

In order to respond to periodic crises, the consumers organized one vacant apartment into a Center of Attention, through which any consumer wanting support could go to the apartment and receive help from peers. (This service has been described in greater detail in Chapters Three and Six.) The Center of Attention was credited by the community with a dramatic reduction in hospitalizations in the first year. Following that success, however, the consumers then decided that they would prefer to organize more outreach-oriented support to one another's homes, and transformed the Center of Attention into a mobile volunteer support system.

Following several years of operation, staff members were asked to expand their efforts to a nearby community that consisted primarily of Southeast Asian refugees with psychiatric disabilities. The staff members chose to organize an autonomous project and to build a second community within the context of these very different cultural needs. Over time, members of the community have built individual connections outside of their own ex-patient community.

Canadian Mental Health Association
(Vancouver, British Columbia, Division)

A third example of a local community effort is neither a program nor a project, but a mutually supportive community that has emerged simply out of the joint involvement of people with psychiatric disabilities and their allies in a common set of advocacy activities. In the last several years, the British Columbia Division of the Canadian Mental Health Association has taken on a number of consumer-operated projects, and hired consumers to staff these activities. In the process, a strong community has developed among people with and without psychiatric disabilities, and the people with psychiatric disabilities have been introduced quite naturally to the social networks of those without labels. This provides an excellent example of how advocates guided by clear values, simply by taking on a variety of other integration and empowerment initiatives, can also advance social integration in both natural and powerful ways.

EMPOWERING CONSUMERS AND THEIR FAMILIES

CHAPTER 10

Sharing Power
with Consumers

Social revolutions occur when people who are defined as the problem seize enough power to redefine the solution.
—S. D. ALINSKY (1971, p. 7)

Empowerment of people with disabilities occurs through three strategies: people having the information and knowledge they need; people having economic opportunities; and people achieving their civil rights.
—W. GRAVES (1990)

From a national policy perspective, mental health and rehabilitation service systems are shifting toward empowerment and choice as core values. This policy shift has already had a significant impact in many parts of North America, including a growing recognition that consumer-directed supports and services are an essential part of the solution to the challenge of community integration; a growing number of studies of the preferences of consumers for housing, work, education, and social support; increased consumer participation in decision making; increased consumer employment in mental health and rehabilitation services programs; increased consumer involvement in the training of professionals and in public education; and increased funding for consumer-operated service programs.

The National Association of State Mental Health Program Directors (NASMHPD, 1989) has issued policy guidelines for all state mental health agencies that make the following clear: Former patients and current consumers have the expertise and experience to make unique contributions to the mental health system; states should include consumers in meaningful numbers and in meaningful ways in program development, policy formulation, quality assurance, system designs, education of professionals, and provision of direct services; states should provide support to facilitate such participation, including financial support, education, and social assistance; and states should support and finance consumer-operated self-help and mutual support services in each locality.

This statement was the product of a work group consisting of consumers and of state and federal mental health representatives, chaired by Paul (Dorfner) Engels, then president of the National Mental Health Consumers Association. Staff members of the Center for Community Change through Housing and Support led by Laurie Curtis and Bill Montague, then worked with several consumer leaders (Howie the Harp and Dayna Caron) to develop a number of specific strategies to implement this new state mental health policy, summarized below (Curtis, McCabe, Montague, Caron, & Harp, 1991). Similar trends are reflected in Canada's provincial mental health systems, fueled in part by growing acceptance of the framework for support (Pape, 1990; see Chapter Two) and in part by the growing National Network for Mental Health, a coalition of consumer-survivor groups across Canada.

This chapter describes strategies that can be used to begin implementing a vision of full and powerful consumer participation in the service system in four critical areas: (1) policy and planning; (2) mental health service delivery; (3) training; and (4) consumer- operated programs. It also discusses the implications for mental health professionals and for organizations of sharing power with consumers, and describes various resource materials available on this subject.

STRATEGIES FOR SHARING
POWER WITH CONSUMERS

Recognizing and Connecting with
the Self-Help Movement

The consumer movement has been growing rapidly. Although as recently as 1987 there were no organized national efforts, there are now two major national groups in the United States (the National Mental Health Consumers Association and the National Alliance of Psychiatric Survivors) and one in Canada (the National Network for Mental Health). Within the larger disability rights movement, people with psychiatric disabilities have begun to play an increasingly visible role. The success of their efforts is attested to by the inclusion of psychiatric disabilities in both of the major recent pieces of disability rights legislation in the United States: the 1990 Americans with Disabilities Act, and the 1989 Federal Fair Housing Amendments Act.

A recent survey of consumer-operated services and consumer organizations (Specht, 1988) identified active groups in every U.S. state, and in some cases dozens of groups in a particular state. Similarly, the National Network for Mental Health (S. Hardie, personal communication, September 1993) has organized consumer and psychiatric groups in every Canadian province into a national organization.

What do these groups do? The groups surveyed by Specht (1988) reported such diverse activities as individual advocacy related to services, entitlements, and consumer rights; advocating for systems change by educating legislators, producing new legislation, pushing for new or increased funding, becoming involved in mental health policy development, promoting research, engaging in class action litigation, and educating the public; providing crisis intervention and short-term crisis shelters; offering peer mutual support through Twelve Step programs, buddy systems, rap groups, and peer counseling; operating drop-in centers and clubhouses; providing case management and housing services; evaluating and monitoring services; and community organizing.

The survey also found that consumers were being employed, that they had formal roles in higher education in many states, and that most states had projects to develop additional consumer-operated services. Chapter Three describes the great variety of community support services that have already been developed by consumers. Nonetheless, while states were spending about $1.3 million for consumer-operated services (Specht, 1988), this amount represented only about 0.25% of their overall budgets. Survey respondents felt that what were most needed were additional technical assistance to states and consumer groups; additional funding; and increased education, training, and systems change efforts within states.

Since the Specht survey was completed, it appears that such efforts have been growing at a rapid pace. Eleven states now support high-level offices of consumer affairs. Consumer-operated services are available in nearly every state and province, and the professional literature has begun to incorporate information on the consumer perspective, on empowerment, and on the consumer movement. Annual consumer conferences ("Alternatives Conferences") now draw thousands of attendees in the United States, and the first national Canadian conference of the National Network for Mental Health was recently held in Toronto. A recent telecast of Self-Help Live, a national interactive teleconference produced for and by ex-patients through White Light Communications, drew 10,000 attendees for a single telecast.

As the movement of people with psychiatric disabilities continues to grow, it is critical for advocates to work closely with this self-help movement both locally and at the state/provincial level—developing collaborative projects, referring individual consumers to become involved, and supporting these groups as they become more visible and influential in the community.

Understanding the Power of Organizing

Advocates, whether they have psychiatric disabilities or not, are greatly in need of new and creative ideas to assist the consumer/ex-patient movement in becoming a more organized and powerful political force. There are many examples of how basic organizing strategies are already having a direct impact in some areas. One such example—the story of a consumer advocate in New Mexico whose self-help group succeeded in overturning a local librarian's policy of not granting library cards to "mental health clients" without a professional's signature—has been described in Chapter Four.

As another example, one community had recently formed a community land trust organization to develop affordable housing. This organization, because of a lack of familiarity with the need, had little interest in working on affordable housing issues as they related to people with psychiatric disabilities. In response, rather than simply using educational or persuasive techniques, one local organizer began encouraging consumers interested in affordable housing first to sign up for membership in the organization, and then to compete, as any member could, for positions on the board of directors. As they did so successfully, the organization became much more interested, and developed a number of limited-equity cooperatives that consumers in that community now own.

The work of M-POWER, a statewide consumer organizing project based in Boston, Massachusetts, provides perhaps the best illustration of effective organizing strategies among people with the most significant psychiatric disabilities (P. E. Deegan, personal communication, June 1994). M-POWER is completely member run, and concentrates on in-depth support of individuals, assisting them to become self-advocates and advocates for change. The approach is to organize local chapters, each of which has a coordinator assigned to work with all members of the group to develop critical thinking about what has happened to them in the mental health system, and, through intensive dialogue in which peers serve as both teachers and learners, to explore ways that they can take back their power. The goal of these efforts is to develop broad leadership, rather than have only a few consumers attempt to represent all others. In these local chapters, people with the most serious disabilities are running the meetings, serving on boards, and participating in various advocacy activities.

Deegan describes this process as a "transformation of consciousness," where people pass through several predictable phases: (1) angry indignation ("Something wrong has occurred that is not my fault"); (2) hope ("There is something that we can do about it—there is strength in our numbers"); (3) personal empowerment and responsibility ("There is a specific contribution I can make").

Deegan describes the process of developing this broad based leadership as very labor intensive and as an indication, if mental health systems are serious about broad consumer representation, of the kinds of resources that will be necessary to make this happen. Agendas for all group meetings, which may involve 30–70 members in a particular chapter, are set well in advance. Organizers, who are paid, well trained, and carefully supervised, meet with *each* meeting participant well before the meeting to provide information about the agenda, to explain the significance of each item, and to help people develop a point of view on every agenda item. Thus, in contrast with many mental health planning meetings where consumers may be silent or unprepared in M-POWER meetings, everyone comes with an opinion on each issue. Thus, the meetings are active and bustling with ideas. Meeting facilitators need to be highly skilled to give everyone air time and to reach consensus on what actions the group will take. When the group is considering a demonstration or other action, they will take the time to work through all possible consequences in advance, so they will be prepared. At times, people come to meetings who are in a crisis and need support, and the group is expected to deal with such issues empathetically, and to also get its work done.

After every meeting, organizers again talk with each member, reviewing how the member felt about their participation in the meeting; any concerns the member had about decisions having gone against their point of view; and how the member would like to approach their role in the next meeting. Through this process, Deegan reports that people who are seen as "much too unmotivated" or "much too disabled" to assume leadership routinely do so (P. E. Deegan, personal communication, June 1994).

Promoting Consumer Roles in Policy and Planning

Who is the System for?
—Popular consumer advocacy button

At a service system level, the behavior of mental health leaders and policy makers is critical in setting a highly visible example for full consumer involvement that will be emulated in agencies and programs throughout the system. Mental health systems should expect, plan for, and facilitate consumer participation in all planning and policy-making bodies at state/provincial, regional and local levels. They should invite and support active consumer participation in setting priorities, making major funding decisions, and developing and evaluating programs.

Some mental health systems are moving toward an explicit goal of 50% consumer membership on planning and policy-making bodies, including agency boards of directors, task forces, study groups, advisory committees, and so forth. Larger numbers of participants help to compensate for changes in individuals' situations that may affect their ability to participate actively. Recent reform plans in Ontario and British Columbia stress that a majority of seats on local mental health planning councils must be filled by consumers and family members. Similarly, Maine is phasing in a new Regional Board structure with 50% consumer and family representation and limited participation by professionals. After intensive training, these boards take over contracting responsibilities for the local mental health service area.

Mental health systems need to provide personal support and resources to consumer participants in order to ensure high levels of involvement. The particular kinds of support that are needed depend on each individual's needs and experience, but they may include in-depth orientation and explanation of the process; clarifying expectations; providing feedback about a person's participation; confidence building; ongoing review of events and issues of concern; and so forth. When the location of a meeting is not convenient, it is important to arrange for transportation. Holding meetings where consumers ordinarily spend time (e.g., at a clubhouse or drop-in center) also increases participation. Whenever professionals are participating in a planning or program development meeting, they should invite consumers along, and then provide transportation, support, and encouragement for future involvement. Money often needs to be advanced for transportation and meal expenses.

Consumers should be provided with financial compensation whenever others are paid to participate. Often professionals attend such meetings as part of their jobs, and are therefore being compensated, but consumers rarely find themselves in that situation. Compensation is a statement that consumers' participation is valued and that their time is valuable.

It is important to plan for a wide range of types and degrees of participation, so that consumers can choose the level of involvement they feel most comfortable with. Consumers often need encouragement, as their needs and willingness to participate change over time.

It is also important to solicit and facilitate the involvement of a wide variety of individuals, not just an identified few; this empowers more consumers to take an active role, and provides for greater diversity of opinion and experience. Elitist practices that involve the same few individuals' being called upon to represent all consumers (usually without financial compensation) can make these people feel like "tokens," can lead to their feeling overextended, and can seriously limit the breadth of consumer perspectives available to a group.

It is important to solicit written information formally and regularly from active ex-patient/consumer organizations regarding their concerns about the current system and their ideas for improving it. This information can then be given to policy makers to be used in implementing needed changes.

Mental health systems can create consumer councils that bring together consumer representatives from all of the mental health programs in a locality, a region, or even a state/province, and thus provide policy makers with regular face-to-face contact with service recipients throughout the system. Vermont has successfully implemented this approach. These councils can provide input to policies and practices; can draw attention to the service, training, and support needs of both providers and consumers; and can function as a program development body—managing a pool of funds for consumer-operated services, reviewing applications, and making decisions about allocation of these funds.

Increasing numbers of mental health systems have established an office of consumer affairs to function as a "watchdog" for the system, and to provide an in-house advocacy presence that represents the concerns of ex-patients and consumers. This office can provide ombudsman services and manage grievance procedures in the system as well. In addition, hiring ex-patients in such senior positions sends a powerful symbolic message to the mental health field.

Finally, one community with whom the Center for Community Change has been working, has begun to formulate a strategy to develop an independent consumer-operated organization that would conduct routine evaluations of consumer satisfaction in all mental health programs in the area. It would then make that information available, along with outcome evaluation data on each of the programs, to prospective consumers. Thus, a consumer who is considering any service in that community would have easy access to information on the effectiveness of the service agency in achieving what it advertises itself as doing (e.g., "88% of the consumers who use this employment program are working within 3 months of beginning the program, and 73% are continuing to work after 12 months"), as well as information on how satisfied consumers are with the service (e.g., "92% of the consumers of this employment service felt strongly that staff members were very respectful of their own preferences and choices, and were effective in helping them find work").

It is important to include consumer involvement in any research and evaluation activities that take place in a system. Too often, the investigation of "what works" is limited to professionals' perspectives. Consumers can play meaningful roles in planning and designing research, in collecting information, in interpreting results, and in disseminating that information. Of vital importance in any program-focused evaluation are (1) soliciting consumers' views on need and preferences before a program is designed; (2) building in monitoring by consumers of any programs that are operating; (3) building in routine collection of information on consumers' satisfaction with the program; and (4) measuring concrete benefits (outcomes) among clients.

Program development efforts, as noted above, should proceed from a systematic gathering of information from consumers focused on the question: "What would you find helpful?" Recently, the Vermont Department of Mental Health and Mental Retardation, which is phasing down its only state hospital and is therefore having to learn what crisis alternatives would be acceptable to consumers who were previously involuntarily committed at the state hospital, organized a series of public forums and a task force to solicit consumer input into the kinds of crisis services consumers felt were needed. The *Final Report of the Vermont Task Force on Crisis Options* (Blanch, 1988) has been influential in creating a number of alternatives to institutionalization.

Finally, agencies and systems should continually examine how they can involve consumers in innovative ways whenever critical policy, hiring, funding, legislative, and other decisions are made. A particularly important locus of power sharing is an agency's board of directors. A real irony exists when service agencies that are organized to support people with psychiatric disabilities have no members of this group in decision-making roles. By way of analogy, imagine the protests that would be heard if organizations formed to meet the needs of women or people with mobility impairments had no women or people with physical disabilities on their boards of directors. In fact, in the case of organizations serving these two groups, it is likely that the boards are either mostly or completely drawn from the groups in question.

Fortunately, there are beginning to be some hopeful signs of greater consumer involvement within mental health programs. Recently, I visited a local chapter of the Canadian Mental Health Association in Dawson Creek, a rural community of British Columbia. When I arrived there, I was delighted to find that the majority of the chapter's board of directors consisted of people who had a psychiatric label. Working with them on developing housing programs provided me with a glimpse of the future of how such services may operate in North America.

It is important to note that, given the great differences in power among policy makers, professionals, and advocates, the road to true consumer involvement, participation, and power sharing is fraught with dangers of co-opting, tokenism, and disappointment. Therefore, it is critical for policy makers and advocates, in soliciting the experience of people with psychiatric disabilities, to be very thoughtful about the process. They need to ask themselves, "Why do we want this involvement?" "How serious are we about acting on consumers' advice?"

Shifting power to consumers is a complicated, difficult, and long-term process. In the final analysis, the success of these efforts often comes down to a question of how much those with power truly value the involvement of consumers; how serious they are about sharing power; how serious they are about making the resources of the system increasingly match what consumers want; and how willing they are to have decisions made increasingly by consumers. If they do hold these values, they will directly support consumer involvement in any way necessary to make it real. They will provide training; invite significant numbers of consumers to participate; accommodate and support consumers; and keep listening even when arguments and anger grow hot. They will continue to focus all discussions on real human needs, and will hold themselves accountable by being clear about whether a group is an advisory or a decision-making group, about how much power consumers actually have in specific decisions, and about what will happen with their input. Similarly, if consumer advocates value their own time and wish to operate with power and integrity, they will participate only in those activities that are valued in these tangible ways, and will say no to any others. They will also work hard to gather information from other consumers who are not present in a particular process, so that they can represent this diversity of views.

The major strategy for building consumer involvement in policy and planning is to listen, listen, and listen some more.

Promoting Consumer Roles in Mental Health Service Delivery

Mental health systems can exercise leadership in overcoming traditional patterns of discrimination against consumers by employing consumers in all aspects of the work force, including clinical and administrative roles at every level of the organization. Some systems and agencies are setting a goal, for example, that a minimum of 10% of their positions should be filled by ex-patients or current consumers after a certain period of time.

A particularly effective strategy is for systems to begin hiring qualified consumers/ex-patients for high-level policy positions. One state mental health department, for example, recently hired an ex-patient, who many years before had been rejected for vocational rehabilitation services as "unemployable." She now directs the state's multimillion-dollar vocational services program. Such an appointment sends a powerful message to the mental health system, to the vocational rehabilitation system, to the state legislature, and to the general public about the capabilities of people with psychiatric disabilities.

Although consumers are being hired in increasing numbers in mental health systems, a recent national survey (Wilson & Mahler, 1991) found that many consumer employees had significant concerns related to their employment in mental health agencies. These concerns included tokenism; the need for role clarification (whether they are seen as professionals or clients); prejudiced attitudes on the part of other staff and clients; job expectations that conflict with their values (e.g., involuntary treatment decisions); segregated jobs or roles (e.g., "consumer case managers"); their jobs' being viewed by other staff members as rehabilitation, rather than as real jobs; lack of comparability in salaries; not being included in social gatherings initiated by other staff members; past or present personal relationships with other service recipients; unclear job descriptions and employer expectations; disability accommodation issues; confidentiality issues; and issues surrounding their personal decisions about disclosing their life experiences. It is critical to create opportunities in the workplace to discuss concerns such as these openly and to resolve them equitably, in ways that improve the overall capacity of the organization to continue to diversify its work force.

It is important to develop an affirmative action policy that will increase consumer employment among those who meet the requirements for a position, and to give recognition to the importance of the added expertise that consumers have gained simply by being service recipients. Consumers need to be made aware that they are eligible for, and desired in these positions. Positions can be advertised, for example, as "Consumer preferred." Such advertisements should be posted and circulated in places where ex-patients and current consumers are likely to see them. It is also important to reach out and hire people from outside the system (i.e., people who are no longer involved in receiving services).

Mental health systems need to define and develop policies for "reasonable accommodations" for people with psychiatric disabilities (see Chapter Eight). They need to ensure, for example, that on-the-job peer counseling and support will be available; to acknowledge the need for leaves for mental-health-related reasons, in addition to physical health problems; to develop schedules with flexible hours; and to make sure that each consumer employee has a place to go and "sound off" when necessary. Whenever possible, liberal and extended leave should be provided as needed, with or without pay. It is also important to guarantee employment security when these leaves occur. Agencies should work with employee assistance programs to make them more sensitive to the needs of consumers, and then make these programs available to consumer employees.

It is important to review the agency's policies for content and language that may represent barriers to consumer employment. These policies need to be fair and respectful toward consumers with regard to pay structures, grievance procedures, personnel qualifications, and evaluation procedures. It is necessary to ensure that individuals have the resources and supports needed to do the work. Consumer employees should also be provided with an extensive orientation to agency procedures and expectations. Cooperative relationships should be developed with external support services that these employees may need, such as mental health services, vocational rehabilitation services, job coaches, interpreters, and so forth.

Consumers should be given the message that their unique skills and expertise are valued in the organization. They should be helped to identify ways to use these skills and expertise in their jobs. For example, consumers/ex-patients who have struggled in the past with substance abuse and being homeless can often be of help to consumers who currently face these challenges. Moreover, at times nondisabled staff members need training and support while they are learning to accept consumer employees and to work with them as peers. Thus, systems and agencies need to affirm the unique contributions and needs of every member of the team in this process, not only those who are consumers.

It is also important to make sure that staff members who happen to be current consumers or ex-patients are included in all informal activities of the organization (meetings, social events, training, etc.). Finally, it should be emphasized that the effort to incorporate consumers into the mental health work force should be viewed as an opportunity to develop a more supportive organization for *all* mental health workers. Often, agencies that begin hiring consumers find that staff members who are not identified as consumers need the same supports or other individualized assistance, and resent it if these same accommodations are not offered to them. Providing equal accommodations serves to promote integration, as well as a healthier and more empowering workplace for the whole staff. Furthermore, such agencies find that hiring consumers encourages other staff members who have had a history of mental health problems, but who were reluctant to disclose this before, to "come out of the closet"; they should be both valued and supported for their courage in doing so. Support groups for current and former consumers among the staff are vital. Because of the need for peer support, it is rarely a good idea to hire just one consumer in an agency. Such practices create an exaggerated sense of "differentness" and encourage special treatment.

It is possible to encourage consumer employment more broadly in a system by developing a capacity to train consumers as mental health workers who are ready to fill positions as these open up throughout a mental health system. This strategy has been successfully employed throughout Colorado by the Psychiatric Rehabilitation Training Program. This program investigates openings in mental health centers throughout the state; analyzes each job; recruits and trains consumers who are interested in these jobs; and then facilitates their transition into the jobs. If an original "match" does not work out, the training program itself hires the consumer until he or she can secure a similar job in another site.

Promoting Consumer Roles in Training

Mental health systems can guarantee significant levels of consumer/ex-patient participation in all training events, both as teachers and as learners. They can fund the participation of consumers in national, state/provincial, and local conferences and training programs for professionals; they can also pay the expenses of consumers to attend meetings set up for consumers.

Consumers/ex-patients can be invited to as many public speaking opportunities as possible, including civic groups, classroom presentations, service clubs, and so forth. If a mental health staff member who is not a consumer is invited to speak on a topic, he or she can insist on sharing the time with a consumer presenter. If this is refused, the staff member should consider not attending the meeting.

Mental health systems and advocates can lobby with higher education professionals to include ex-patients/consumers as teachers in programs focused on human services and mental health, particularly in the core mental health disciplines (psychology, psychiatry, nursing, and social work). Consumers can make presentations in a class, or serve as adjunct faculty members, and thereby teach or coteach one or more courses. Similarly, mental health systems should work with higher education to ensure that consumer empowerment and self-help content are incorporated into relevant parts of the curriculum. (See Chapter Six.) Finally, it is important to develop ways for those consumers/ex-patients who wish to return to college to do so with support.

Promoting Consumer-Operated Programs

Again, Chapter Three gives examples of consumer groups providing the full range of community support services. Unfortunately, as noted above, public mental health funding for consumer-operated services typically constitutes far less than 1% of the total mental health budget in a system (Specht, 1988). By comparison, state hospital services usually consume about 70% of the budget, while community support services are allocated 30% or less. Mental health systems can designate a set percentage of funding (e.g., 10%), to be achieved over a certain number of years, to be allocated to consumer-operated services. To begin this process, they can document the amount of funding currently allocated to these services. They can then invite broad consumer input into the types of services and alternatives they would like to see available (e.g., hot lines/"warm lines"; drop-in centers; safe houses; consumer crisis services; assistance with basic needs, such as benefits counseling, housing, and work; and peer support). This input can be used to design an implementation plan for consumer-operated services in the system.

In many cases, funding consumer-operated services is not a simple proposition. Many systems have found that existing rules, regulations, and reporting procedures tend to be less applicable to small grassroots consumer groups than they are to some of the large, well-established organizations that systems often fund to provide mental health services. New procedures typically have to be worked out, including decision-making procedures, methods for holding grantees accountable, provisions for substantial up-front payments, streamlined reporting requirements, different monitoring procedures, and so forth. Even traditional ethical guidelines about relationships and staff–client boundaries in professionally operated programming may need to be adapted to peer and self-help initiatives.

Systems and agencies can pursue grant funding from a variety of sources to expand these services. They can also provide or arrange technical assistance to consumer groups on applications for funds, the management of services and administrative functions, and other needed areas of expertise.

It is important to encourage the growth of free-standing, autonomous support groups. One strategy for developing them is to invite consumer leaders from outside the system to advise on their formation, to visit newly started groups, and to provide technical help and encouragement to them. Organizing a local or regional conference for consumers to make contact with one another is also a very effective strategy. Finally, it is helpful to provide resources for new consumer groups to visit other such groups in different areas, in order to facilitate skills building and networking. A variety of such resources are available from the National Mental Health Self-Help Clearinghouse in Philadelphia (see below).

IMPLICATIONS OF SHARING POWER
FOR MENTAL HEALTH PROFESSIONALS

The Importance of Client-Based Planning
and of Consumer Choice

Developing life opportunities based on individuals' own choices and preferences is the essential element both of consumer empowerment and of a rehabilitation approach. In a rehabilitation approach, consumers are seen as being "in the driver's seat" with regard to setting goals for where and how to live, to work, to learn, and to socialize and recreate. Plans based on a process that assists each individual to choose his or her own directions in these areas are more likely to succeed than plans in which professionals or family members are deciding on such directions. Simply put, continuing to have others make decisions about the individual's life promotes the traditional patient role.

Overcoming the patient role is not simply a matter of educating consumers/ex-patients or of adopting a new clinical approach. To be effective, this effort also requires a restructuring of power relationships between professionals and consumers, and changes in the ways services are provided. This is true whether services are provided by mental health professionals, by other consumers/ex-patients, or by family members. Approaches that do not acknowledge the need for such changes can encourage dependency, or can limit services only to those individuals who are "motivated" or "ready to take charge of their lives." Such approaches can abandon many of the individuals who have been most disabled by years of institutional care and by the effects of a psychiatric disability. These individuals need, above all, people who can work with them on a basis of hope and of positive appreciation for their strengths, and who have the skills to help them overcome the patient role.

Therefore, it is critical that mental health organizations with a general commitment to integration and empowerment also make a specific commitment to retrain their staff members in skills related to rehabilitation: skills in planning goals, teaching skills, and organizing resources. It is also critical that staffs be retrained in the full range of issues related to integration and empowerment.

The basic posture of an empowerment-oriented professional toward a consumer involves a clear understanding of what one has to offer the other, and the posing of such basic questions as "Who are you?" "What are your hopes and aspirations?" and "How can I be of help?" Professionals try to connect their clients with self-help options, and maintain a personal commitment to having consumers leave every professional–client interaction with more power than when they entered it.

Changing Power Relationships

Much has been written in this book about the need to allocate resources so that they are accountable to consumers themselves. To the extent that mental health services are expected to achieve specific and concrete outcomes, and to the extent to which ongoing funding of these services or ongoing employment of staff members is based on achieving these outcomes, accountability must be present. Typically, this means that consumers will take on increasing roles of responsibility in serving on boards of directors of these service programs, in being hired as staff members, and in planning and monitoring the services themselves. Increasing "consumer voice" in this way has a powerful effect on perceptions of personal power and opportunity for each individual client served by these programs.

Working Effectively with the Issue of Choice

The core of empowerment is returning to consumers the responsibility for choices about their lives and their lifestyles. Making choices is at once a simple and an extremely complicated matter. Each individual, with or without a disability, is at a very different point in his or her willingness and ability to make clear choices about different issues. Although everyone makes a multitude of choices every day, having the ability to make effective choices for oneself about major life goals requires the availability of specific skills, as well as the presence of a variety of resources to implement these choices. In considering what needs to be in place for consumers' choices to be meaningful, it is important to focus at least on the following elements.

Having Real Options and Knowing about Them

Increasing the number of housing, work, or education options that consumers prefer, and offering the supports that will allow them to use these options, greatly facilitate choice. It is also important to inform consumers about these options, to encourage them to visit or experience different examples of options, and to offer help in figuring out whether any of these represent what they really want.

Knowing One's Own Preferences

Consumers who have been in dependent positions for some time, where their specific preferences have not mattered, often lose sight of what they want or need. This may also be an effect of having missed out on a number of typical developmental experiences, which in the normal course of events provide a valuable learning base for making future decisions. Ironically, these individuals are often described by staff members as "unmotivated." They may also see themselves as incapable of making major decisions. Changing consumers' sense of themselves as incompetent, and helping them to learn or relearn what is personally important, can be a major undertaking. This process is greatly facilitated by continually encouraging choices, no matter how small, and then supporting successively more important life choices.

Having the Ability to Make Tradeoffs

The ability to make tradeoffs is critical in the day-to-day world, in which few people have unlimited resources to make all of their choices a reality. In fact, every person has to decide which personal values are more important than others in making a particular major life choice, and consumers are no different in this regard. For one person, privacy may be such an important value that the individual is willing to pay a disproportionately large amount of disposable income for it, through living alone. Another person may be comfortable in sharing housing, and thus may have more disposable income for social activities. Learning to make these tradeoffs based on personal preferences is a major part of successful decision making.

Having Access to Supports, Regardless of What Choices Are Made

Often consumers will choose from a very narrow range of options (e.g., a group home or a boarding home) because of their past experience of only being offered support in a very narrow range of settings. A powerful strategy for increasing choice is to offer consumers support *wherever* they choose to live, work, or learn, and to assume that working out the complexities of offering services in this way is the *service provider's* responsibility, not an obstacle that should be used to force consumers to choose only from among those places where services are traditionally available. At times, this offer of support may be met with skepticism by family members or even by consumers themselves, given past experiences. In this case, it is the task of the service provider to build trust that the supports will be there, and to be diligent about providing them.

Having Successful Role Models Available

Recently, in conducting a consumer housing preference research study in a state hospital, one of the Center for Community Change's staff members who used to be a patient in that hospital returned there to interview several patients. As staff and patients alike recognized him and began asking, "What are you doing here?", he replied "I'm conducting research for the University of Vermont." The response on the part of hospital staff and patients was extremely powerful, as they compared the only way they had known this individual in the past—as a patient in serious crisis—with the present reality of a worker, a researcher, and a competent professional.

In another recent project, in which the Center for Community Change was asked to help a state hospital and a set of community programs work more effectively together, we heard frequent complaints that neither the hospital staff nor the community staff was "able to get patients motivated" to consider leaving the hospital. In response, a consumer self-help group began organizing meetings in which successful ex-patients in the community began visiting groups of people still in the hospital, in order to "demystify" the process of finding places to live and to work in the community (K. Kangas, personal communication, June 1989). Soon after this program began, staff members reported a much higher level of interest among patients in considering community options.

If professionals simply encourage consumers to make major changes, their efforts are sometimes met with skepticism, because the consumers may not have sufficient self-confidence to believe that they can succeed. It is extremely helpful, particularly for people who are currently in hospitals, in group homes, or in other dependent situations, to have available other consumers who have taken the next steps and who can provide encouragement and problem solving about how they too might take the next steps in their lives.

Adopting Empowering Practices

Empowering practices begin with listening to the individual consumer's personal experience and accepting the value of this experience, no matter how different it is from that of the helper or advocate. Listening from the perspective of the other person's premise communicates respect, in addition to giving the listener insight into the person's preferences and needs. These preferences then guide the process of offering support services. It is critical to provide each individual with as much information as possible, in order for him or her to make informed choices. It is also important to support the individual through a succession of choices, even if some of the choices are not "successful"; it is only through choosing and then seeing the consequences that one becomes more effective at choice. It is important to identify and reinforce the person's strengths, and to help the person reframe disability as ability. Professionals who convey an attitude of "people first" are those with whom consumers will prefer to work. Staff members need to nurture hope and help consumers implement their dreams. In their own lives, they need to be as inclusive as they want society to be. They need to be willing to share their own experiences in ways that are helpful to consumers, and to "come out of the closet" when they are ready to do so about any experiences they may have had with the mental health system. Finally, staff members, as allies of people with psychiatric disabilities, need to be willing to fight injustice in their communities and in the larger society.

IMPLICATIONS FOR ORGANIZATIONS OF SHARING POWER

Empowering Staff Members

Fostering consumer empowerment in organizations, if it is to be welcomed by staff, requires a strong focus on empowering staff members as well. In fact, organizations that have become involved in the effort to share power with consumers often find themselves redefining the nature of power itself in their agencies, and developing an ethic of holding power *with* staff and consumers, not holding power *over* either or both groups. In such an approach, staff members are encouraged to increase their power over their jobs, and to decrease their power over their clients.

What are some effective ways to increase empowerment among staff members? Curtis (1990) has summarized a number of successful strategies: listen to staff members, motivate them, and support them; encourage staff members to speak up about any and all aspects of the agency's functioning, and then make changes based on this input; solicit input from the staff regularly (perhaps anonymously at first or through peer interviews), to bring to the surface major themes about what the agency is doing well and what needs changing; reward staff members by putting them in the spotlight when they succeed or perform in some special way; recognize and celebrate the work and worth of the staff regularly; assume a posture of not knowing all of the answers, of not being able to solve all of the problems, and of needing the staff's help to figure out solutions; respect and build on the strengths of each individual staff person; and create "win–win" situations with the staff.

Creating Healthy Organizations

Simply encouraging staff members to offer input, and providing recognition for the staff's work, may not be enough if the goal is to create a truly empowered staff and clientele in an agency. Typically, it is important to examine the structure and functioning of the organization itself, in order to identify ways in which it can become clearer about its purposes, and ways in which it can support healthy, powerful behavior on the part of all involved. Previous chapters of this book have described the importance of mission and values in an organization; however, true empowerment strategies must also focus on who is making decisions and on how decisions are made. What is needed is an effort by consumers, staff, managers, and board members to create practices that support diversity; that keep the agency true to its integration and empowerment values; that insist on staff competence; that provide reasonable accommodations to all staff members, not just those with identified disabilities; and that support nonhierarchical decision making. Staff members who are actively taking on their own empowerment are of much more value to consumers in this process than are staff members who feel disempowered and "burned out."

The goal of many such efforts is to redefine the responsibilities of each component of the organization. For instance, the board of director's role becomes supporting the management of the agency; management's role becomes supporting the staff of the agency; and the staff's role becomes supporting the consumers of the agency. Each of these partners is ultimately focused on consumer outcomes, since these are the *raison d'être* of the agency. Such an effort redefines management, administration, and supervision as support functions, rather than principally as accountability or decision-making functions. In addition, it clearly defines authority and responsibility; allocates resources accordingly; makes management accountable; sees all key organizational functions as opportunities for increased consumer and staff decision making; creates decision-making teams of consumers and staff that have authority over resources and are accountable for their performance; and commits the organization to effective communication strategies that keep everyone informed and involved.

RESOURCES

There are a number of excellent resources related to consumer empowerment. Fortunately, the number of materials being produced directly by consumers/ex-patients is increasing dramatically. These include information on self-help programs and organizing approaches; a number of newsletters; various books and articles providing personal testimony and experiences; and policy or conceptual materials.

Three major resources for a variety of materials related to consumer empowerment and organizing are: The National Empowerment Center (20 Ballard Road, Lawrence, MA 01843-1018; [800] POWER-2U); Project Share (311 S. Juniper Street, Room 902, Philadelphia, PA 19107; [215] 735-6367); and the National Network for Mental Health (490 York Road, Building A, Room 212, Guelph, Ontario N1E 6V1 [519] 766-1032). The National Empowerment Center and Project Share have both been designated as national technical assistance centers by the Center for Mental Health Services.

Information on Self-Help Programs and Organizing Approaches

Specht (1988), as noted earlier in this chapter, has summarized the activities of self-help groups across the United States. Toff, Van Tosh, and Harp (1990) describe a number of self-help programs serving people who are homeless. A similar description of programs is available from the National Resource Center on Homelessness and Mental Illness (262 Delaware Avenue, Delmar, NY 12054; [800] 444-7415). Project Share and the National Mental Health Self-Help Clearinghouse, Mental Health Association of Southeastern Pennsylvania (311 S. Juniper Street, Room 902, Philadelphia, PA 19107; [215] 735-6367), have a large number of materials, as well as an active technical assistance program focused on organizing and change efforts. The Center for Community Change through Housing and Support also has a variety of relevant materials available.

The manual by Zinman et al. (1987) is a practical and thorough guide to organizing self-help efforts, with many detailed chapters on such issues as developing an organization, creating a newsletter, managing public relations, conducting self-help groups, and so forth. This book also contains an extensive listing of resources related to self-help.

Newsletters

The *Community Support Network News* (Boston University, Center for Psychiatric Rehabilitation, 730 Commonwealth Avenue, Boston, MA 02215; [617] 353-3549), consistently has consumer-oriented content in each of its issues; it has also published a special issue on consumer demonstration projects. *Access* is an excellent newsletter produced by the National Resource Center on Homelessness and Mental Illness (see address on page 167). Its December 1989 issue focuses on "helping people help themselves." This center also has a wide variety of materials on homelessness available. *Resources* is the newsletter of the Human Resource Association of the Northeast (187 High Street, Suite 302, Holyoke, MA 01040; [413] 536-2401). It frequently has consumer-oriented content, and has a special issue on consumer employment (Spring 1990), an excellent article by Meg Simon (1990) on ex-patients as staff, and a special issue on empowerment and recovery (Spring 1993).

Listen is published by the Alabama Department of Mental Health, Office of Consumer and Ex-Patient Relations (P.O. Box 3710, 200 Interstate Park Drive, Montgomery, AL 361099-0710; [800] 832-0952). It has excellent content on recovery, on organizing strategies, and on consumer-operated services.

OMH News is the newsletter of the New York State Office of Mental Health (44 Holland Avenue, Albany, NY 12229; [528] 474-8910). This newsletter also has consistent content focused on a consumer perspective, and a special issue (July 1990) explores a number of projects and perspectives on consumer empowerment. Other state mental health departments, such as those of Oregon, Hawaii, and North Carolina, produce high-quality newsletters as well; these frequently incorporate a consumer perspective, and several special issues have focused on consumer projects. *In Sites,* the newsletter of the Robert Wood Johnson Foundation Program on Chronic Mental Illness (74 Fernwood Road, Boston, MA 02215; [617] 738-7774), periodically has information on consumer activities in the nine urban sites funded to develop comprehensive community support systems. *Madness Network News,* the first national newsletter produced by consumers, provides a radical perspective on ex-patient issues (2054 University Avenue, Berkeley, CA 94704; [415] 548-2980). *Disability Rag,* which unfortunately has only a very minor focus on psychiatric disabilities, is an excellent source of information about the larger disability rights movement (Box 145, Louisville, KY 40201).

Finally, the Center for Community Change through Housing and Support, publishes a quarterly newsletter, *In Community* (Institute for Program Development, Trinity College of Vermont, 208 Colchester Avenue, Burlington, VT 05401; [802] 658-0000). This newsletter provides up-to-date information on innovative community integration and empowerment projects focused on housing and supports for people with psychiatric disabilities.

Personal Testimony and Experiences

The book by Hutchison et al. (1985) is an excellent summary of ex-patients' views, based on an information-gathering effort throughout Canada's provinces. Leete (1988) summarizes her perceptions and management strategies for coping with her disability. Blackbridge and Gilhooly (1985) present a searing perspective on the experience of hospitalization, with a specific reference to lesbian concerns.

A number of prominent public figures have recently published books or articles about their experiences with a major mental illness or psychiatric disability. These include Kate Millett (1990), William Styron (1990), Art Buchwald (1990), and Patty Duke (1992).

Ridgway (1988a) quotes the views of a number of national consumer leaders on the issue of housing and supports. The meeting that produced this document also resulted in the production of a popular videotape, *Coming Home,* available from the Center for Community Change through Housing and Support (1989).

Deegan (1988, 1989, 1990, 1992) has produced a very moving series of papers on the experience of fellow ex-patients, on recovery, and on the rehabilitation process. Many of her papers are available from the National Empowerment Center and from the Center for Community Change through Housing and Support

Policy or Conceptual Materials

Chamberlin (1978), in a classic book on the ex-patient perspective, describes a variety of self-help efforts; she also presents a strong conceptual approach to the experience of consumers, calling for consumer-controlled alternatives to the mental health system. Estroff (1981), in the first ethnographic study of ex-patients, has described the experience of a number of consumers participating in a "model community support program"—the Program in Assertive Community Treatment

(Madison, Wisconsin). Leete (1988) presents an overview of the emerging consumer movement, and changing conceptualizations of the role of consumers. Ridgway (1988b) provides a detailed bibliography of consumer perspectives on mental health services. Wilson et al. (1987) present a summary of consumer perspectives on the emerging human resource development agenda in mental health for the 1990s. NASMHPD (1989) has issued a policy statement on consumer contributions to mental health systems, which has been summarized earlier in this chapter; this statement is useful in state and local advocacy.

Over 50 studies of consumer preferences for housing, services, and other supports have now been conducted in North America, and these are summarized in Tanzman (1993). Consumer perspectives on the need for crisis response services are summarized in Blanch (1988).

Since so many materials are emerging, it makes sense to get on the mailing list of each of the national organizations mentioned above, to subscribe to newsletters, and to subscribe to the relevant electronic bulletin boards. Since much of this information is simply not available through such traditional media as journals or books, it is well worth the effort to keep abreast of emerging knowledge through these other media. Searching out such materials also represents a great opportunity for "networking" with those individuals whose work and thinking is influencing the field most significantly. Now that we have focused on strategies for sharing power with consumers, it is time to focus on the other major constituency group in mental health, family members.

CHAPTER 11

Involving Families
as Partners
in the Process of Change

As mental health systems experience rapid and far-reaching changes in the way they view people with psychiatric disabilities, one of the most exciting developments is the growth of an increasingly articulate and powerful advocacy movement among families who have members with this disability. Since so much of my own learning about the nature of psychiatric disabilities and about mental health systems has occurred in the context of having a family member with this disability, I have been particularly gratified with the growth of this movement. Families are a centrally important constituency whose needs are an essential focus for all mental health planning, program development, and evaluation.

From its modest beginnings in Madison, Wisconsin in 1979, the National Alliance for the Mentally Ill (abbreviated in this chapter as NAMI) has become a force to be reckoned with at every level of mental health systems in the United States, from local agencies to the halls of Congress. There are Alliance for the Mentally Ill affiliates in every state, and over 1000 local chapters.

Hatfield (1988), in a review of NAMI's progress and a perspective on how families should be involved in the process of rehabilitation and treatment, points out that professionals initially assumed that family members would simply be advocates for more funding and services. Instead, families have articulated their views on virtually every issue facing mental health systems, including assuming a dominant role in defining mental illness itself as a distinct brain disease, uniquely different from mental health problems or adjustment difficulties. Hatfield (1988) points out eloquently:

Families see themselves as "customers" who as a matter of right and good economics, insist on knowing the nature of the services offered, evidence as to their effectiveness, their inherent risks, and an accurate assessment of cost–benefit. They insist that professionals live up to the stated ethical principles of their professional organizations, and that they become vigorous in policing their organizations' members.

Families of the mentally ill want the power of informed choice. They want safe, efficacious, cost-effective help for their relatives and for themselves. They want increased control over their own lives. Families want providers who are willing and able to explain their theories and practices, the risks and benefits of their procedures, and a description of alternatives that might be considered. (p. 84)

Hatfield (1992) also notes that the family movement has operated with clear assumptions that have directly affected its ability to influence mental health systems. These include a commitment to autonomy and independence; an assumption that ordinary people can take charge and help one another; and a belief that families should not be abandoned to the role of long-term care providers. She notes the strong focus on illness, and what she calls the "medicalization" bias, as well as the bias toward research. According to Hatfield, families want to acquire knowledge and information, not to be seen as clients. Families have strengths, and when they have to meet difficult struggles, their competency emerges. Language is important as professionals seek to communicate respectfully with families. Finally, families want to share in decision making as equals with professionals, not just to be involved.

To be sure, this movement has faced many challenges. Not the least of these is incorporate the enormous diversity of opinion within its membership on many issues, including community integration; the role of community support systems and of hospitals; strategies for working with (or not working with) consumer/ex-patient groups; the research agenda that needs to be pursued; and the extent to which the family movement speaks for individuals with psychiatric disabilities, or simply on behalf of families and their needs. Nonetheless, the movement grows stronger each year. It is increasingly taking its rightful place as a full partner in planning, implementing, and monitoring public mental health services, educating the public about psychiatric disabilities, and insisting that the needs of families themselves are a high priority.

Hatfield (1992), in a recent address in Toronto, has summarized the ways in which mental health systems have changed by virtue of family involvement in recent years. She notes that in the United States family involvement is now mandated for anything important that happens in mental health systems, and that families are increasingly involved in monitoring services, since they feel that they cannot rely on professionals to police themselves. She notes that although families now have increased access to policy making, they continually struggle to overcome "tokenism." Hatfield concludes that the family movement is a well-structured movement that has staying power. The movement in Canada, principally represented by the organization Friends of Schizophrenia is at a much earlier stage of development, and is only beginning to emerge as a political force.

This chapter describes some of the current challenges that the family movement faces; describes strategies for engaging families in treatment and rehabilitation; presents emerging strategies for fully involving families as partners in mental health service systems, as well as in systems change; and describes resource materials available on this subject.

THE FAMILY MOVEMENT AT THE CROSSROADS

The family movement's growing power is something to celebrate. Now that the initial explosion of growth and influence has passed through its beginning stages, however, family groups are beginning to take stock and to thoughtfully address a number of "second-generation" questions related to change. One such issue involves whether the movement will adhere only to biological and genetic explanations for mental illness, or will also be willing to engage in active dialogue about related environmental factors (e.g., physical or sexual abuse), or even about alternative explanations for many behaviors that have been labeled as symptomatic of mental illness. Viewing the national advocacy agenda, some family members (e.g., M. Schneier, personal communication, September 1992) have expressed concerns about a singular emphasis on brain research; the powerful partnerships that have developed with the psychiatric research community; the relative lack of leadership on the need for dramatic expansion of community support services and community integration approaches; the conflicts between the family movement and the ex-patient/consumer movement; and what many feel is an unwillingness to work with a broad spectrum of advocates on some critical national issues.

There are also internal disputes within the family movement, focused on such questions as the extent to which families speak for their own needs or also for the needs of individuals with psychiatric disabilities. Partly because of the emphasis of family groups on biological explanations of mental illness, there has been some real tension between many consumer advocates and family advocates; these disputes generally center on the issue of who is speaking for whom. Some family leaders decry the "radical" perspective of consumer leaders, who are described as "not representative" or "not as ill" as their own disabled relatives. These leaders often contend that they speak for consumers who are "too ill" to speak for themselves, and who therefore need their families to speak for them. And it is certainly the case that many significantly disabled individuals who are not at all involved in the consumer movement receive their major support from their families. But in extreme cases, this contention in effect discounts the potential of recovery by asserting that if someone with a psychiatric disability gets better, it must be a sign that the person never had a serious mental illness. Consumer leaders, on the other hand, more typically focus on the commonality of their experience with those who are described as too disabled to speak for themselves. They will note that their own recovery from a very similar set of circumstances speaks to the potential of those who are currently more seriously disabled to take on their own recovery. They also point out the need of very disabled individuals for peer support as part of the recovery process, and conclude that other consumers are the most appropriate spokespersons for these very disabled individuals.

Such concerns ultimately raise questions for the community integration movement about whom various groups do speak for. They also raise questions about successful strategies for directing the power of the family movement toward the needs of families, and simultaneously toward support for the autonomy and independence of individuals with psychiatric disabilities. Finally, these concerns raise questions about whether families should independently be advocating for broad systems changes that will have a profound effect on the lives of people with psychiatric disabilities, in the absence of those individuals' speaking for themselves, and whether families rather than consumers should have the primary role in defining the nature of mental illness. Failure to resolve these questions may well pit family advocates against consumer advocates in a struggle that inevitably both will lose. Given North American society's pervasive lack of support for community support services, and especially for the rights of people with psychiatric disabilities to full community membership, any advocacy efforts, if they are to be effective, must focus on the common ground among consumers, family members, and progressive professionals.

STRATEGIES FOR ENGAGING FAMILIES IN TREATMENT AND REHABILITATION

Understanding the Experience of Families

For years, the mental health literature related to families focused almost exclusively on the role or "responsibility" of families in creating or exacerbating mental illness, or on therapeutic approaches to be pursued with "pathological" families. Only recently, and primarily because of the advocacy of the family movement, have family members come to be seen in the literature as people who face serious challenges in coping with the disability of a relative, and as people with the strengths and capacities to support themselves and others. Thus, in recent years, a growing literature is articulating the needs of families, presenting findings on successful interventions with individuals that also support families, and describing strategies to meet the needs of families directly.

Although the family movement has focused strongly on self-help, families have pressed increasingly to become full partners in the process of rehabilitation (Lefley, 1990b). Hatfield (1988) points out, however, that perhaps as few as 15% of people with psychiatric disabilities actually participate in an organized mental health program; this leaves families themselves as the major agents of rehabilitation and community support. Since so many families are, in effect, the primary caregivers, many family members serve in lieu of professionals as they attempt to help their disabled relatives set goals, learn skills, and organize the supports they need to get on with their lives. Hatfield points out the critical need to begin gathering information on the strategies these families use both to cope with psychiatric disabilities, and to assist in the rehabilitation of disabled individuals.

Hatfield (1988) also notes that though many families would prefer much broader availability of community programs, many people with psychiatric disabilities may find it more advantageous *not* to become involved with the formal mental health system, with its demand for compliance, its "preoccupation" with disability, and its lack of models for roles other than the traditional patient role. And she reminds us that it can be harder to reintegrate people with disabilities into the community, once they have been removed from the community in order to become a part of the "client world" in mental health systems. She goes on to point out the need for research on the coping strategies of individuals who never enter the mental health system.

Among those families that do have access to community treatment programs, many wish to collaborate directly with professionals in the process of community support and rehabilitation. Hatfield (1988) points up some of the major barriers to this collaboration. These include the difficulty of overcoming the hierarchically defined relationship between professionals and nonprofessionals, as well as state confidentiality laws that complicate the process of collaboration— laws that are unlikely to change if clients' rights are to remain intact. This latter issue points out the difficult course professionals must navigate in giving families the information they want, and at the same time respecting consumers' right to privacy. Although it is often difficult, however, meeting both consumer and family needs is an important responsibility of professionals. Finally, Hatfield points out that the field seems to have an insufficient understanding of the process of separation between families and consumers, and a lack of resources and skills for making the transition a smooth one. To make matters more difficult, many professionals seem unprepared to handle the normal, inevitable conflicts that arise in the process of collaboration with families.

Lefley (1993) emphasizes that for collaboration to be effective, families need to see what professionals are offering as credible. They also need to see that professionals' attitudes toward them are positive, and that the work of professionals is shaped by knowledge about families and about working effectively with them. Finally, they need to see that the work of professionals is based on those core competencies necessary for effective work with people with significant psychiatric disabilities.

Lefley (1993) goes on to point out that families are central to the process of treatment and rehabilitation. In the United States, approximately 65% of all psychiatric patients are discharged to their families. At any given time, between 40% and 50% of individuals with psychiatric disabilities live with their families; in addition, many others have significant contact with their families. According to a recent survey conducted by NAMI (Kasper et al., 1992), most families that are in contact with their disabled members supplement the individuals' income, at an average of about $300 per month. In spite of their centrality, families are often excluded from treatment; as a result, clinicians are excluded from the perspective, experience, and knowledge of families.

Hatfield (1988) points out that professionals are often overly concerned about the "dependence" of adult clients on their families. They may fail to understand that it is natural for any family to want to protect one of its members, and that this tendency is even more pronounced among families with disabled members. Mental health workers who are still engaged in the developmental process of separating from their own families may be particularly unhelpful in understanding the normal balance of dependence and independence in families. Hatfield points out that families should not be scorned for this natural tendency. Similarly, she points out that it is natural for professionals to promote a higher level of risk among individuals with disabilities, and that the inevitable tension between these perspectives can be a healthy and productive one, if it is managed with respect.

Part of understanding the barriers to working effectively with families involves an appreciation of the barriers to developing smooth working relationships. Lefley (1993) reminds us that because of past aversive experience with professionals (including the experience of being blamed for their relatives' disabilities), many family members are still resentful, but have not worked through their resentment to the point that they are prepared to work smoothly with professionals. Many feel "burned out" by their experience of the disabilities, and withdrawing from involvement may feel adaptive to them. Others may be too far removed from ongoing involvement with their disabled relatives. In still other families, one individual (usually the mother), is the only family member who has continued contact with the disabled person, and therefore feels very burdened.

Lefley acknowledges that some family environments are chaotic and dysfunctional, but that their numbers are far fewer than many clinicians might believe. In fact, according to Lefley, dysfunction in families appears to be independent of serious mental illness, occurring as frequently in familes without a psychiatrically disabled member. Families struggle with "double messages" from clinicians who now involve them because they are supposed to, but may still not have changed their fundamental negative assumptions about families. Finally, a disabled individual may not want his or her family involved. Lefley points out that what is needed is a vigorous outreach and follow-up approach with families, in which they are given the consistent message that they are needed and valued.

Using a Collaborative Teamwork Approach

Lefley (1993) suggests a model of collaborative teamwork with families. She also points out that for such an approach to be effective, a professional, a family, and a client all need to agree that they want to work together. Such an approach is focused on recovery and on the development of an independent lifestyle for the client. In this process, all parties hold one another accountable for progress on goals. Collaborative teamwork reduces battles for control through joint problem solving, and helps overcome any denial about the disability itself. It also incorporates psychoeducational approaches, particularly with family members who have coped with a relative's psychiatric disability over an extended period of time. Psychoeducation may be less effective with family members during the early onset of the disability, according to Lefley, since many find the idea that they may need to learn long-term or even lifelong coping skills related to the disability very discouraging.

Lefley suggests that a variety of characteristics will help the clinician assess the readiness of the family–client relationship for such collaborative work. These include the level of stability or disruption in the family process; the extent to which family members appear committed to one another's welfare; the current orientation of the other family members toward the disability, and their expectations; the level of congruence between the client's goals and those of the rest of the family; the level of problem-solving ability within the family; and the level of impairment in the individual with the disability.

Similarly, a number of characteristics of the clinician suggest relative readiness for collaborative teamwork. These include the attitude toward the family, and the nature of prior training related to families; a willingness to accept the knowledge and expertise of families; an ability to understand the variety of positive and negative reasons why a client may not want to be involved with his or her family, and a willingness to talk through these issues with the client; an understanding of the purposes and limits of confidentiality; an understanding that most clinical interventions are very short events in a lifelong process of disability, with which the family is involved over the long haul; and the willingness to be a leader and a guide in navigating the changing relationship between the family and the individual, while keeping the control over that relationship in the individual's hands, and emphasizing his or her control over the process.

Confidentiality is perhaps the most frequent source of conflict among clinicians, families, and disabled individuals. Lefley (1993) points out that family members generally respect confidentiality, and do not want private communications between a client and a clinician revealed. Instead, they want information about treatments, medications, ways to cope with certain behaviors, and ways to take care of themselves. She encourages the clinician to fulfill his or her responsibility to structure the parameters of confidentiality, and to let the client draw the boundaries. For example, the clinician might point out to the client that the family wants to be involved, and encourage the family and individual to meet together to discuss how to make this work. In the process, the clinician supports the client in deciding what he or she does and does not want to have shared.

Many families may want to be involved in their disabled relatives' treatment teams. Lefley (1993) points out that all families need education and the opportunity to participate in support groups. She contends, however, that only some families should be directly involved in treatment teams. Lefley reminds us that some family members are disruptive or may have their own agendas; such members should be excluded if a client wishes it. Similarly, at times a client may want the family members involved and the family may be very reluctant. In such cases, the clinician needs to continue holding the door open for family involvement, while understanding why some family members may want to distance themselves. Finally, Lefley points out that clinicians need to focus on practical barriers to collaboration, such as transportation or the need for child care, and to help address these needs.

In summary, then, professionals have begun to respond to families' needs in many communities. Through the increased participation of families in the process of system change (see below), far more of such responses are in store. In an excellent summary of some of the positive steps that professionals can take in working with families, Spaniol, Zipple, and Fitzgerald (1984) point out that families need information, practical advice, and support from professionals. They recommend the following strategies for professionals: (1) clarifying mutual goals; (2) learning rehabilitation/educational approaches; (3) not forcing families to fit professional models; (4) acknowledging their own (the professionals') limitations; (5) working with family members as a team; (6) pointing out families'' strengths; (7) learning to respond to intense feelings; (8) encouraging family enrichment; (9) learning about psychiatric disabilities and medications; (10) learning to provide practical advice; (11) learning about the community's resources; (12) meeting local family support groups; (13) making a personal commitment to support families; (14) learning to acknowledge diverse beliefs; and (15) developing their own (the professionals') support systems.

STRATEGIES FOR INVOLVING FAMILIES
IN MENTAL HEALTH SYSTEMS
AND IN SYSTEMS CHANGE

Many family members have begun to advocate for major changes in mental health systems, so that more effective supports will be made available. Systems should expect, plan for, and facilitate meaningful involvement of families in all aspects of policy and program development, as well as evaluation and monitoring of the outcomes of the system for individuals and communities. One initial but major step in this direction is to establish a clear policy (to be implemented at all levels of the system, and within any agencies or programs with which the system contracts) that there will be substantial involvement of families in all governance, advisory, or other bodies responsible for the development and improvement of the mental health system. Just as Chapter Ten has encouraged setting specific goals for consumer involvement in such bodies (at least 50% of the membership), a good definition for "substantial" involvement of families is about one-third of the total membership of any planning group.

Service settings that do not have a clear commitment to this kind of involvement may complain that they are not aware of eligible family members, but such claims simply emphasize their lack of connection with family interests. They may also caution that they are agencies serving many groups, and that people with psychiatric disabilities and their families are, after all, only one "constituency." Since people with psychiatric disabilities are, however, the major priority of public mental health funding, these individuals and their families should always be represented on governing bodies. If the presence of other "constituencies" prevents majority or substantial representation, then separate advisory or program oversight groups should also be formed. The continued presentation of concerns about consumers and their families constituting only one "interest group" in an agency should prompt a serious examination of whether an agency that has so many varied commitments can be responsive to the specific needs of consumers and family members.

Of course, advocates for community support systems have been debating for some years now whether it is desirable to have all services for people with psychiatric disabilities flow only through specialized agencies that may be particularly skilled at providing relevant services to this population, or whether these services are best provided through a more generic mental health organization. There is no hard and fast answer to this question, since it involves many complex factors (the potential for integration, the unique context of how each community organizes services, etc.). What is critical, however, is to keep an eye on the specific extent of an agency's commitment to people with the most severe disabilities; the level of leadership it assumes in fully involving consumers and their families; and the extent of its commitment to integration.

Systems and agencies that are committed to substantial family involvement can make great strides in the areas of policy and planning, mental health service delivery, training, and development of family-operated services. A recent series of planning processes in Vermont illustrates this potential. The Vermont Department of Mental Health and Mental Retardation asked the Center for Community Change through Housing and Support to convene a planning process intended to improve the competence of the mental health work force throughout the state. Families were heavily involved, and brought to the planning meetings a strong sense of each local agency's accountability for staff competencies and for consumer outcomes. They also insisted on independent mechanisms through which families could participate in the assessment of local staff competence and the identification of staff training needs. Finally, they insisted that family members be involved as learners and trainers in all training events; that key family concerns be included in the knowledge and skill competencies being prepared for all staff; and that family members be powerfully involved in oversight of a Mental Health Training Institute that the state was developing. They also insisted on similar involvement for people with psychiatric disabilities themselves. This input was provided through a process that attempted to identify the common ground among families, consumers, and professionals, and was both highly useful and very effective. As a result, the role of families in all human resource development activities in the state will substantially increase.

Involving Families in Policy and Planning Activities

First, it is important to draft an explicit policy on family involvement throughout the mental health system—one that affirms the role of families as essential partners in the planning and delivery of mental health services. This policy should specify the expectations of the system about membership on governing bodies, boards of directors, task forces, advisory groups, and so forth. A system often finds it helpful to designate an individual or office that will be responsible and accountable for family involvement throughout the system.

Many factors interfere with true family involvement in the actual provision of mental health services, including strong negative views about families among many clinicians, and the crisis-oriented nature of so many service delivery systems. To illustrate the latter problem, I recall a late-night conversation I had with an emergency room psychiatrist in New York City, regarding whether my mother would be involuntarily committed. I struggled to collaborate with this obviously harried clinician; finally, however, sensing that my concerns were not being taken seriously, I firmly announced, "The family does not want her committed." There was a silence, and then the clinician responded, "But what does the family have to do with it?"

Other constraints on meaningful family involvement are based in pervasive concerns about confidentiality—concerns that are sometimes used as an excuse for avoiding such involvement. Finally, the reality is that, for a variety of reasons, many consumers may not want their families involved. The following policy statement on family involvement, recently adopted within the Vermont mental health system, was developed by a working group of family members and policy makers, and then reviewed by a multiconstituency planning group involving consumers. To be sure, this policy is likely to be quite controversial. Some advocates who strongly support family involvement have expressed concern that this statement may not articulate strong enough values about consumer autonomy, and that it may imply that therapists should use their influence to change consumers' legitimate decisions about how they want their families involved. Nonetheless, it is presented here in its entirety, since it is one of the very few examples of an attempt to provide guidance regarding family involvement to clinicians throughout a system.

The policy of the Department of Mental Health and Mental Retardation is that family involvement is to be encouraged because it is presumed that such involvement has important therapeutic benefits. It is essential that this policy be applied, and confidentiality laws do not bar its application.

What this means in individual cases is that families (first degree relative or other significant others whom the client defines as family) are to be made part of the treatment process, absent the expressed refusal of the client or compelling evidence that such involvement would be counter-therapeutic. There obviously may be questions in individual cases about what material might be revealed, but, as a general rule, confidentiality laws do not bar family involvement in efforts to treat clients and such involvement should be the norm rather than the exception.

Families in the role of caregivers should know, at a minimum, the importance of ensuring that clients take their medication and what side effects might occur. Families also should be told what signs or symptoms to look for if the client does not comply with treatment or take prescribed medication, or if his or her condition begins to deteriorate. Caregivers, including families, should know the special needs of clients who are living with them while receiving follow-up outpatient or day care treatment. Any perceived potential for dangerous behavior to self or others should be discussed. Mental health professionals should also encourage family members and other caregivers to report to the treatment source—the treating psychiatrist, other mental health professional, or outpatient clinic—any changes in the client that may be significant and relevant to future behavior. A clinician should actively enlist the family with whom the client is most involved as a source of information about compliance because the family may be the best source of information.

On the other hand, we do not suggest that details of conversations between clinician and client should be revealed, nor do we suggest that other material not relevant to the families' role as caregiver be divulged. Such details lie at the heart of the confidentiality principle.

The disclosures to and exchanges with families would be preceded by a discussion with the client on the value of these communications and by obtaining the client's consent. We do not suggest that families be involved regardless of client's choice; however when the client withholds consent to share information, the therapist should work with the client to understand the reasons for the refusal and help the client accept family collaboration. (Vermont Department of Mental Health and Mental Retardation, 1993, pp. 1–2)

In setting goals related to family involvement in planning and policy making, it is important to be aware of the diversity of family members, and to avoid involving only a small number of people from similar educational, economic, and/or ethnic backgrounds. The family movement at the national level in the United States, for example, has faced major challenges in fully involving family members of color, those who come from culturally diverse groups, and those who live in poverty. Similarly, family advocates hold a variety of different perspectives with regard to the impact that their relatives' psychiatric disabilities have had on them individually and on their families. Parents tend to have somewhat different interests from siblings, who, in turn, tend to have interests distinct from those of adult children of people with disabilities. NAMI has organized a strong siblings network to respond to these differences. Finally, parents of children and adolescents with severe emotional disturbances tend to have a different set of concerns, as contrasted with parents of adult children with disabilities. For this reason, in fact, a new U.S. national organization, separate from NAMI, was recently formed to advocate for the needs of children and adolescents—the Federation of Families for Children's Mental Health (1021 Prince Street, Alexandria, VA 22314; [703] 684-7710). This group is a strong advocate for "wrap-around" services that include a variety of involved professionals (education, social services, mental health, corrections) and services that are child centered and geared toward the goal of family preservation. The Federation also focuses strongly on "transition issues" (i.e., service needs of adolescents who are shifting from service systems organized for children to those organized for adults).

It is critical to make an effort to involve the full diversity of family members in roles throughout the system, in order to assure that the system is responsive to this diversity of concerns.

Family members often need support in getting to meetings of the groups they join. This may take the form of scheduling meetings on evenings or weekends so that people will not have to miss work; some families will also need assistance with child care or transportation. Family members will need an in-depth orientation to the purposes of the group and to the expectations for participation. The group will need to make a serious effort to avoid the typical mental health "jargon" or "alphabet soup" of abbreviations and acronyms that makes the work almost unintelligible for a newcomer. Families should be made to feel welcome, and to feel that their ideas and input are valued.

Systems should regularly solicit input and feedback from family groups about their concerns and their perceptions of service needs, particularly those services that can help families to support one another and to cope with psychiatric disabilities.

It is helpful to thoughtfully consider the extent to which each of the key constituencies (consumers, families, professionals, and other advocates) will provide separate input to the system, as contrasted with the extent to which they will work together, and to base future directions for the system on a process of identifying common ground. Thus, although some systems or family advocates may initially see it as helpful to call for the establishment of a family advisory committee, systems that are focused on integrated planning will also develop a larger planning and advisory group consisting of consumers, family members, professionals, and other advocates who do most or all of their work *together,* rather than only having multiple advisory groups representing different perspectives. In the latter case, families may feel they have power because they have their own advisory group, but the reality may be that they have *less* power, since pulling together the perspectives of each of these separate groups and establishing a course of action becomes more centrally the role of mental health policy makers and staff members. On the other hand, if all groups are represented in a common planning body, the process can be more difficult and consensus can be harder to reach. But once consensus is reached, it becomes very difficult for mental health policy makers or staff members to create their own separate directions for action. This is not an "either–or" situation, however. All mental health systems in the United States have a state-level multiconstituency planning body by federal law (Comprehensive Mental Health Systems Planning Act, 1987), and many also have separate advisory committees reflecting the interests of each constituency. Increasingly, this is the case in Canada's provinces as well.

It is particularly important to stress the need for full involvement of families in the research, evaluation, and program-monitoring activities of a system. In a growing number of communities and systems, it has become routine practice to include families on site visit teams, and to seek their involvement in all planning for research on the behavior and effects of the system. Focused studies of family perspectives and family needs are essential. Before any services are developed for families, there needs to be an organized effort to solicit families' views as to what they would find helpful. Collection of information on families' satisfaction with services should also be a routine component of program operations. On a national level, a recent major research program undertaken by NAMI and funded by the MacArthur Foundation (Kasper et al., 1992) is adding significantly to our understanding of the needs and experiences of families, by gathering in-depth information from families across the United States. At both the local and state levels, systems are beginning to organize routine collection of information from families.

Finally, many systems, after clarifying their overall policy on family involvement, have found it helpful to start with several specific steps: (1) providing partial or full funding for an initial family education and training effort geared toward developing local support groups throughout a state or community; (2) organizing an initial survey of family needs throughout a system; and (3) partially or fully funding, often for a time-limited period, an advocacy organization through which families can begin organizing on a system-wide basis. Typically these efforts, with "seed" funding, will flourish increasingly on their own; this is important, since their autonomy and independence from the formal operations or control of the mental health system are vital. This need for autonomy, however, should not be used as an excuse to abdicate an essential responsibility of mental health systems, which is to serve as a major catalyst for the development of effective advocacy by families.

As with consumers, agencies and systems need to continually develop creative ways to involve families whenever critical policy, programmatic, and funding decisions are about to be made. And as with consumers, the major tool for fully involving families is to listen, listen, and listen some more.

Involving Families
in Mental Health Service Delivery

There are two major areas in which family involvement can be pursued with regard to directly providing services: (1) encouraging the development of services explicitly intended to support families, including family education and training, respite, counseling, outreach, crisis services, and other vital community supports; and (2) recruiting family members to staff these and other community support services.

Families are the most vital source of knowledge about how services intended to meet family needs should be organized. Their guidance in the development of these services should be sought in the variety of ways described above.

An explicit set of strategies also needs to be employed to let families know they are valuable and sought after as potential employees of the mental health system. It is helpful to develop an affirmative action policy that explicitly promotes employment of family members and recognizes their unique contributions, based on their experiences with psychiatric disabilities in their families and with the mental health service system. Position descriptions should indicate that experience with psychiatric disabilities is a preferred qualification, and positions should be advertised in ways that assure that families will be aware of these openings and encouraged to apply. Similarly, system and agency policies that may inadvertently discriminate against families—for example, in required job qualifications—need to be examined and changed.

Like consumers, some family members will need reasonable accommodations on the job to ensure successful employment—not only with regard to their own needs, but also as they provide support to their relatives with disabilities. Particularly at these times, family members will need flexibility in their schedules.

As with consumers, systems can develop explicit programs to train family members for service delivery roles, and can also vigorously pursue roles for family members in training programs as they are developed (e.g., roles as case managers or other new service personnel).

Involving Families in Training

Mental health systems should guarantee significant involvement of family members in all training events in the system, both as learners and as teachers. They should fund, as needed, the participation of families in relevant national, state/provincial and local conferences.

Family members should be encouraged to make as many public presentations as possible, since these are valuable in educating the public and in improving public attitudes. When mental health professionals are invited to meetings, they should insist that family members be included; if necessary, they should refuse to attend meetings to which families have not been invited.

Mental health professionals can lobby with higher education institutions to include content about families and their needs in the curriculum. Similarly, family members should be encouraged to teach in these settings, whether they give lectures in a course, coteach a course with a professional, or are themselves recruited for faculty positions. Current faculty members who have relatives with psychiatric disabilities should be encouraged to "come out of the closet," and to use their influence to promote change in higher education. Finally, individuals whose higher education plans were interrupted because of a relative's psychiatric disability should be supported in returning to school.

Developing Family-Operated Services

To support families, systems can typically begin by funding family education and training services. There are now a number of "models" for accomplishing this, and substantial information about these is available from NAMI. Often, once local groups are given information, and family members have an opportunity to support one another, people's coping skills improve dramatically; many members of these groups then choose to become active advocates.

The decision as to whether a family group should target its energies toward advocacy, or should also try to develop services, should be made with great care. In many communities, families, seeing the lack of decent services, housing, education, or employment opportunities for consumers, will decide to organize and operate a set of services themselves (e.g., a group home). This can often be a very taxing decision for family members, who may invest several years of very hard effort in developing a single housing setting, for example, only to find that their own relatives with psychiatric disabilities have little interest in living there. In such cases, it is extraordinarily hard for those family members to maintain enthusiasm for working on broader advocacy for housing. Thus, such an experience often also saps the vital energy needed for ongoing advocacy, rather than service delivery itself.

Family members, on the other hand, may well want to consider developing and offering support services to other family members (e.g., outreach, respite, or participation in crisis response services). The core of these services, for which family members are uniquely qualified, is a strong program of self-help and mutual support among families themselves.

RESOURCES

There are a number of excellent resources for families who wish to become more involved in systems change. Many are available from NAMI, which has an ever-growing set of materials, books, and films.

Some of the items available from NAMI (2101 Wilson Boulevard, Suite 202, Arlington, VA 22201; [703] 524-7600) at this writing include titles in areas as diverse as science and research; public policy; unipolar depression; bipolar disorder (manic depression); schizophrenia; other diagnoses; children and adolescents; families and coping strategies; legal and financial considerations; services and facilities; information for professional service providers; personal narratives; publications produced by NAMI itself; an annotated bibliography (NAMI, 1990); and a series of videotapes. Readers are encouraged to call or write NAMI for its latest publications list.

Several items can be highly recommended as introductory reading in this area. A book by Torrey and Flynn (1990) rates U.S. state programs on the extent to which they support people with psychiatric disabilities; this is a very controversial book, and one that is important to review. It evaluates each state mental health system on such issues as hospital services, community services, rehabilitation, housing, and services to people in jails.

Three books on coping with psychiatric disabilities have been especially popular: those by Torrey (1988), Walsh (1986), and Hatfield (1990). Two works written for a professional audience that are particularly useful are Hatfield and Lefley (1987) and Lefley (1990b). Finally, a moving set of first-person set of accounts is found in NAMI (1989).

As the family movement grows in numbers and influence, and as more and more professionals are successful in working collaboratively with families, so will the potential correspondingly increase for creating truly effective partnerships among policy makers, professionals, family members, and people with psychiatric disabilities—partnerships that will accelerate the movement for community inclusion, empowerment, and recovery.

CONCLUSION

CHAPTER 12

Future Challenges and New Directions

Community integration and empowerment for people with psychiatric disabilities are ideas whose time has come. Putting the ideas and strategies in this book into practice in communities, however, will require more than mere information. Individuals with these disabilities, their family members, other citizens, professionals, and policy makers face major challenges in the process—challenges that will need to be overcome if community integration is to become the norm rather than the exception.

Family members face unique challenges: to work as allies with consumers for changes that reflect their aspirations, and to avoid having the power of the family movement overshadow or supplant the smaller, more fragile movement of consumers themselves; to embrace the concept of recovery and to celebrate those who have taken responsibility for moving on with their lives, not as heroic exceptions, but as role models for all people with psychiatric disabilities; and to insist on high-quality community support services for consumer and their families, on the full protection of the rights of consumers, and on full partnerships with families in every community.

People with psychiatric disabilities face special challenges in this process as well: daring to hope and to dream; joining with others to speak out for what they need; being willing to be held responsible for their lives; and, as they move on with their own recovery, not abandoning those who are left behind. These challenges are especially difficult, given the day-to-day struggle of most consumers simply to meet their basic needs, while also coping with their disabilities.

Citizens without obvious disabilities face the challenges and opportunities of letting go of the negative attitudes that have made segregation a reality, and replacing them with real relationships; becoming neighbors, coworkers, coworshipers, employers, and friends to people with psychiatric disabilities; and, in the process, creating communities that are more inclusive and more supportive of all members.

Professionals and policy makers, like the other partners in this process, will need the courage and the support to look deeply within and to undertake a process of personal transformation; they need to acknowledge how little they currently know about successful integration and empowerment, and (for those who are not consumers themselves) how little they know about the actual experience of psychiatric disabilities. They will need the courage to take what is essentially a personal journey, through which they come to understand that all they have to offer others in this struggle is themselves as people—without magical cures, without the tools of coercion, without power over others. In the process, they will need to continue striving to see mental health systems through the eyes of those whom they are expected to serve, and to see both the potential and the real limitations of those systems and services. In acknowledging the limitations of mental health programs, they must continue to press for fundamental change in the attitudes and behaviors of every individual associated with services for people with psychiatric disabilities, and of every citizen in our communities.

What is needed, above all, is personal leadership. As advocates, we can fill the vacuum of leadership by daring to imagine a world in which people with psychiatric disabilities are truly in charge of their own destinies, and are supported to assist one another in the process of recovery, of healing, and of reintegration into communities. We can dare to imagine a mental health system in which consumers are making the key decisions about programs, funding, and accountability; a system in which family members are respected and supported as partners; in which professionals, with and without histories of psychiatric disability themselves, are respected as valuable resources; and in which policy makers are held accountable, while they are supported for visionary and risk-taking leadership. Guided by that vision, we can work together to make integration a reality on a daily basis.

Achieving community integration and empowerment will not be an easy task for any of the allies in this movement. We are challenged by the legacy of the 1980s, in which the U.S. national leadership promoted a culture of self-interest and marginalization of all citizens who were neither white, male, nor privileged. We are just emerging from a period of sustained assault on all of those seen as different: women; people living in poverty; people of color; gay, lesbian, or bisexual people; and people with disabilities. We are moving out of a time in which we were sold a bill of goods about the "politics of scarcity"—

one in which we've been warned that there will never be enough to go around to meet the basic needs of all citizens for decent housing, full employment, and affordable health care. The deep recession of the last several years, and the continuing prospect of real economic constraint, provide serious challenges to the kind of expansive and visionary approach we need to take to become truly inclusive communities.

But the United States, Canada, and indeed the rest of the world are also in a time of ferment—of attempting to shift course from the politics of the 1980s, and of insisting on real change. In a parallel way, the fields of mental health and rehabilitation are in the midst of a revolution about who people with psychiatric disabilities really are, what they need, and what our collective human responsibility should be for one another. As mental health consumers themselves, professionals, family members, policy makers, and the public at large make the shift from viewing consumers not as patients who need supervision, nor as passive service recipients whose potential for success is limited to "maintenance" in the community, but instead as citizens with disabilities—people who have the capacity for recovery and for contributions to all of our lives in the community—this sea change in attitudes will fundamentally alter every aspect of mental health and rehabilitation services, and ultimately every aspect of community life.

Thus, I believe that this period provides more opportunity for leadership, for creative ideas, and ultimately for hope than has been the case for some time. The times seem especially ripe for a large-scale movement of advocates interested in basic change in society's approach to mental illness. Such a movement can insist at the national level, in North America and elsewhere, that community integration and independent living for people with psychiatric disabilities are rights rather than privileges; that federal programs and policies be oriented toward creating integrated housing, work, learning, and program environments; that federal policies and funding be shifted toward assuring the full range of community support and rehabilitation services that are needed to replace the institutional and sheltered approaches of the past; and that federal policies and funding be shifted to support independent living services provided by individuals with disabilities themselves.

In the final analysis, of course, we cannot limit ourselves to acting only when the times are most opportune. We have a responsibility to act regardless of the quality of the current political leadership, the current mood of the populace, or the relative certainty of success. After all, the struggle for self-determination for people with psychiatric disabilities is a historic one that is unlikely to be fully won in any of our lifetimes. I believe, however, that the shift toward community integration and empowerment is inevitable; the only real question is whether we yet have the collective courage and wisdom to embrace this new vision, and thereby to imagine and foster new possibilities in people's lives. It does take courage to make a commitment to the simple idea of putting people first—to advocate for the dangerous idea that, regardless of their level of disability, all people have the right to determine their own destinies, choose their own lifestyles, and control their own services. And it takes courage because those who are the pathfinders, in the forefront of this movement, are those who are most often discounted and criticized.

The choice that each of us has to make about community integration is no less critical than the choice that people with psychiatric disabilities, or with any conditions or labels that have been targets of social marginalization, have had to make throughout history. This is the choice that must be made at the crucial point when individuals finally take responsibility for their own lives and their own recovery. I recently attended a "street theater" production in Vancouver, British Columbia, by Kate the Great, an ex-patient and actress who presents her life in the mental health system with incredible humor and pain. Kate recounts her experience of that moment of choice—sitting alone in her hospital room, looking back at her life of multiple hospitalizations, homelessness, medications, and shock treatments, and then looking forward and seeing nothing but more of the same. In the telling of it, there is a long, almost deafening silence. Then Kate shouts out: "I choose to live." She has never been hospitalized again, and has recently phased herself off medications.

Like Kate, change agents choose *life* in the community. They choose community support that helps to integrate and empower them over the slow and quiet death of endless patienthood in outdated mental health programs. They choose hope and recovery over the addiction of helplessness, terminal dependence, and despair—an addiction so deep that it has led them to discount those who take on their own recovery and speak out. Instead of the "mental health world," they choose the real world, in which the essential task is to get on with their lives. They choose health, and they make a commitment to pursuing wellness for themselves and for each of their allies in this enterprise, as they collectively pursue change. Advocates choose to accept the responsibility that each member of a community has for supporting others, and for building community. They remember that everyone is destined for some kind of greatness, but that as they pursue their individual destinies, they also choose to have fun. I have a favorite button that I keep above my desk, with the words of Emma Goldman: "If I can't dance, I don't want to be part of your revolution."

Advocates remember that the forces opposed to integration are significant, but that their strength lies in the common ground that people with psychiatric disabilities share with all other marginalized groups. They remember that in spite of their small numbers change agents will succeed, because they are on the side of life. They will succeed because they understand that in the final analysis, there are many voices but only one real struggle—the struggle for life.

Finally, advocates choose *faith* in people with psychiatric disabilities, in families, in one another, and in themselves—faith that high-quality services reflecting what consumers want, and caring communities, can both become realities across North America and elsewhere. They choose the faith that there is a whole new world out there for everyone to understand, and that the key to entering that world is a new set of partnerships among individuals with disabilities, their families, and professionals—partnerships based on mutual respect and on the right to self-determination. With such faith, they understand that each time they reach the end of their current knowledge and step off together into the unknown, either there will be an ally there to assist them, or they will learn how to fly.

REFERENCES

The Center for Community Change through Housing and Support (Institute for Professional Development, Trinity College of Vermont, 208 Colchester Avenue, Burlington, VT, 05401; [802] 658-0000) has extensive resource materials on consumer perspectives, family involvement, community opposition, community support systems, employment, housing, public mental health systems, program approaches, research and evaluation, and training, all of which are related to community integration. The Center has videos available, and sponsors a graduate training program, the Program in Community Mental Health. The program offers certificates, a master's degree, and continuing education, which focus on adults with psychiatric disabilities, wrap-around services for children and adolescents with serious emotional problems, and management of community programs. References followed by an asterisk (✱) are available from the Center.

Alinsky, S. D. (1971). *Rules for radicals.* New York: Vintage Books.

Alisky, J. M., & Iczkowski, K.A. (1990). Barriers to housing for deinstitutionalized psychiatric patients. *Hospital and Community Psychiatry, 41,* 93–95.

Americans with Disabilities Act of 1990, Public Law No. 101-336.

American Psychiatric Association. (1987). *Diagnostic and statistical manual of mental disorders* (3rd ed., rev.). Washington, DC: Author.

Anthony, W. A. (1979). *The principles of psychiatric rehabilitation.* Amherst, MA: Human Research Development Press.

Anthony, W. A. (1982). Explaining psychiatric rehabilitation by an analogy to physical rehabilitation. *Psychosocial Rehabilitation Journal, 5,* 61–65.

Anthony, W. A. (1990a, July). *What are the "bottom lines" that family members should expect from mental health service agencies?* Keynote address to the annual meeting of the National Alliance for the Mentally Ill, Chicago.

Anthony, W. A. (1990b). *The philosophy and practice of psychiatric rehabilitation.* Boston: Boston University, Center for Psychiatric Rehabilitation.

Anthony, W. A., & Blanch, A. K. (1987). Supported employment for persons who are psychiatrically disabled: An historical and conceptual review. *Psychosocial Rehabilitation Journal, 11,*(2), 5–23.

Anthony, W. A., & Blanch, A. K. (1989). Research on community support services: What have we learned? *Psychosocial Rehabilitation Journal, 12*(3), 5–14.

Anthony, W. A., Cohen, M. R., & Cohen, B. (1984). *The characteristics and principles of psychiatric rehabilitation programs.* Boston: Boston University, Center for Psychiatric Rehabilitation.

Anthony, W. A., Cohen, M. R., & Farkas, M. (1982). A psychiatric rehabilitation treatment program: Can I recognize one if I see one? *Community Mental Health Journal, 18,* 182–192.

Anthony, W. A., Cohen, M. R., & Farkas, M. (1990). Curriculum for the core disciplines for professional preservice training in working with the long-term mentally ill. In D. L. Johnson (Ed.), *Service needs of the seriously mentally ill: Training implications for psychology* (pp. 51–57). Washington, DC: American Psychological Association.

Anthony, W. A., & Jansen, M. A. (1984). Predicting the vocational capacity of the chronically mentally ill: Research and policy implications. *American Psychologist, 39,* 537–548.

Aviram, U., & Segal, S. P. (1973). Exclusion of the mentally ill: Reflection on an old problem in a new context. *Archives of General Psychiatry, 29,* 126–131.

Bachrach, L. L. (1980). Model programs for chronic mental patients. *American Journal of Psychiatry, 137,* 1023–1031.

Bachrach, L. L. (1982). Young chronic patients: An analytic review of the literature. *Hospital and Community Psychiatry, 33,* 189–197.

Bassuk, E. L. (1984). The homelessness problem. *Scientific American, 251,* 40–45.

Baxter, E., & Hopper, K. (1984). Troubled in the streets: The mentally disabled homeless poor. In J. A. Talbott (Ed.), *The chronic mental patient: Five years later* (pp. 49–62). New York: Grune & Stratton.

Belcher, J. R. (1988). Defining the service needs of homeless mentally ill persons. *Hospital and Community Psychiatry, 39,* 1203–1205.

Benda, B. B., & Datallo, P. (1988). Homelessness: Consequence of a crisis or a long-term process? *Hospital and Community Psychiatry, 39,* 884–886.

Bertsch, E. F., & Dolan, J., Jr. (1990, May). *Consumer controlled funding of services through a voucher system in Nassau County, New York.* Keynote presentation at the 13th Annual Educational Conference of the New York State Chapter of the Association of Mental Health Administrators, Albany.

Biss, S. M., & Curtis, L. C. (1993). Crisis service systems: Beyond the emergency room. *In Community, 3*(1), 1–4. (∗)

Blackbridge, P., & Gilhooly, S. (1985). *Still sane.* Vancouver, BC: Press Gang.

Blanch, A. K. (1988). *Final report of the Vermont Task Force on Crisis Options.* Burlington, VT: Center for Community Change through Housing and Support. (∗)

Blanch, A. K. (1990). Issue paper: Stigma and discrimination in mental health. *Community Support Network News, 6*(4), 12–15.

Blanch, A. K. (1993). Involuntary commitment. *OMH News* [Office of Mental Health, New York State], *5*(8), 1–4.

Blanch, A. K., Carling, P. J., & Ridgway, P. (1988). Normal housing with specialized supports: A psychiatric rehabilitation approach to living in the community. *Rehabilitation Psychology, 32*(4), 47–55. (∗)

Blaska, B. (1990). The myriad medication mistakes in psychiatry: A consumer view. *Hospital and Community Psychiatry, 41*(9), 993–998.

Bond, G. (1987). Supported work as a modification of the transitional employment model for clients with psychiatric disabilities. *Psychosocial Rehabilitation Journal, 11*(2), 55–73.

Braun, P., Kochansky, G., Shapiro, R., Greenberg, S., Gudeman, J., Johnson, S., & Shore, M. F. (1981). Overview: Deinstitutionalization of psychiatric patients—A critical review of outcome studies. *American Journal of Psychiatry, 138,* 736–749.

Breakley, W. R., & Fischer, P. J. (1990). Homelessness: The extent of the problem. *Journal of Social Issues, 46,* 31–47.

Brown, M. A., Ridgway, P., & Anthony, W.A. (1991). Comparison of outcomes for clients seeking and assigned to supported housing services. *Hospital and Community Psychiatry, 42,* 1150–1153.

Brown, M. A., & Wheeler, T. (1990). Supported housing for the most disabled: Suggestions for providers. *Psychosocial Rehabilitation Journal, 13*(4), 59–68.

Buchwald, A. (1990, October). Buchwald on Styron. *Vanity Fair,* p. 174.

Budson, R. D. (Ed.) (1981). *New directions for mental health services: Issues in community residential care* (Vol. 11). San Francisco: Jossey-Bass.

Bush, C. T., Langford, M. W., Rosen, P., & Gott, W. (1990). Operation outreach: Case management for severely psychiatrically disabled adults. *Hospital and Community Psychiatry, 41*(6), 647–649.

Campbell, M. (1981). The three-quarterway house: A step beyond the halfway house toward independent living. *Hospital and Community Psychiatry, 32,* 500–501.

Carling, P. J. (1978). Residential services in a psychosocial rehabilitation context: The Horizon House model. In J. Goldmeier, F. V. Mannino, M. F. Shore (Eds.), *New directions in mental health care: Cooperative apartments* (pp. 52–64). Adelphia, MD: National Institute of Mental Health. (∗)

Carling, P. J. (1981). Nursing homes and chronic mental patients: A second opinion. *Schizophrenia Bulletin, 7,* 574–579. (∗)

Carling, P. J. (1984). *Developing family foster care programs in mental health: A resource guide.* Rockville, MD: National Institute of Mental Health. (∗)

Carling, P. J. (1987). *Final report of the Vermont Consumer Advocacy Task Force.* Burlington, VT: Center for Community Change through Housing and Support. (∗)

Carling, P. J. (1990a). Major mental illness, housing, and supports: The promise of community integration. *American Psychologist, 45*(8), 969–975. (∗)

Carling, P. J. (1990b). Supported housing: An evaluation agenda. *Psychosocial Rehabilitation Journal, 13*(4), 95–104. (∗)

Carling, P. J. (1990c). Strategic attempts of a psychology department to promote community integration: The University of Vermont experience. In D. L. Johnson (Ed.), *Service needs of the seriously mentally ill: Training implications for psychology* (pp. 129–134). Washington, DC: American Psychological Association. (∗)

Carling, P. J. (1990d). Principles for promoting community integration of people with psychiatric disabilities: The challenge to the academic psychology community. In D. L. Johnson (Ed.), *Service needs of the seriously mentally ill: Training implications for psychology* (pp. 37–41). Washington, DC: American Psychological Association. (∗)

Carling, P. J. (1992). Community integration of people with psychiatric disabilities: Emerging trends. In J. W. Jacobson, S. N. Burchard, and P. J. Carling (Eds.), *Community living for people with developmental and psychiatric disabilities* (pp. 20–32). Baltimore: Johns Hopkins University Press. (*)

Carling, P. J. (1993). Reasonable accommodations in the workplace for people with psychiatric disabilities. *Consulting Psychology Journal: Practice and Research, 45*(2), 46–62. (*)

Carling, P. J. (1994, May). *New Service approaches, empowerment, and the future of involuntary intervention.* Paper presented at the First National Conference on Involuntary Interventions: The call for a national legal and medical response, Houston, TX. (*)

Carling, P. J., Miller, S., Daniels, L., & Randolph, F. (1987). Operating a state mental health system without a state hospital: The Vermont feasibility study. *Hospital and Community Psychiatry. 38*(6), 617–623. (*)

Carling, P. J., Randolph, F. L., Blanch, A. K., & Ridgway, P. (1987). *Rehabilitation research review: Housing and community integration for people with psychiatric disabilities.* Washington, DC: DATA Institute. (*)

Carling, P. J., & Ridgway, P. (1987). Overview of a psychiatric rehabilitation approach to housing. In W. A. Anthony, & M. Farkas (Eds.), *Psychiatric rehabilitation: Turning theory into practice* (pp. 28–80). Baltimore: Johns Hopkins University Press. (*)

Carling, P. J. & Wilson, S. F. (1988). *Strategies for state mental health directors in implementing supported housing.* Burlington, VT: Center for Community Change through Housing and Support. (*)

Carling, P. J., Wilson, S. F., McCabe, S. S., & Curtis, L. C. (1990). *Flexible services: A key to supported housing implementation.* Burlington, VT: Center for Community Change through Housing and Support. (*)

Carpenter, M. D. (1978). Residential placement for the chronic psychiatric patient: A review and evaluation of the literature. *Schizophrenia Bulletin, 4,* 384–398.

Center for Psychiatric Rehabilitation. (1989). *Coming Home* [Videotape]. Boston, MA: Producer.

Center for Psychiatric Rehabilitation. (1990, Spring). *Community support network news.* Special issue on supported education. Boston, MA.

Center for Mental Health Services. (1993). *Mental health statistics.* Rockville, MD: Author.

Chamberlin, J. (1978). *On our own: Patient controlled alternatives to the mental health system.* New York: McGraw-Hill.

Chamberlin, J. (1987). The case for separatism: Ex-patient organizing in the United States. In I. Barker, & E. Peck (Eds.), *Power in strange places: User empowerment in mental health services* (pp. 24–28). London: Good Practices in Mental Health.

Chatetz, L., & Goldfinger, S. M. (1984). Residential instability in a psychiatric emergency setting. *Psychiatric Quarterly, 56,* 20–34.

Cherniss, C. (1980). *Staff burnout: Job stress in human services.* Beverly Hills, CA: Sage.

Cioffari, A. T., Blanch, A. K., Wilson, S. F., Carling, P. J., & Pierce, J. (1988). Building a vision of community support: A collaborative colloquium series. In *Innovation in collaboration: Vignettes of state/university collaboration to improve mental health systems* (pp. 79–88). Boulder, CO: Western Interstate Commission on Higher Education. (∗)

Cioffari, A. T., Burchard, J. D., Carling, P. J., & Copeland, R. E. (1993). Creating a competent workforce in Vermont: Promoting public–academic linkages and human resource development. In P. Wohlford, H. F. Myers, & J. E. Callan (Eds.), *Serving the seriously mentally ill: Public–academic linkages in services, research, and training* (pp. 111–117). Washington, DC: American Psychological Association. (∗)

Ciompi, L. (1980). Catamnestic long-term study on the course of life and aging in schizophrenia. *Schizophrenia Bulletin, 6,* 606–608.

Comprehensive Mental Health System Planning Act of 1987, Public Law No. 99-660.

Cohen, C. I., & Thompson, K. S. (1992). Homeless mentally ill or mentally ill homeless? *American Journal of Psychiatry, 6,* 816–822.

Cohen, D. (1989). Biological basis of schizophrenia: The evidence reconsidered. *Social Work, 34,* 255–257.

Cohen, M. D., & Somers, S. (1990). Supported housing: Insights from the Robert Wood Johnson Foundation Program on Chronic Mental Illness. *Psychosocial Rehabilitation Journal, 13*(4), 43–50.

Cometa, M. S., Morrison, J. K., & Ziskoven, M. (1979). Halfway to where? A critique of research on psychiatric halfway houses. *Journal of Community Psychology, 7,* 23–27.

Coulton, C. L., Holland, T. P., & Fitch, V. (1984). Person–environment congruence and psychiatric patient outcome in community care homes. *Administration in Mental Health, 12,* 71–88.

Cousins, N. (1979). *Anatomy of an illness as perceived by the patient: Reflections on healing and regeneration.* New York: Norton.

Culhane, D. P. (1992). Ending homelessness among women with severe mental illness: A model program from Philadelphia. *Psychosocial Rehabilitation Journal, 16,* 63–76.

Curtis, L. C. (1990). *Training package on consumer empowerment.* Burlington, VT: Center for Community Change through Housing and Support.

Curtis, L. C. (1992). Boundaries and ethics in community services: Guidelines for decision making. *In Community, 2*(4), 5.

Curtis, L. C., McCabe, S. S., Montague, W., Caron, D., & Harp, H. the. (1991). *Strategies for increasing and supporting consumer involvement in mental health planning, management, and service delivery.* Burlington, VT: Center for Community Change through Housing and Support.

Daniels, L., & Carling, P. J. (1986). *Housing and service need of mental health consumers in Kitsap county, WA: A needs assessment.* Boston, MA: Center for Psychiatric Rehabilitation.

Danley, K. S., & Mellen, V. (1987). Training and personnel issues for supported employment programs which serve persons who are severely mentally ill. *Psychosocial Rehabilitation Journal, 11*(2), 87–102.

Davis, K. (1990, July). *Public mental health/academic linkages.* Paper presented at the annual meeting fo the National Alliance for the Mentally Ill, Chicago.

Dear, M. (1977). Impact of mental health facilities on property values. *Community Mental Health Journal, 13,* 150–158.

Deegan, P. E. (1988). Recovery: The lived experience of rehabilitation. *Psychosocial Rehabilitation Journal, 11*(4), 10–19.

Deegan, P. E. (1989, November). *A letter to my friend who is giving up.* Keynote presentation to the Connecticut Conference on Supported Employment, Wenham, MA.

Deegan, P. E. (1990). Spirit breaking: When the helping professions hurt. *Humanistic Psychologist, 18*(3), 301–313. (*)

Deegan, P. E. (1992). The independent living movement and people with psychiatric disabilities: Taking back control of our lives. *Psychosocial Rehabilitation Journal, 15*(3), 3–19. (*)

Dellario, D., & Anthony, W. A. (1981). On the relative effectiveness of institutional and alternative placements of the psychiatrically disabled. *Journal of Social Issues, 37,* 21–33.

Dion, G., & Anthony, W. A. (1987). Research in psychiatric rehabilitation: A review of experimental and quasi-experimental studies. *Rehabilitation Counselling Bulletin, 30,* 177–203.

Downs, M. (1989). *The perspective of ex-psychiatric patients on employment.* Unpublished master's thesis, University of Vermont. (*)

Downs, M. (1990). *Report on the case manager data collection project.* Waterbury: Vermont Department of Mental Health and Mental Retardation. (*)

Drake, R. E., Wallach, M. A., & Hoffman, J. S. (1989). Housing instability and homelessness among aftercare patients of an urban state hospital. *Hospital and Community Psychiatry, 40,* 46–51.

Duke, P. (1992). *A brilliant madness: Living with manic-depressive illness.* New York: Bantam.

Edgar, E. (1989). Family and case manager perspectives on consumers' housing and support needs. *Journal of the California Alliance for the Mentally Ill, 3,* 10–11. (*)

Estroff, S. E. (1981). *Making it crazy: An ethnography of psychiatric clients in an American community.* Berkeley: University of California Press.

Estroff, S. E. (1987). No more young adult chronic patients. *Hospital and Community Psychiatry, 38*(1), 5.

Estroff, S. E. (1989). Self, identity, and subjective experiences in schizophrenia: In search of the subject. *Schizophrenia Bulletin, 15*(2), 189–196.

Everett, B., & Nelson, A. (1992). We're not cases and you're not managers: An account of a client–professional partnership developed in response to the "borderline" diagnosis. *Psychosocial Rehabilitation Journal, 15*(4), 49–60.

Fair Housing Amendments Act of 1989, Public Law No. 100-430, May 1989.

Fair Housing Amendments Act of 1992, as Amended, Public Law No. 100-430, May 1989.

Fairweather, G. W. (Ed.). (1980). *New directions for mental health services: No. 7. The Fairweather Lodge: A twenty-five year retrospective.* San Francisco: Jossey-Bass.

Fields, S. (1990). The relationship between residential treatment and supported housing in a community support system. *Psychosocial Rehabilitation Journal, 13*(4), 105–113. (*)

First, R. J., Rife, J. C., & Kraus, S. (1990). Case management with people who are homeless and mentally ill: Preliminary findings from an NIMH demonstration project. *Psychosocial Rehabilitation Journal, 14*, 87–91.

First, R. J., Roth, D., & Arewa, B. (1988). Homelessness: Understanding the human dimensions of the problem for minorities. *Social Work, 33*, 120–124.

Fisher, D. (1994, May). *The damage to citizenship and personhood by involuntary interventions.* Paper presented at the First National Conference of Involuntary Interventions: The call for a national legal and medical response, Houston, TX.

Flanagan, J. C. (1978). A research approach to improving our quality of life. *American Psychologist, 33*, 138–147.

Fleming, M., & York, J. (1989). Implementing a community support system in an urban setting. *Psychosocial Rehabilitation Journal, 12*(3), 41–53.

Franklin County Mental Health Board. (1987). *Providing safe, affordable housing for persons with severe and long-term mental illness: A plan for local action.* Columbus, OH: Author.

Freire, P. (1970). *Pedagogy of the oppressed.* New York: Herder & Herder.

Friedan, B. (1963). *The feminine mystique.* New York: Norton.

Gelberg, L., & Linn, L. (1988). Social and physical health of homeless adults previously treated for mental health problems. *Hospital and Community Psychiatry, 39*, 510–516.

Geller, M. P. (1982). The "revolving door": A trap or a life style? *Hospital and Community Psychiatry, 33*, 388–389.

Goering, P., Durbin, J., Trainor, J., & Paduchak, D. (1990). Developing housing for the homeless. *Psychosocial Rehabilitation Journal, 13*(4), 33–42.

Goldman, H. H., Gatozzi, A. A., & Taube, C. A. (1981). Defining and counting the chronically mentally ill. *Hospital and Community Psychiatry, 32*, 21–27.

Goldmeier, J., Shore, M. F., & Mannino, F. V. (1977). Cooperative apartments: New programs in community mental health. *Health and Social Work, 2*, 119–140.

Graves, W. (1990, October–November). *Empowerment of people with disabilities.* Keynote presentation to the National Institute on Disability and Rehabilitation Research State of the Art Conference on Rehabilitation Research, Bethesda, MD.

Grunberg, J., & Eagle, P. F. (1990). Shelterization: How the homeless adapt to shelter living. *Hospital and Community Psychiatry, 41*, 521–525.

Hall, G. B., Nelson, G., & Fowler, H. S. (1987). Housing for the chronically mentally disabled: Part I. Conceptual framework and social context. *Canadian Journal of Community Mental Health, 6*(2), 65–78.

Halter, C. A., Bond, G. R., & Graaf-Kaser, R. D. (1992). How treatment of persons with serious mental illness is portrayed in undergraduate psychology textbooks. *Community Mental Health Journal, 28*(1), 29–42.

Harding, C., Brooks, G., Ashikaga, T., Strauss, J., & Brier, A. (1987). The Vermont longitudinal study of persons with severe mental illness: I. Methodology, study sample, and overall status 32 years later. *American Journal of Psychiatry, 144*(6), 718–726.

Harp, H. the (1991). *A crazy folks' guide to reasonable accommodation and psychiatric disability.* Oakland, CA: Independent Living Support Center. (∗)

Hasazi, J. E., Burchard, S. N., Gordon, L. R., Vecchione, E., & Rosen, J. W. (1992). Adjustment to community life: The role of stress and support variables. In J. W. Jacobson, S. N. Burchard, & P. J. Carling (Eds.), *Community living for people with developmental and psychiatric disabilities* (pp. 111–124). Baltimore: Johns Hopkins University Press.

Hasazi, S., & Collins, M. (1988). *Supported employment technical assistance manual.* Burlington: University of Vermont, Supported Employment Technical Assistance Project.

Hatfield, A. B. (1988). The role of the family in the rehabilitation process. In L. Perlman (Ed.), *Proceedings of the 1988 Switzer Memorial Seminar on rehabilitation support systems for persons with long-term mental illness* (pp. 48–65). Washington, DC: National Rehabilitation Association.

Hatfield, A. B. (1990). *Coping with mental illness in the family: A family guide* (2nd ed.) Baltimore: Mental Hygiene Administration.

Hatfield, A. B. (1992, October). *On the role of families.* Keynote address to the Annual Mental Health Conference, Queen Street Mental Health Centre, Toronto.

Hatfield, A. B., Fierstein, R., & Johnson, D. (1982). Meeting the needs of families of the psychiatrically disabled. *Psychosocial Rehabilitation Journal, 6*(1), 27–40.

Hatfield, A. B., & Lefley, H. (1987). *Families of the mentally ill: Coping and adaptation.* New York: Guilford Press.

Hellkamp, D. T. (1993). The Cincinnati consortium: Training for services to seriously mentally disabled adults and their families. In P. Wohlford, H. F. Myers, & J. E. Callan, (Eds.), *Serving the seriously mentally ill: Public–academic linkages in services, research, and training* (pp. 137–142). Washington, DC: American Psychological Association.

Hogan, M., & Carling, P. J. (1992). Normal housing: A key element of a supported housing approach for people with psychiatric disabilities. *Community Mental Health Journal, 28*(3), 215–226. (∗)

Holmes-Eber, E. L., & Riger, S. (1990). Hospitalization and the composition of mental patients' social networks. *Schizophrenia Bulletin, 16,* 157–164.

Housing Committee of the California Alliance for the Mentally Ill, Castaneda, D., & Sommer, R. (1986). Patient housing options as viewed by parents of the mentally ill. *Hospital and Community Psychiatry, 37*(12), 1238–1242.

Huber, G., Gross, G., & Schuttler, R. (1980). Longitudinal studies of schizophrenic patients. *Schizophrenia Bulletin, 6,* 592–605.

Hutchison, P., Lord, J., Savage, H., & Schnarr, A. (1985). *Listening to people who have directly experienced the mental health system.* Toronto: Canadian Mental Health Association.

Jones, J. (1993). *Movement toward empowerment: Living our words.* Kitchener, Waterloo: Canadian Mental Health Association.

Joyce, S. (1994a). *Discovery: A facilitator's guide to personal planning with people who receive support.* Kitchener, Waterloo: Canadian Mental Health Association.

Joyce, S. (1994b). *Discovery: An introduction to personal planning with people who receive support.* Kitchener, Waterloo: Canadian Mental Health Association.

Karoff, D., & McCabe, S. S. (1992). Housing development corporations in mental health: The pro and cons. *In Community, 2*(3), 3–4. (∗)

Kasper, J. D., Steinwachs, D. M., & Skinner, E. A. (1992). Family perspectives on the service needs of people with serious and persistent mental illness: Part II. Needs for assistance and needs that go unmet. *Innovations and Research in Clinical Services, Community Support and Rehabilitation, 1*(4), 21–33.

Kent County Community Mental Health Center. (1987). *Principles for community support.* Warwick, RI: Author.

Kiesler, C. A. (1982). Mental hospitals and alternative care: Noninstitutionalization as potential public policy for mental patients. *American Psychologist, 37,* 349–360.

Knoedler, W., Carpenter, E., McCabe, S. S., Rutkowski, P., & Allness, D. (1992). Supporting people with mental illness regardless of their environment: The Wisconsin experience. In J. W. Jacobson, S. N. Burchard, & P. J. Carling (Eds.), *Community living for people with developmental and psychiatric disabilities* (pp. 53–66). Baltimore: John Hopkins University Press. (∗)

Koegel, P., & Burnham, M. A. (in press). Problems in the assessment of homelessness: An empirical approach. In M. J. Robertson, & M. Greenblatt, (Eds.), *Homelessness: The national perspective.* New York: Plenum Press.

Kohen, W., & Paul, G.L. (1976). Current trends and recommended changes in extended care placement of mental patients: The Illinois system as a case in point. *Schizophrenia Bulletin, 2,* 575–594.

Kozol, J. (1988). *Rachel and her children: Homeless families in America.* New York: Crown.

Kübler-Ross, E. (1969). *On death and dying.* New York: Macmillan.

Kuhn, T. (1970). *The structure of scientific revolutions* (2nd ed.). Chicago: University of Chicago Press.

Lamb, R. H., (1984). *The homeless mentally ill.* Washington, DC: American Psychological Association.

Lamb, R. H., & Lamb, D. M. (1990). Factors contributing to homelessness among the chronically and severely mentally ill. *Hospital and Community Psychiatry, 41,* 301–305.

Lapp, R. E. (1964, August 2). The Einstein letter that started it all. *New York Times Magazine,* 14–39.

Leete, E. (1988). The role of the consumer movement and persons with mental illness. In L. Perlman (Ed.), *Proceedings of the 1988 Switzer Memorial Seminar on rehabilitation support systems for persons with long-term mental illness* (pp. 66–84). Washington, DC: National Rehabilitation Association.

Leete, E. (1989). How I perceive and manage my illness. *Schizophrenia Bulletin, 15,* 197–200.

Lefley, H. P. (1990a). Rehabilitation in mental illness: Insights from other cultures. *Psychosocial Rehabilitation Journal, 14*(1), 13–20.

Lefley, H. P. (Ed.). (1990b). *Families as allies in treatment of the mentally ill.* Washington, DC: American Psychiatric Press.

Lefley, H. P. (1993, November). *The role of families in treatment and rehabilitation: Keynote address to the Vermont Alliance for the Mentally Ill Conference on Collaboration between Families and Professionals,* Rutland, VT.

Linn, M. W., Caffey, E. M., Klett, J., & Hogarty, G. (1977). Hospital vs. community (foster) care for psychiatric patients. *Archives of General Psychiatry, 34,* 78–83.

Linn, M. W., Klett, J., & Caffey, E. M. (1980). Foster home characteristics and psychiatric patient outcome. *Archives of General Psychiatry, 37,* 129–132.

Lipton, A. A., & Simon, F. S. (1985). Psychiatric diagnosis in a state hospital: Manhattan state revisited. *Hospital and Community Psychiatry, 36*(4), 368–372.

Livingston, J., & Srebnik, D. (1991). States' strategies for promoting supported housing for persons with psychiatric disabilities. *Hospital and Community Psychiatry, 42*(11), 1116–1119. (*)

Low-Income Housing Information Service. (1988). *Low Income Housing Bulletin No. 12.* Washington, DC: Author.

Lutfiyya, Z. (1988). *Reflections on relationships between people with disabilities and typical people.* Syracuse, NY: Syracuse University, Center on Human Policy.

Mancuso, L. L. (1990). Reasonable accommodations for workers with psychiatric disabilities. *Psychosocial Rehabilitation Journal, 14*(2), 15–16.

Mandiberg, J. M., & Telles, L. (1990). The Santa Clara County Clustered Apartment Project. *Psychosocial Rehabilitation Journal, 14*(2), 21–28.

McCabe, S. S., Edgar, E. R., Mancuso, L. L., King, D., Ross, E. C., & Emery, B. D. (1993). A national study of housing affordability for recipients of supplemental security income. *Hospital and Community Psychiatry, 44*(5), 494–495. (*)

McKnight, J. (1987). Regenerating community. *Social Policy, 18*(3), 54–58.

Mental Health Law Project. (1992). *Mental health consumers in the workplace: How the Americans with Disabilities Act protects you against employment discrimination.* Washington, DC: Author.

Millett, K. (1990). *The loony bin trip.* New York: Simon & Schuster.

Milstein, B. (1986). *The myth of mentally ill people as dangerous: An annotated bibliography.* Washington, DC: Mental Health Law Project.

Milstein, B. (1988). *The effects of group homes on neighboring property: An annotated bibliography.* Washington, DC: Mental Health Law Project.

Molinaro, L. (1988). *Housing for people with mental disabilities: A guide for development.* Boston: Robert Wood Johnson Foundation Program on Mental Illness.

Montague, W. J. (1989). Who would care to be homeless? *Journal of the California Alliance for the Mentally Ill, 2,* 1–5. (∗)

Morrison, J. (1989). Correlations between definitions of the homeless mentally ill population. *Hospital and Community Psychiatry, 40,* 952–954.

Morse, G., & Calsyn, R. J. (in press). Mental health and other human service needs of homeless people. In M. J. Robertson, & M. Greenblatt (Eds.), *Homelessness: The national perspective.* New York: Plenum Press.

Mosher, L. R., & Menn, A. Z. (1978). Community residential treatment for schizophrenia: Two-year follow-up. *Hospital and Community Psychiatry, 29,* 715–723.

Mulkern, V., & Bradley, V. (1986). Service utilization and service preferences of homeless persons. *Psychosocial Rehabilitation Journal, 10,* 22–30.

Nader, R. (1990, October). An interview. *Vanity Fair,* pp. 41–44.

Nagy, M. P., & Gates, H. M. (1992). Decongregating residential programs in mental health: Staff and client impact. In J. W. Jacobson, S. N. Burchard, & P. J. Carling (Eds.), *Community living for people with developmental and psychiatric disabilities* (pp. 201–218). Baltimore: John Hopkins University Press. (∗)

National Alliance for the Mentally Ill (NAMI). (1989). *Experiences of patients and families: First person accounts* (NAMI Publication No. 2, Second Series). Arlington, VA: Author.

National Alliance for the Mentally Ill (NAMI). (1990). *Annotated reading list 1990* (NAMI Book No. 4). Arlington, VA: Author.

National Association of Home Builders, National Research Center (1989). *Financing housing for people with disabilities: The financing mechanisms.* Upper Marlboro, MD: Author.

National Association of State Mental Health Program Directors (NASMHPD). (1986). *Position statement on community support systems for people with severe and persistent mental illnesses.* Alexandria, VA: Author. (∗)

National Association of State Mental Health Program Directors (NASMHPD). (1987). *Position statement on housing and support for people with long term mental illness.* Alexandria, VA: Author. (∗)

National Association of State Mental Health Program Directors (NASMHPD). (1988). *Financing of state mental health care.* Alexandria, VA: Author.

National Association of State Mental Health Program Directors (NASMHPD). (1989). *Position paper on consumer contributions to mental health service delivery systems.* Alexandria, VA: Author. (∗)

National Association of State Mental Health Program Directors (NASMHPD). (1990). *Position statement on employment of persons with psychiatric disabilities.* Alexandria, VA: Author. (∗)

National Housing Institute. (1988) *A status report on the American dream.* Princeton, NJ: RL Associates.

National Institute of Mental Health (NIMH). (1987a). *Guidelines for meeting the housing needs of people with psychiatric disabilities.* Rockville, MD: Author. (∗)

National Institute of Mental Health (NIMH). (1987b). *Guidelines for comprehensive state mental health plans: P.L. 99-660.* Rockville, MD: Author.

National Institute of Mental Health (NIMH). (1990). *National plan of research to improve care of severe mental disorders.* Rockville, MD: Author.

New York Times. (1990, April 15). The new Calcutta [Editorial], p. 34.

Ohio Department of Mental Health, Mental Health Housing Task Force. (1986). *Final report.* Columbus: Ohio Department of Mental Health. (∗)

Ohio Department of Mental Health, Office of Housing and Service Environments. (1989). *Financing the development of supported housing.* Columbus, OH: HDK Associates.

Pace, S., & Turkel, W. (1990). Participants, community volunteers and staff: A collaborative approach to housing and support. *Psychosocial Rehabilitation Journal, 13*(4), 81–83.

Pandiani, J. A., Edgar, E. R., & Pierce, J. E. (in press). A longitudinal study of the impact of changing public policy on community mental health client residential patterns and staff attitudes. *Journal of Mental Health Administration.*

Pape, B. (1990). *Building a framework for support for people with mental disabilities* (CMHA Social Action Series). Toronto: Canadian Mental Health Association.

Peck, M. S. (1985). *People of the lie: The hope for healing human evil.* New York: Simon & Schuster.

Peck, M. S. (1987). *The different drum: Community making and peace.* New York: Simon & Schuster.

Protection and Advocacy for Mentally Ill Individuals Act of 1993, as amended, Public Law No. 99-319, May 1986.

Racino, J. A. (1993). Madison mutual housing association and cooperative. In J. A. Racino, P. Walker, S. O'Connor, S. & S. J. Taylor (Eds.), *Housing, support, and community: Choices and strategies for adults with disabilities.* (Vol. 2, pp. 31–63). Baltimore: Paul H. Brookes.

Randolph, F. L., Sanford, C., Simoneau, D., Ridgway, P., & Carling, P. J. (1988). *The state of practice in community residential programs: A national survey* (Monograph Series on Housing and Rehabilitation in Mental Health). Boston: Boston University, Center for Psychiatric Rehabilitation. (∗)

Rapp, C. (1990). *Strategies for change in higher education.* Address to the annual meeting of the National Alliance for the Mentally Ill, Chicago, IL.

Reidy, D., & Shea, K. (1990). *Community organizations as a vehicle for social integration for people with disabilities.* Paper presented at the Seventh Annual Community Psychology Conference, American Psychological Association, Burlington, VT.

Reidy, D. (1992). Shattering illusions of difference. *Resources, 4*(2), 3–6.

Ridgway, P. (1986). *Meeting the supported housing and residential services needs of Americans with psychiatric disabilities: A state by state review* (Monograph Series on Housing and Rehabilitation in Mental Health). Boston: Boston University, Center for Psychiatric Rehabilitation. (∗)

Ridgway, P. (1987). *Avoiding zoning battles.* Washington, DC: Intergovernmental Health Policy Project. (∗)

Ridgway, P. (1988a). *Coming home: Ex-patients view housing options and needs.* Burlington, VT: Center for Community Change through Housing and Support. (∗)

Ridgway, P. (1988b). *The voice of consumers in mental health systems: A call for change.* Burlington, VT: Center for Community Change through Housing and Support. (∗)

Ridgway, P. & Carling, P. J. (1988). *A user's guide to needs assessment* (Monograph Series on Housing and Rehabilitation in Mental Health). Boston: Boston University: Center for Psychiatric Rehabilitation. (∗)

Ridgway, P., & DeSisto, M. (1987). *Community support systems workbook.* Augusta: Maine Department of Mental Health and Mental Retardation, Office of Community Support Systems.

Rose, S., & Black, B. L. (1985). *Advocacy and empowerment: Mental health care in the community.* Boston: Routledge & Kegan Paul.

Rose, S., Peabody, C., & Strategias, B. (1990, Summer) Overcoming double jeopardy: Childhood trauma as a major factor in distress. *National Association of Psychiatric Survivors News,* 5–7.

Roth, D., Toomey, B. G., & First, R. J. (in press). Homeless women: Characteristics and service needs. *Affilia: Journal of Women and Social Work.*

Ryan, W. (1976). *Blaming the victim.* New York: Vintage Books.

Schutt, R. K., Goldfinger, S. M., & Penk, W. E. (1992). The structure and sources of residential preferences among seriously mentally ill homeless adults. *Sociological Practice Review, 3,* 148–156.

Segal, S. P., & Aviram, U. (1978). *The mentally ill in community-based sheltered care: A study of community care and social integration.* New York: Wiley.

Segal, S. P., Baumohl, J., & Moyles, E. W. (1980). Neighborhood types and community reaction to the mentally ill: A paradox of intensity. *Journal of Health and Social Behavior, 21,* 345–359.

Segal, S. P., & Specht, H. (1983). A poorhouse in California, 1983: Oddity or prelude? *Social Work, 28,* 319–322.

Sigelman, C., Spankel, C., & Lorenzen, C. (1979). Community reactions to deinstitutionalization: Crime, property values and other "bugbears." *Journal of Rehabilitation, 52,* 1–4.

Simon, M. (1990, Spring). Consumers as staff. *Resources,* p. 6.

Spaniol, L., Zipple, A. M., & Fitzgerald, S. (1984). How professionals can share power with families: A new approach to working with families of the mentally ill. *Psychosocial Rehabilitation Journal, 18*(2), 77–84.

Specht, H. (1988). *Findings of the national survey on state support of consumer/ex-patient activities in mental health.* Holyoke, MA: Human Resource Association of the Northeast.

Stastny, P. (1994, May). *Involuntary interventions by psychiatrists: A breach of the Hippocratic Oath?* Paper presented at the First National Conference of Involuntary Interventions: The call for a national legal and medical response. Houston, TX.

Stein, L. I., & Test, M. A. (Eds.). (1985). *New directions for mental health services: No. 26. The training in community living model: A decade of experience.* San Francisco: Jossey-Bass.

Strauss, J. (1989). Subjective experiences of schizophrenia: Toward a new dynamic psychiatry. *Schizophrenia Bulletin, 15,* 179–188.

Styron, W. (1990). *Darkness visible.* New York: Random House.

Tabor, M. A. (1980). *The social context of helping: A review of the literature on alternative care for the physically and mentally handicapped.* Rockville, MD: National Institute of Mental Health.

Tanzman, B. H. (1990). *Researching the preferences of people with psychiatric disabilities for housing and supports: A practical guide.* Burlington, VT: Center for Community Change through Housing and Support. (*)

Tanzman, B. H. (1993). Researching the preferences for housing and supports: An overview of consumer preference surveys. *Hospital and Community Psychiatry, 44*(5), 450–455. (*)

Tanzman, B. H., Wilson, S. F., King, D., & Voss, W. J. (1990). *The Vermont State Hospital cohort study.* Burlington, VT: Center for Community Change through Housing and Support. (*)

Tanzman, B. H., Wilson, S. F., & Yoe, J. T. (1992). Mental health consumers' preferences for housing and supports: The Vermont study. In J. W. Jacobson, S. N. Burchard, & P. J. Carling (Eds.), *Community living for people with developmental and psychiatric disabilities* (pp. 155–166). Baltimore: Johns Hopkins University Press. (*)

Taylor, E. H. (1989). Schizophrenia: Fire in the brain. *Social Work, 34,* 258–260.

Taylor, S. J., Racino, J., Knoll, J., & Lutfiyya, Z. (1987). *The nonrestrictive environment: A resource manual on community integration for people with the most severe disabilities.* New York: Human Policy Press.

Teplin, L. A. (1985). The criminality of the mentally ill: A dangerous misconception. *American Journal of Psychiatry, 142,* 593–596.

Test, M. A. (1981). Effective community treatment of the chronically mentally ill: What is necessary? *Journal of Social Issues, 37,* 71–86.

Test, M. A., & Stein, L. (1978). Community treatment of the chronic patient: Research overview. *Schizophrenia Bulletin, 4,* 350–364.

Thompson, K. S., Griffith, E. H., & Leaf, P. J. (1990). A historical view of the Madison model of community care. *Hospital and Community Psychiatry, 41*(6), 625–634.

Toff, G. E., Van Tosh, L., & Harp, H. the (1990). *Self-help programs serving people who are homeless and mentally ill.* Washington, DC: Intergovernmental Health Policy Project, George Washington University.

Toffler, A. (1970). *Future shock.* New York: Random House.

Torrey, E. F. (1988). *Surviving Schizophrenia: A family manual* (rev. ed.). New York: Harper & Row.

Torrey, E. F., & Flynn, L. (1990). *Care of the seriously mentally ill: A rating of state programs* (3rd ed.). Washington, DC: Public Citizen Health Research Group/National Alliance for the Mentally Ill.

Torrey, E. F., Wolfe, S. M., & Flynn, L. (1988). *Care of the seriously mentally ill: A rating of state programs* (2nd ed.). Washington, DC: Public Citizen Health Research Group/National Alliance for the Mentally Ill.

Trainor, J., & Church, K. (1984). *A framework for support for people with severe mental disabilities.* Toronto: Canadian Mental Health Association.

Trainor, J., Pomeroy, E., & Pape, B. (1993). *A new framework for support for people with serious mental health problems.* Toronto: Canadian Mental Health Association.

Tsuang, M., Woolson, R., & Fleming, J. (1979). Long-term outcome of major psychoses: I. Schizophrenia and affective disorders compared with psychiatrically symptom-free surgical conditions. *Archives of General Psychiatry, 36,* 1295–1301.

Turner, J. E., & TenHoor, W. J. (1979). The NIMH Community Support Program: Pilot approach to a needed social reform. *Schizophrenia Bulletin, 4*(3), 319–344.

Unger, K. V., Danley, K. S., Kohn, L. & Hutchinson, D. (1987). Rehabilitation through education for young adults with psychiatric disabilities on a university campus. *Psychosocial Rehabilitation Journal, 10*(3), 35–50.

U.S. Department of Health and Human Services. (1980). *Toward a national plan for the chronically mentally ill: Report to the Secretary by the DHHS Steering Committee on the Chronically Mentally Ill.* Rockville, MD: Author.

U.S. Department of Health and Human Services. (1983). *Report to Congress on shelter and basic living needs of chronically mentally ill individuals.* Washington, DC: U.S. Government Printing Office.

U.S. General Accounting Office. (1988). *Estimating the size and location of homeless persons with mental illness.* Washington, DC: U.S. Government Printing Office.

U.S. Senate Special Committee on Aging, Sub-Committee on Long-Term Care. (1976). *The role of nursing homes in caring for discharged mental patients (and the birth of a for-profit boarding home industry)* (Supporting Paper No. 7). Washington, DC: U.S. Government Printing Office.

Vermont Department of Mental Health and Mental Retardation (1991). *Mental health directions for the future, 1991–1996.* Waterbury: Author.

Vermont Department of Mental Health and Mental Retardation (1993). *Policy statement on family involvement.* Waterbury: Author. (∗)

Virginia Department of Mental Health, Mental Retardation and Substance Abuse. (1990). *Policy on housing and supports.* Richmond: Author. (∗)

Wallace, A. (1992). *Mothers with mental illness: Unheard voices, unmet needs.* Burlington, VT: Center for Community Change through Housing and Support. (∗)

Walsh, M. (1986). *Schizophrenia: Straight talk for families and friends.* New York: Warner Books.

Wasow, M. (1982). *Coping with schizophrenia: A survival manual for parents, relatives, and friends.* Palo Alto, CA: Science and Behavior Books.

Wasow, M. (1986). The need for asylum for the chronically mentally ill. *Schizophrenia Bulletin, 12,* 162–167.

Watterson, B. (1988). *The essential Calvin and Hobbes.* Kansas City, MO: Andrews & McMeel.

Wehman, P., & Kregel, J. (1985). A supported work approach to competitive employment of individuals with moderate and severe handicaps. *Journal of the Association for Severe Handicaps, 10*(1), 3–11.

Wilson, S. F. (1988). Implementation of the CSS concept statewide: The Vermont experience. *Psychosocial Rehabilitation Journal, 12*(3), 27–40. (∗)

Wilson, S. F. (1989). *Outcome research and its relevance to case managers.*

Unpublished manuscript, Center for Community Change through Housing and Support, Burlington, VT. (∗)

Wilson, S. F. (1992). Community support and integration: New directions for outcome research. In S. Rose (Ed.), *Case management: An overview and assessment* (pp. 113–129). White Plains, NY: Longman. (∗)

Wilson, S. F., Blanch, A., & Quinn, K. (1987). *The role of ex-patients and consumers in human resource development for the 1990's.* Burlington, VT: Center for Community Change through Housing and Support. (∗)

Wilson, S. F., & Mahler, J. (1991). *The role of consumers/ex-patients in housing and community support services.* Burlington, VT: Center for Community Change through Housing and Support. (∗)

Winokur, G., Morrison, J., & Clancy, J. (1972). The Iowa 500: II. A blind family history comparison of mania, depression, and schizophrenia. *Archives of General Psychiatry, 27,* 462–464.

Witheridge, T. (1990). Assertive community treatment as a supported housing approach. *Psychosocial Rehabilitation Journal, 13*(4), 69–75.

Yankelovich, D., & Associates. (1990). *National survey of public attitudes toward mental illness.* Boston: Robert Wood Johnson Foundation.

Yoe, J. T., Carling, P. J., & Smith, D. J. (1991). *A national survey of supported housing for persons with psychiatric disabilities.* Burlington, VT: Center for Community Change through Housing and Support. (∗)

Zinman, S., Harp, H. the, & Budd, S. (1987). *Reaching across: Mental health clients helping each other.* Sacramento: California Network of Mental Health Clients.

Zipple, A. M., Carling, P. J., & McDonald, J. (1988). A rehabilitation response to the call for asylum. *Schizophrenia Bulletin, 13,* 539–546. (∗)

Zipple, A. M., & Ridgway, P. (1990). The paradigm shift in residential services: From the linear continuum to supported housing approaches. *Psychosocial Rehabilitation Journal, 13*(4), 11–31. (∗)